Palliative Care for People with Cancer

Palliative Care for People with Cancer

Edited by

Jenny Penson and Ronald Fisher

Edward Arnold
A division of Hodder & Stoughton
LONDON   MELBOURNE   AUCKLAND

© 1991 Jenny Penson and Ronald Fisher

First published in Great Britain 1991

British Library Cataloguing in Publication Data

Palliative care for people with cancer: A guide for nurses.
 I. Fisher, R.   II. Penson, J.
 616.99

  ISBN 0-340-53198-3

Typeset in Ehrhardt by Rowland Phototypesetting Limited
Bury St Edmunds, Suffolk
Printed and bound in Great Britain for Edward Arnold
a division of Hodder and Stoughton Limited, Mill Road,
Dunton Green, Sevenoaks, Kent TN13 2YA by
Biddles Limited, Guildford and King's Lynn

Contents

Acknowledgements

It was not an easy time when we introduced Hospice Care into the National Health Service but we were inspired by our patients and families and sustained by the dedication and loyalty of those colleagues who pioneered with us. We would like to thank all of them and particularly Frances Alders, Mary Brookes, Olga Craig, Henry Garnett, Charles Hall, Gill Hambling, Maurice Harker, Julia Hopper, Pat Jones, Anne Newbury, Penny Megg, Margaret Rapson, Pat Rushton, Sue Stone, Elaine Walker and Ronnie Whitlock-Smith. We are also greatly indebted to Paul Manners, Managing Director of Napp Pharmaceutical Group who, because of his interest and enthusiasm for further education in Palliative Care, has sponsored and is continuing to sponsor our educational programmes for nurses, not only in this country but abroad.

We also thank profoundly those who have contributed to this book for their wise words and amenability.

Finally, we thank our families for their love and support and patience, without them little would have been achieved.

Ronald Fisher
Jenny Penson

'A Physician [or Nurse] does not violate etiquette even if, being in difficulties on occasions over a patient and in the dark through inexperience, he [she] should urge the calling in of others in order to learn by consultation the truth about the case and in order that there may be fellow workers to afford abundant help. For when a diseased condition is stubborn and the evil grows, in the perplexity of the moment most things go wrong.'

Corpus Hippocraticum

List of Contributors

The Editors

Ronald A Fisher, MA, MRCS, LRCP, FFARCS
Lecturer in Palliative Care, and formerly Consultant Physician in Continuing Care at the first Macmillan Unit, Christchurch Hospital, Dorset.

Ronald Fisher introduced Hospice Medicine into the National Health Service at Christchurch Hospital in January 1975. This included the first N.H.S. Home-Care Service for cancer patients, the fore-runner of the present Macmillan Nursing Service, and a Support and Advisory Team for the district general hospitals. In 1977 a Day Care service was started.

From 1977–80 he was Chairman of a Select Committee of Experts at Strasbourg at the invitation of the Council of Europe to study "Problems related to death".

He has been long associated with Cancer Relief, was its Honorary Consultant, and is now a Vice President of that charity.

Jenny Penson, MA(ed), SRN, HV Cert, Cert. Ed, RNT
Lecturer in Higher Education. Consultant and writer on nursing and health topics. Former Macmillan Nurse who was part of the first domiciliary team in the National Health Service for patients with advanced cancer and their families.

The Contributors

Sally Anstey, RGN, Dip N (Wales), Cert Counselling, Oncological Nursing Certificate
Specialist in Palliative Nursing, Llandough Hospital, Penarth, South Glamorgan.

Ray Corcoran, FRCOG
Consultant Medical Director, Hayward House, Macmillan Palliative Care Unit, City Hospital, Nottingham.

Olga M Craig, SRN, SCM, Dip Soc Studies (Edinburgh), Cert in Child Care (Birmingham)
Formerly Senior Medical Social Worker and a lecturer at the Macmillan Unit, Christchurch Hospital; with 30 years experience in social work in the community and in hospitals.

Ilora Finlay, MRCGP
Consultant in Palliative Medicine and Director, Holme Tower Marie Curie Centre, Penarth, South Glamorgan.

Dawn Foxley, RGN, NDN Cert, NBS PSII (Care of the Dying)
Macmillan Sister, Fife Macmillan Team.

Charlette Gallagher-Allred, PhD, RD, LD
Nutritionist for Kobacker House Hospice at Riverside, Columbus, Ohio, USA.

Denise Hodson, SRN, RSCN
Clinical Nurse Specialist, Paediatric Oncology Unit, Seacroft Hospital, Leeds.

Tim Hunt, MD, DSc, MRCP
Consultant Physician in Palliative Medicine, Arthur Rank Home, Macmillan Continuing Care Unit, Cambridge.

Bill Kenny
Psychiatric Social Worker, Formerly Head of Department, Nursing and Social Service, Dorset Institute of Higher Education.

Kathryn A Mannix, MB, BS, MRCP
Senior Registrar in Palliative Medicine, Saint Oswald's Hospice, Newcastle upon Tyne.

Pat Mathers, BSc (Hons), PhD, CBiol, MIBiol
Senior Lecturer in Biological Sciences, Department of Nursing, Health and Community Studies, Bournemouth Polytechnic, Dorset.

Ann Newbury, SRN, SCM, NDN Cert, FAETC
Team Leader, Home Care Service, Macmillan Unit, Christchurch.

Morna Rutherford, BSc (Soc Sc/Nurs), RGN, NDN Cert, Cert Dip Couns (PCP Britain), Oncol, CCNS (930)
Macmillan Sister, West Lothian, Scotland, also a Person-Centred Therapist.

The Reverend David Stoter
Senior Chaplain, Queen's Medical Centre, Nottingham and Co-ordinator of Chaplains, Nottingham Health Authority.

Valued care

1

Introduction: Palliative care – a rediscovery

Ronald Fisher

'There are indeed two things, knowledge and opinion, of which the one makes its possessor really to know, the other to be ignorant.'

Corpus Hippocraticum

The words 'terminal care' are the most insensitive ones in our medical jargon. They obscure rather than clarify, they mislead, they are inadequate. So why add to the distress of patients and families by using such ill-chosen words?

'Words are the vehicles of thought and feeling, the wires that stretch between us', said the late Lady Violet Bonham-Carter when addressing the Royal College of Physicians (Lloyd-Roberts, 1951). 'I love words,' she said, 'because words used properly can make a blank sheet of white paper glow with all the colours of a Turner sky – because they can fill the air with music in a silent room.' These two words that we use – terminal care – are drab and discordant and diminish the care we are trying to give. The expression 'Palliative Care', though not perfect, is far more acceptable and carries with it a hint of hope. And yet doctors and nurses, and others associated with cancer, add to the confusion by using both phrases as if they are synonymous.

I appreciate it can be argued that, since incurable cancer is a terminal disease, then the care given must also be terminal. But to carry this argument to its logical and perhaps ridiculous conclusion then all care is terminal since life is made up of partial deaths and we begin to die from the moment we are born:

'death borders upon our birth and our cradle stands in our grave'.

Joseph Hall, Epistles (1608) 3.2

We are destined to die, it is a fact of life. Death, as the philosopher Martin Heidegger (1889–1976) said, is the culminating point of both pathology and normality. But too much logic bores, so let us not

'starve the best parts of our minds by leaning on logic.'

J. B. Yeats

Let us instead take poetic licence and firmly declare that Palliative Care and Terminal Care are *not* the same.

Palliative Care is a broad band of care of indeterminate length which should start the moment the cancer is diagnosed or even before, when there is a gleam of apprehension in the patient's eye. I would suggest that it is at this point that the District Nurse should be introduced to the family concerned, even though the care required initially might only be intermittent. Terminal Care is only a *part* of the palliative care programme and comes at the end of life, that is in the last hours or days. Important and demanding though it is, it is usually the least difficult part of our total care. Perhaps 'ultimate care' would be a better expression.

Sir Thomas Browne, a 17th century Physician of some repute, said 'death is the cure of all diseases', in which case doctors and nurses always lose-out in the end. If we accept this, it follows that our endeavours should be to increase the quantity and improve the quality of the preceding years. If we now re-arrange those words in the context of the patient with advancing malignant disease and say that our endeavours should be to *improve the quality of the preceding days, weeks, months and years*, and by so doing quite possibly increase the quantity of those weeks, months and years, then we have an acceptable philosophy for Palliative Care. We can now go on to define Palliative Medicine as being 'to relieve suffering when cure is impossible, suffering which can be physical, psychological, social and spiritual and which involves both the patient and the family'. A more precise but still acceptable definition is

'to do away with the sufferings of the sick, to lessen the violence of the disease'.
Corpus Hippocraticum

The reader may be surprised to know that this was written before the birth of Christ, probably by Hippocrates, but then, as it says in the book of Job,

'with the ancient is wisdom'.

It is not inappropriate to enrich these definitions with the words of Barbara McNulty, who was once the nurse in charge of the Home-Care service at St Christopher's Hospice in London. In the early seventies I was privileged to accompany her on her round in the community. She taught me so much.

'In caring for the dying patient one cannot separate his needs from those of his family – they are a unit whose individual members interact; what affects one will react upon another. One cannot treat a dying patient's physical symptoms and ignore his emotional needs. The home with all its problems, the patient with all his fears and pain are the objects of our concern.'
By permission of Barbara McNutty

I have already pointed out that Palliative Care may well start the moment the patient is informed of the diagnosis of cancer. Peter Maguire has written that the emotional upheaval that occurs at this time often goes unrecognised (Maguire and Faulkner, 1988). Consequently there is no psychological intervention and the psychiatric morbidity goes untreated.

'It should not be forgotten either that death from cancer is never instantaneous. It occurs in stages, it is a process, and there are variations in the rate at which the final point approaches. Total final death is merely the last in a series of functional, organic partial deaths, since although the organs live together they die separately.'
European Public Health Committee report

What I am suggesting is that dying from cancer can be a prolonged affair which means the period of Palliative Care can be very variable in length. Nor should it be forgotton that Medicine is not an exact science, we are not always sure what will happen next, therefore a miracle is always possible. Like other colleagues, I have cared for patients with established cancer over periods ranging from one to three to five and even nine years. By improving the quality of a patient's life, by helping the patient to *live* through his or her cancer, every so often a '*little*' miracle happens. Janet McCusker of the University of Massachusetts reviewed 2989 patients dying of cancer during the years 1976–78 and showed that the length of the 'terminal care period' varied from one month to over four years (McCusker, 1983). One must again question the appropriateness of the blanket use of the label 'terminal care'. An interesting observation arising out of McCusker's study is the relationship between the length of time that elapses from the diagnosis to the death of the patient and the place of death. As the length of the survival period increased so did the percentage of patients dying at home.

It is encouraging also to know that, in Britain, 90% of the last year of life of the patient with cancer is spent at home, and, according to a survey of 703 patients by Derek Doyle, during that year surprisingly 14% are bed-bound for less than one week, 27% for 1–4 weeks, 10% for 3 months, and only 4% of the dying are in bed for 3–6 months (Doyle 1982, 1986). As drug therapy improves we can be cautiously optimistic that these figures will improve and though cure may not be achieved the progress of the disease will be slowed and life prolonged. So we should always give hope, as long as it is reasonable to do so. Hope, not for the cure of the cancer, but to enable the patient to achieve goals and live a life full of meaning in whatever environment that patient may be. Without hope there is no endeavour.

Medical historians will report in due course that it wasn't until well into the second half of the 20th century that the fortunes of the chronic cancer patient began to improve. Until then many patients with advancing malignant disease had suffered unnecessarily. For example millions had unalleviated cancer pain, and many tragically died in pain. This is now generally accepted with regret, but then history is full of regrets. Why was this? Why has this been such a neglected area of medicine?

It has been said the fault lies with the education nurses and doctors have received or have not received. An education that has been orientated to cure, so that when we failed to cure we did not know how to cope with our failures and tended therefore to retreat from the situation. What I call the 'Eeyore Syndrome' takes over: (with apologies to A. A. Milne)

Said Eeyore – 'I make it seventeen days come Friday since anyone spoke to me'.
Said Rabbit: 'I was here myself a week ago.'
'Not conversing', said Eeyore. 'Not first one and then the other. You said "Hallo" and *flashed past*'!

From A. A. Milne

Life sustaining treatments ranging from antibiotics to organ transplants, it is argued, have caused us to concentrate on the disease rather than on the patient. Ivan Illich, the philosopher, calls it 'the medicalization of life', and the opening sentence of his book *Medical Nemesis* rather startlingly states 'the Medical Establishment has become a threat to life' (Illich, 1974). By this he means Health Care professionals have taken over so completely that the patient loses his or her independence. Professor Ziegler of Switzerland, also commenting on the omnipotence of doctors, has coined the word 'thanatocrats' who have the power to prolong life or terminate it.

Another interesting thought is that doctors and nurses have inherited this attitude of neglect over the centuries, that it is a 'hangover' from the past. Is this theory so wild? After all we have inherited and accepted much that is in the Corpus Hippocraticum (Hippocratic collection). Hippocrates is universally known as the 'Father of Medicine' and many of the clinical observations in use today are all there, clearly stated in these ancient manuscripts. As W. H. S. Jones writes,

'there is within the corpus the work of a medical genius, perhaps the greatest genius among all the physicians whose writings have come down to us. He inherited much from his predecessors but either personally or through his pupils he bequeathed far more to his successors. Whether or not his name was Hippocrates the inheritance is still ours'.

W. H. S. Jones (1945)

Over the centuries contributions by Galen, William Harvey, John Hunter, Edward Jenner, Joseph Lister, Alexander Fleming, Frederick Banting and Charles Best, Richard Bright, Thomas Addison, William Osler, Florence Nightingale, Cicely Saunders, to name but a very very few, have added to that inheritance to create medicine as it is today.

Let us now look at a part of that inheritance, at one of the bequests.

'First, I will define what I conceive Medicine to be. In general terms it is to do away with the sufferings of the sick, to lessen the violence of their disease, *and to refuse to treat those who are overmastered by their disease realizing that in such cases such medicine is powerless'*.

Corpus Hippocraticum

We have totally accepted the first half of that definition, but did we not also accept the second half and is it not until recently that we have begun to reject it?

Fascinating though these theories are, the fact remains – we were ignorant of what could be done.

'Wisdom is prevented by ignorance and delusion is the result.'

Bhagaradgta, 5 tr P Lal

And delusion certainly was the result because generations of nurses and doctors deluded themselves into believing that nothing could be done for the patient with an incurable cancer with the result that we took refuge in those all too familiar statements 'We have done all we can' or 'There is nothing more to be done'. In retrospect I suppose we should be grateful for such delusions because if there had been no doubts there would have been no questioning, and if there had been no questioning there would have been no enlightenment. And so we had a neglected area of medicine. Health services world-wide were failing to improve the care of these unfortunate patients, failing to satisfy their physical, emotional, social and spiritual needs. It wasn't until we were alerted by Dr Cicely Saunders to this famine of care that Hospices and Continuing Care Units began to appear in this country. We (the editors) were privileged to introduce Continuing Care into the National Health Service in January 1975 at Christchurch Hospital in Dorset. At the same time we started a Home-Care service which was the prototype of to-day's Macmillan Nursing Service and a peripatetic 'support team' for the hospitals in the district. Two years later we introduced Day-Care. From these Specialist Units with their growing expertise and scientific approach was born Palliative Medicine, now recognised by the Royal College of Physicians as a Speciality. The emergence of Palliative Medicine is one of the best things that has happened to medicine in the 20th century.

When lecturing in the early seventies I used to remind audiences that since dying is a part of living then *care of the dying is care of the living.* This may well have been said by others at that time but I never heard it and it was certainly original to me. It is a vital statement which follows the aphoristic style adopted by the early Greek philosophers. An aphorism is capsulated wisdom, a device used 'to arrest attention and assist the memory'. *Care of the dying is care of the living* – an aphorism which is totally acceptable to-day, but in those earlier days there was much more talk of helping people to die well, to die with dignity, to have a good death. To my puzzled mind this thanatological terminology was deceptive, full of promise but signifying very little. Better surely to speak of 'a tranquil death'.

Nursing care of the dying patient is care for the patient who is still living, it is helping that patient to live his or her life to the fullest whether at home or in hospital. It is care that is not just centred on the individual but includes members of the family. The nurse in a Palliative Care team, whether in the community or hospital, is just as important as the doctor. He or she is in the unique position of being able to spend most time with the patient and the family and, by virtue of this intimacy, acquire a wide knowledge of the patient. This knowledge can be shared with other members of the caring team and in this way the patient and the family receive total harmonious care. As Lisbeth Hockey (1989) says, the nurse is the main communicator between the patient, the relatives and the doctors and has the function of not only giving care but of coordinating the care of others.

I remember saying in 1974, prior to the opening of the Macmillan Unit at Christchurch, that I considered we were a short-term concept in a neglected area of Medicine and that a measure of our success would be when we had made ourselves redundant. Obviously I have modified this view over the years but I still believe that if all nurses, whether working in a hospital or the community, receive adequate education in Palliative Care then most patients, most of the time, can be cared for by the family doctor and family nurse and the hospital team. The relief of cancer pain is an excellent example of this because there are now standard procedures of pain control, that are well within the scope of any nurse or doctor. Surveys have demonstrated that total or acceptable relief can be achieved in 71–97% of patients (Twycross, 1989).

What then is the role of the Specialist Unit and the Specialist Nurse? Both are of vital importance. They are there to advise on difficult problems, to take over the care of the patient if necessary, preferably on a temporary basis, to research and evaluate, and to teach. Given the tools, the community and hospital nurses will be able to play their natural roles. It is important that, as far as the 'family nurse' is concerned, this role should not be stolen from them. After all, nurses have worked in the community for some considerable time, in fact from 1859 when that socially conscious philanthropist William Rathbone started the District Nursing Service in Liverpool (Hardy, 1981). There is a wealth of 'know-how' inherent in this service.

This book is primarily for nurses. The contributors have tried to look at the problem through the nurses' eyes and then give the information which will enable them to give the comprehensive care which will satisfy the needs of the patient and the family, and indeed their own needs should the occasions arise. Medical Social Workers, Physiotherapists, Medical Students, Occupational therapists, teachers, administrators and others will also find much to interest them. The contributors are all experts in their various fields and are, or have been, associated with Palliative or Continuing Cancer Care over many years. Their involvement in undergraduate and particularly postgraduate education has been extensive. Indeed, many have been members of my teams, who have travelled not only in this country but overseas teaching and advising on new Palliative Care programmes. We have tried to include the more important aspects but inevitably there will be omissions in a book of this size. Ethical issues, Symptom Control, Confusional States, Communication, Counselling skills, Bereavement, Nutrition and Complementary Therapies have all been highlighted.

One omission is Day Care, and since Day Care has become a part of the network of Domiciliary care a brief mention should be made.

Day Care is for those patients who do not need in-patient care but who still need support. Symptoms can be controlled, the patients progress monitored and Physio-therapy and Diversional therapy provided. A Day Unit provides a 'day-out' for the patient and a 'day-off' for the caring relative. Volunteers can be used extensively particularly those with special skills. A Day Unit can be purpose-built, an ordinary house can be converted or an unwanted hospital ward or building can be used. It does not have to be attached to or be a part of a Palliative Medicine Unit or Hospice. Indeed, there is no reason why such units or conversions should not be managed by nurses in the community and groups of family doctors. According to Spooner (1986) one place per 10 000 head of population is a rough working guide-line. It is an economical way of supervising and giving care, and it is interesting to note that, according to Spooner's costings, about five purpose-built Day-Care units could be built for the price of just one Palliative Medicine Unit or Hospice, and of course even more conversions. This also applies to the revenue consequences.

I will conclude with yet another telling passage from the Corpus, hoping that I have made the point that, apart from technology, there is little that is new in our medical philosophy.

> 'With regard to disease, the circumstances from which we form a judgement of them are
> – by attending to the general nature of all, and the peculiar nature of each individual, to the disease, the patient, and the applications;
> – to the person who applies them, and that makes a difference for better or for worse;
> – to the patients habits, regimens and pursuits;
> – to his conversation, manners, taciturnity, thoughts, sleep, or absence of sleep, and sometimes his dreams;
> – to his picking and scratching;
> – to his tears, alvine discharges, urine, sputa and vomitings, and to the changes of disease from the one into the other;
> – to the deposits, whether of a deadly or critical character;
> – to the sweat, coldness, rigor, cough, sneezing, hiccup, respiration, erudation, flatulence, whether passed silently or with a noise;
> – to haemorrhage and haemorrhoids;
> – from these and their consequence, we must 'form our judgement''
>
> *Corpus Hippocraticum*

We must indeed and we cannot be more holistic than that!

It should be remembered also that Palliative Care does not necessarily end with the death of the patient. Until life begins to glow again some surviving relatives may need support during the bereavement period. Likewise for those patients whose disease has been controlled as a result of treatment, there may be a transition period during which the family nurse and the family doctor will need 'to map the middle ground of survivorship and provide psycho-social support' (Loescher *et al.*, 1989). As Mullen (1985) reflects 'there is no moment of cure but rather an evolution from the phase of extended survival into a period when the activity of the disease or the likelihood of its return is sufficiently small that the cancer can now be considered permanently arrested'. It is only then that Palliative Care can end.

I cannot close without these final and relevant words of advice from our 'Father':

> 'The Physician (and Nurse) must have a certain degree of sociability, for a morose disposition is inaccessible both to those who are well and those who are sick'.
>
> *Corpus Hippocraticum*

How true!

References

DOYLE, D. (1982). *Journal of the Royal College of General Practitioners*, **32**, 285–91.

DOYLE, D. (1986). Domiciliary care – a doctor's view. In *International Symposium on Pain Control*, pp. 61–7. Royal Society of Medicine.

European Public Health Committee. *Problems related to Death: Care of the Dying.* Report of the European Public Health Committee, Council of Europe, Strasbourg. Chairman of Committee and Editor of Report, Ronald Fisher.

HARDY, GWEN (1981). *William Rathbone and the Early History of District Nursing.* G. W. and A. Hesketh (Publishers), Ormskirk, Lancashire.

HOCKEY, LISBETH (1989) Medical education. In *The Edinburgh Symposium – Pain Control*, pp. 3–15. Royal Society of Medicine International Congress – Symposium Series.

ILLICH, IVAN (1974). *Limits of Medicine: Medical Nemesis.* Penguin, Harmondsworth.

JONES, W. H. S. (1945). Hippocrates and the Corpus Hippocraticum. In *Proceedings of the British Academy*, Vol. XXXI, communicated June 6th, 1945. Geoffrey Cumberledge, Amen House, London EC4.

LLOYD-ROBERTS (1951). The power of words. Lecture at the Royal College of Physicians, November 1951. Reported in the *Lancet*, December 1st, 1951.

LOESCHER, L. J., WELCH-MCCAFFREY, D., LEIGH, S. A., *et al.* (1989). Surviving adult cancers. Parts 1 and 2. *Annals of Internal Medicine*, **111**, 411–32, 517–24.

MCCUSKER, JANET (1983). Where cancer patients die: an epidemiological study. *Public Health Reports*, March–April 1983, **98(2)**, 170–6. University of Massachusetts.

MAGUIRE, P. and FAULKNER, ANNE (1988). How to communicate with cancer patients. Part 2. Handling uncertainty: collusion and denial. *British Medical Journal*, **297**, 972–4.

MILNE, A. A. (1928). *The House at Pooh Corner.* Methuen & Co. Ltd.

MULLEN, F. (1985). Seasons of survival: reflections of a physician with cancer. *New England Journal of Medicine*, **313**, 270–3.

SPOONER, D. (1986). *American Journal of Hospice Care.* January 1986, pp. 24–40.

TWYCROSS, R. (1989) Medical education. In *The Edinburgh Symposium – Pain Control.* Royal Society of Medicine International Congress – Symposium Series.

2

Ethical issues

Tim Hunt

'One must have studied much to know that one knows little.'

Anon

Nurses and doctors are entrusted with caring for the sick; this is a privilege. Today, in a hectic world, there is little time to think and nurses and doctors are under increasing pressure to make decisions. They find themselves faced with increasing and conflicting demands in attempting to give good care and, in their caring role, may forget what is right and what is wrong and this may result in forgetting their duties to both their patients and to their professions. Such considerations introduce thoughts on the ethics and morals of patient care. Ethics can be considered as the theory of morals, and morals as the practice of ethics. There are many approaches to outlining the principles of ethics and morals; one simple outline or pattern is to consider three broad principles:

  (*i*) justice and fairness;
 (*ii*) autonomy – respecting the choice of the patient;
(*iii*) beneficence – kindness to patients.

Justice and fairness

The practice of justice and fairness may depend on political decisions, often at government level. For example, should limited funds be directed to the care of the elderly or to transplant surgery? But the carer may also need to make difficult decisions. Does the carer give more time and effort to one patient at the expense of another patient? Which patient should be expected to pay for a private night nurse when there is only one Marie Curie nurse and two patients with equal need? Frequently there is no way of being fair because the carers efforts are constrained by matters outside their control. Nevertheless, these principles are pertinent to patient care.

Autonomy – respecting the choice of the patient

In an ideal world each person ought to have complete personal freedom to decide how they want to be looked after. However, this is not often possible. At one extreme there is the comatosed, confused or demented patient; these patients cannot express their wishes. At the other extreme is the articulate patient who is very able and knows what he or she wants but his or her requirements cannot be fitted into the rigid system of care. If the principle of autonomy is recognised then problems do arise in considering the wish of any patient who wants to die.

Beneficence – kindness to our patients

It is fundamental to a caring profession that the carers are beneficent; their aim is to do good, to be kind and charitable in feeling. If the need for doing good is accepted then maleficence, that is the doing of evil or ill-will to another, must be prevented. Even when a patient or his or her relatives are displeasing, aggressive or do not want to follow the advice which has been given, carers must refrain from being spiteful or acting with vengeance. When speaking to patients doctors and nurses should not frighten them or abuse their position of apparent authority.

In looking after patients with advanced cancer, while many of the problems are different from those seen, for example, in obstetrics or intensive care units, the principles of ethical and moral thought remain the same.

There are three areas which provoke much thought in the care of the patient with advanced cancer:

(*i*)   what to tell and not to tell the patient and relatives;
(*ii*) not striving officiously to keep a patient alive; and
(*iii*) euthanasia.

What to tell and not to tell

'What a distance there is between what people say and what they think.'
Jean Racine, 1639–1699

There is no doubt that a decade ago patients were given limited information about their illness and this, especially, was the case with patients with cancer. With immense social and educational changes, no longer is it embarrassing to discuss disease and death; these topics feature frequently on radio and television and in print. Therefore, public awareness about illness and cancer is considerable. In the United States the present trend is to disclose nearly every possible aspect of a disease, and although this is not yet evident in Europe, the caring professions must take into account such trends when communicating with patients and their families.

The fundamentals to help decide on what to tell and not to tell are first, the autonomy or rights of the patient; and second, kindness and beneficence to the patient.

The earlier approach of being frugal with the truth was considered kinder to the patient. The arguments in favour of this policy may be on the following lines. If an ill person is given unfavourable or disturbing information, the problems for that already troubled person are increased. Further, it may be felt that telling the truth will remove the often underlying hope that the disease will regress or that treatment will bring about a complete cure. Hope is a necessary requirement for survival, so that if the hope of the patient is removed or diluted, so too may the will for survival be removed. These considerations rest mainly on being kind to the patient, they do not consider truth. Here there is a conflict between kindness and truth, and what may be meant by truth is difficult to define as will be mentioned later.

There are examples where the carer, in telling the truth, can be unkind; a frequent criticism of busy out-patient clinics is that honest information is given to patients but in a hurried and seemingly cold and curt manner. This may impart truth but cannot be condoned as it violates the principles of beneficence. Therefore, in certain situations, if truth negates beneficence then truth may not be of such importance.

There are other areas where truth may underline ethical consideration for the patient. For example, a patient may enter a state of denial, rejecting what he or she has been told about his illness. Some carers cannot accept this and strive to breach this denial because they believe that denial does not help the patient. But denial may be a normal coping mechanism for some people and if a patient wishes to continue denial then that wish should be respected. To force information on a patient against their wish is contrary to the principles of autonomy and beneficence.

> 'Before you tell the "truth" to the patient, be sure you know the "truth", and that the patient wants to hear it.'
>
> *Richard Clarke Cabot, 1868–1939*

In broad moral terms the importance of truth cannot be denied, but it is the application of truth as an obligatory principle that is often unclear. The professional carer cannot speak in terms of absolute or whole truth because they often do not know what is happening and what will happen to a patient. When they think they are speaking the truth to a patient what they are expressing is an opinion based on their experience, and opinion may be some distance from the truth. The logic and thought as to what is truth is a subject of its own with far reaching consequences, but the carer must be cautious about making claims on the importance of truth and prudent when they think they are speaking the truth to the patient.

It will be of value to examine some of the practical issues. Why do doctors and nurses hesitate to give a patient information about his own illness?

● It takes both time and patience to explain an illness in terms that can be understood. It may be difficult to create an opportunity which is unhurried so that there is time to answer questions and support the distress that may result in what will be a sensitive discussion.

● Sometimes the carer may find discussion difficult because it requires a mental agility and sensitivity to feel the nuances from the patient. At other times the carer may have become so close to the patient that it is painful to disclose disturbing information because one does not want to further upset the patient. A further reason may be that the discussion may encroach on the personal problems of the carer.

● Relatives often feel that to disclose too much information could be injurious to the mental health of the patient, and may request the carer to filter information given to the patient. Some of the ethical considerations have been mentioned earlier, but carers may find themselves in a difficult position between patient and relative because if they accede to such requests they may remove the autonomy of the patient. Some relatives fear disclosure of information because they do not know how to respond to the patient once additional and more pertinent information is given, and although the ethical principles of the caring profession apply to the patient, carers may have to give equal support to a distressed relative.

● Inter-professional communication problems do arise. For example, if information is disclosed to a patient, will it upset other professionals who are also involved in the case? A patient often asks a nurse about his or her illness; the nurse may vacillate because he or she is uncertain of the views of the general practitioner, and if pertinent information is disclosed it may fall on the next carer who visits the patient to provide emotional support to help the distressed patient. It is often not possible to avoid such problems but there is a responsibility on each carer to try and enhance communication.

There is no single or correct way to communicate with a patient. Each patient is individual as are carers, but all carers need considerable sensitivity to establish what the patient wishes to know. This will help determine what to tell, when to tell and how to tell. Sensitivity requires flexibility for good communication.

There are a few guidelines to supplement the ethical principles; in general the greater the request for information from a patient the more information should be provided, likewise the greater the patient's ability to understand the greater is the need to disclose information at a depth in keeping with his or her mental ability, and the information given must be within the comprehension of the patient.

Ethical considerations embrace the subject of confidentially, and professional codes have evolved in this subject to help the patient. In simple terms if doctors and nurses need honest and unrestricted information from the patient then they must provide an implied assurance that the information will not be disclosed. Otherwise the patient will give partial or even misleading information which may hamper correct diagnosis and treatment of an illness. The patient may need to be assured of this aspect.

Problems may arise in considering what to tell and what not to tell relatives. If a patient has a competent mind the carer's duty is to discuss first with the patient his or her illness and plans for his or her care. In practice the first discussion often takes place with the closest relatives. This may be done to try and unravel the thoughts and known wishes of the patient, but no person other than the patient (except in the case of children) has the right to consent or decide on treatment for that patient. Voluntary disclosures about the illness should not be made to a third party without the consent of the patient; third parties, in a technical sense, include relatives and friends. If the patient is denied information and it is given to others, or if relatives are allowed to make decisions, the carer may be removing autonomy from that patient. If patients and relatives are not equally informed there is a risk of considerable misunderstanding. The ideal is to discuss sensitive matters with the patient and relative at the same time.

As professionals, carers need to re-examine what they communicate to a patient. Perhaps they should establish what their patients want to know and what element of truth they require and not tell them what they think they should be told. But this is difficult and often impossible.

Not striving officiously to keep a patient alive

'Thou shalt not kill; but need'st not strive
Officiously to keep alive.'

Arthur Hugh Clough, 1819–1861
The Latest Decalogue

The last decade has heard many voices speaking for the quality of life instead of the length or quantity of life for those patients with advanced illness. This view has been promoted by the hospice movement. Sometimes these doctrines are considered as the quality of life and the sanctity of life and may be the subject of considerable debate. Belief in the sanctity of life would seem very finite and implies, in its strictest sense, that every step should be taken to keep the patient alive; it is thought that this belief stems from early religious codes. On the other hand, the quality of life views are based on subjective and compassionate assessments. Awareness of the need to consider the quality of life came about 30 years ago when studies of patients dying in hospital wards showed that carers should work to enable a patient to die peacefully and to live until he or she dies. Those who have cared for the very sick know that it is possible to maintain a policy of continual and sometimes aggressive intervention, without conviction that it will help, sometimes at extreme psychological and physical distress to the patient and relatives. It is to overcome such suffering that caring trends today are towards the quality of life concept.

At first it may seem that the extreme interpretation of the sanctity of life doctrine is irreconcilable with the quality of life concept. However, in 1957 Pope Pius XII put forward the view that doctors were not obliged to give extraordinary medical measures to keep a patient alive, and in 1977 the Archbishop of Canterbury expressed support for this principle. This brought about discussion as to what are 'extraordinary measures' and related expressions as 'heroic treatments'. It is difficult to make a list of such measures and perhaps every case must be considered on its own, but others may argue that it is impossible to make such distinctions. But extremist views are not only found in religious teachings, because 20 years after the declaration by Pope Pius XII, Lord Hailsham, when Lord Chancellor, said 'The law, at the moment, is perfectly plain; if you have got a living body, you have got to keep it alive, if you can'.

Extending from this discussion as to what professional carers should and should not do to allow an acceptable quality of life in the very sick patient, there has evolved debate on the subtle distinction between carrying out some deliberate act that leads to the death of a patient and not taking action that leads to the same result. In practical terms simple examples include giving a lethal injection or even smothering a patient with a pillow with, of course, the intention of killing him or her; not taking some action would be the withholding of treatment as a result of which a patient dies. In moral terms most will regard the first two examples as unacceptable and the third example as acceptable. This concept is referred to as the 'acts and omissions doctrine'. But the apparent distinction between what is an act and what is an omission becomes blurred if the thinking behind the original thought is considered: if treatment is withheld with the intent of killing then this passivity is as guilty as if the carer had decided to smother the patient.

The concept of acts and omissions is complex and, because it leads to considerable confusion, some argue that it should be rejected partly because of the enormous scope as to what is an acceptable omission. If a person knows that they will benefit from the death of a patient, and if they then fail to treat the patient and he or she dies, this type of omission is as immoral as if the person had smothered the patient. But sometimes omission is because of carelessness, ignorance or laziness and there is no motive to kill the patient. To illustrate the problems that arise in considering the acts and omission doctrine there is the well known dilemma of the old-age pensioners. If pensioners have insufficient means to keep themselves warm they will die of hypothermia, and Society may view this as an omission by those responsible for making available funds to old age pensioners; but if the same numbers of pensioners were machine-gunned in the streets there would be a very different response from Society. Sometimes omissions are unavoidable because carelessness and ignorance will always exist; but most acts can be avoided.

If a person takes on the duty of caring for a patient then that person may be guilty of an offence if they fail to carry out that duty. But in carrying out that duty the problem may be how far should one treat or not treat? The principle of autonomy makes it obligatory to discuss proposed treatment with the patient if he or she so wishes; often patients who have seen many miles of hospital corridors do not wish for further uncomfortable intervention. The carer may have to discuss with the patient what is the aim of further treatment? Will it cause pain or distress? Will it help the extension of life, and will the functioning of that continued life be in any way impaired? The law cannot define the professional carers' precise responsibilities and the carer cannot look for definitive guidelines, but they can consider the principles of justice, autonomy and kindness in each case. But, as professionals, carers may be asked to give their opinion and where they know that there are two or more alternatives on some aspect of treatment then, whenever possible, these should be explained to the patient so as to help him or her to decide on the merits or otherwise of further treatment.

The law does not insist that doctors and nurses should persist indefinitely in treating someone; even in general medicine, following a cardiac arrest, it is not necessary to persist indefinitely in efforts to resuscitate a patient. Where there are cases where the circumstances are changing, it may be that an earlier decision on treatment requires reappraisal. For example, if nutrition is first provided by a naso-gastric feeding line and other problems arise in the progression of the disease there is no continuing obligation to continue with such feeding. Therefore there is, in practice, and in general thoughts about this subject, no compulsion to continue with any treatment, but if the carer deliberately withholds what is reasonable and acceptable treatment from the patient then this may be an offence.

There are instances where a competent patient refuses further treatment and, recalling the principle of patient autonomy, the carer should respect this request even if they disagree with it. In these cases there is still a moral obligation to continue to provide care for the patient as required by the principle of beneficence. Of course the duties of the carer may be different if the patient is demented or in some other way unable to comprehend the advantage of therapy, as would be the case if he or she is a danger to him or herself, relatives or other patients. It is good practice to sedate these sad cases by the use of medication.

A person's views on when to treat and not to treat must be influenced by their upbringing, spiritual attitude, professional background and private conscience. The aim of care is to provide an optimum living for the remaining weeks or months of the patient's life. Where treatment may cause further mental or physical distress then it must be viewed with circumspection, taking into account the wishes of the patient.

Euthanasia

'Euthanasia is a long, smooth sounding word, and it concedes its danger as long, smooth words do, but the danger is there nevertheless.'

Pearl Buck, 1892–1973

In 1989 an Austrian nurse was charged with the murder of 17 elderly patients in West Germany. She admitted using large doses of drugs to provide 'mercy killing'. This nurse may have cared very much for her patients, to the extent that she found their suffering incompatible with living. She decided to practice euthanasia which some may describe as 'mercy killing', but the law in most countries views such action as murder, and we can frequently read about similar cases. Increasingly people are more open in speaking and writing about the suffering of someone they love thereby giving some support to the concept of euthanasia.

What is euthanasia? The word is derived from the Greek – eu meaning easy, and thanatos meaning death – easy death. But the meaning of the word today is used to describe the hastening of death of a patient to prevent further suffering; and within this broad meaning are a number of terms used to describe different forms of euthanasia, although there is no agreement on the precise meaning of these terms. In general three forms are described – voluntary, involuntary and non-voluntary euthanasia.

Voluntary euthanasia is where the patient has expressed a wish to die and either they or someone else carries out an action to enable this. It is this form that is the basis of attempts to legalise euthanasia.

There is little difference between this and suicide, even though it may be thought to be a great source of comfort (Frederich Nietzcke). Whatever views are held by professional carers, there are both legal and professional constraints why they should not encourage a patient to commit suicide. Since the Suicide Act 1961 it is no longer a criminal offence for a person to attempt to take his or her own life, but it *is* an offence to advise another person on how to set about this.

Involuntary euthanasia is where a competent patient who has the ability to make decisions is not consulted, and his or her life is ended by the action of another person. This is murder.

Non-voluntary euthanasia is where a patient is unable to make a decision, for example he or she may be in coma, and their life is ended by the action of another. The press often describe this as 'mercy killing' and it is this form of euthanasia that causes considerable problems in medical ethics.

There is another distinction in considering euthanasia: this is the use of the terms '*active euthanasia*', where death would not have taken place without certain steps being taken as with the giving of a drug; and '*passive euthanasia*' where certain steps to prolong life have been discontinued as with the withdrawal of drugs. This is the basis of the 'acts and omissions doctrine' which was considered earlier.

It is difficult to encompass these varied descriptions of euthanasia and one attempt to describe the present meaning of the word was the definition adopted by the Linacre Report in 1981. This report concludes: 'In euthanasia a persons death is brought about on the ground that, because of his present mental condition and quality of life, and sometimes in consideration also of the quality of life of his family, it would be better for him, or at least no harm, if that person were dead.'

Euthanasia is a silent subject and discussion of it is avoided, even among professional carers. Professional carers have all faced the patient who asks for their help to die, and the relatives who challenge why someone should endure such suffering and not be allowed to die. In these conversations carers feel inadequate and may remain silent or move the conversation elsewhere. Why is it awkward to talk about this subject? As with sensitive subjects, the roots of the carers' thinking are difficult to untangle and their thoughts result from professional influences and principles, social concern, respect for life and religious screeds, some of which have evolved over the last two thousand years.

It is no coincidence that the Christian churches, nor indeed the Jewish and Islamic faiths, do not support the taking of ones own life or the lives of others who are in pain or suffering. Probably it is from the early religious teachings that our present thoughts have evolved. The origins are obscure but may arise from the battle between the Philistines and the Israelites after which King Saul was found dead. It is unknown whether Saul was slain in battle or whether he took his own life because of the ignomy of losing the battle. David, who succeeded Saul, may have found it inconceivable that the leader of the Israelites committed suicide, and it may be that from about that time to take one's own life was considered sinful. Later rabbinical teachings forbade the taking of one's life or assisting the ill who wished this. In simple terms, the belief evolved that man was not the owner of his body and that no person should interfere with the natural life span, because to shorten life may prevent receiving absolution which may be given at any time up to the actual moment of death. These early thoughts and teachings probably provided a basis for present religious and professional views on euthanasia, and it was often these views that formulated early civil and criminal laws.

There are examples in early societies where suicide was practiced for social or economic reasons. Nomadic tribes, as in the Sudan, could not carry around their very sick, and at times of war and famine the very sick may have burdened the survival of a tribe, and rituals developed to practice some form of euthanasia. In Roman times suicide was sometimes a demonstration of patriotism, and this 'self-sacrifice' is seen in recent wars and fighting.

What is the present legal situation in Britain? The background to recent views dates from 1957 when Dr John Bodkin Adams, an Eastbourne general practitioner, was charged with using excessive doses of drugs to bring about the deaths of some patients. The conclusions of the Adams case should be considered alongside the judgement in the more recent case of Dr Arthur who, in 1981, was charged with the death of a child with Down's Syndrome that was given dihydrocodeine. In both cases the doctors concerned were acquitted, but the views of the trial judges provide important guidelines to all carers. First, no person whether a doctor, nurse or other carer is above the law and even a professional code is unable to override the law. Second, it is unlawful for any person to bring about euthanasia or carry out some act with the intention of killing a person. Third, that the proper practice of medicine is to relieve pain and suffering, and adequate doses of drugs may be used to achieve such relief, even if the use of those drugs may shorten life. These views contain important practical considerations.

There are movements for and against euthanasia. In England the Voluntary Euthanasia Society, sometimes known as Exit, was founded in 1935 and now has more than 10 000 members; its counterpart in Holland claims over 36 000 members while the related organisation in the USA has over 300 000 members. One of the first opinion polls on this subject was carried out in 1969 by Mass Observation and this reported that just over half the population in England favoured euthanasia; in

1976 and 1985 research by National Opinion Poll showed 69% and 72% respectively supporting euthanasia. There have been attempts in Parliament to introduce
legislation on euthanasia, the most recent being in 1990, but these moves have been
unsuccessful. Groups in favour of euthanasia have encouraged the idea of Living
Wills or Advance Declarations. This is a declaration completed and signed by an
adult that requests that their life is not prolonged in certain circumstances. This
declaration provides no exception to current law in Britain, but it is recognised in
many of the states of the USA.

Holland is often mentioned as allowing voluntary euthanasia; but this is incorrect
– it is still illegal in Holland. Doctors are not prosecuted in Holland for practicing
euthanasia partly because of the manner in which a death is certified and partly
because the Supreme Court recommended that euthanasia on medical grounds
should be the responsibility of the medical profession. But the position in Holland is
far from stable because these concepts are continually being debated.

But the movement for voluntary euthanasia is not unchallenged; even in Holland
there are groups against euthanasia, including the Christian Democrat political
party and other groups with strong representations of the Church. In Britain groups
such as 'Life' and the World Federation of Doctors who Respect Human Life are
reminders that there are social, religious and professional groups that do not support
euthanasia.

Hospice philosophy does not favour euthanasia, and had it favoured euthanasia it
may be that the hospice concept would never have been born, because one aim was
that by giving adequate care there would be no requests for euthanasia. But it can be
argued that the majority of suffering patients are not looked after in hospices.
Further, there are patients even within hospices who request a foreshortening of
their life; who find the side effects of medicines to control symptoms remove their
mental faculties and independence, and who feel a weariness and tiredness and want
to leave this world. It could be further argued that, because the hospice movement
was founded on religious creeds, it follows the views of the main churches which
oppose euthanasia, and may not represent the actual views of all those working in the
hospice field.

Some of the religious aspects that relate to euthanasia have been mentioned
earlier, and while the official doctrines of the main churches oppose euthanasia it is
difficult to generalise the contemporary and future views of religious groups. For
example while the Declaration on Euthanasia by the Vatican in 1980 declared
suicide to be as wrong as murder, a National Opinion Poll in 1985 suggested that
54% of English catholics favoured euthanasia. This may reflect the uncertainty
whether any official body represents the views of its members. What has become
clear is that there is not a single religious concensus on this subject, because while
only 54% of Catholics in England supported euthanasia, such support was given by
75% of Protestants and 84% of Jews. The opinions of these religious groups fifty
years ago is not known but these findings support the view that a person's ethical and
moral views are influenced by their religious upbringing and that these views may be
changing.

The implications of attempting to legalise euthanasia are immense because the
present laws and professional codes are designed to protect everyone. This subject
does not concern only the very ill patients with advanced cancer, it also concerns the
mentally and physically infirm, those born with congenital abnormalities and even
those who have a poor quality of life. In an ideal world it could be argued that care of

the living should be so good that euthanasia is unwarranted, but sadly we are not in an ideal world. The problem remains – how can the law protect everyone and yet recognise the individual right to foreshorten a suffering life? Afterall this is a principle of patient autonomy. But can this be reconciled with professional ethics and social conscience?

Conclusions

Ethical and moral considerations are often the forgotten keystone of professional practice in caring for patients. Perhaps it is easier to overlook such considerations, but those people who are able to embrace this subject will experience a unique insight and a means to examine their own thinking and reasoning in making decisions and, at the same time, recognising the wishes of their patients.

Further reading

BURNARD, P. and CHAPMAN, C. M. (1988). *Professional and ethical issues in nursing.* John Wiley, Chichester.
GLOVER, J. (1977). *Causing death and saving lives.* Penguin, Harmondsworth.
MELIA, K. M. (1989). *Everyday nursing ethics.* Macmillan, Basingstoke.
SKEGG, P. D. G. (1984). *Law, ethics, and medicine.* Clarendon Press.

From cure to care: the role of the nurse

3

The management of pain

Ray Corcoran

'All pain is subtle, variable and shifting. We are all unskilled in describing our pain. Few patients talk with their doctors, rather doctors and patients talk at each other. Of all health professionals, the nurse is unique in having close, trusted, prolonged contact. This position is one of enormous responsibility and opportunity. At a minimum, the nurse is in the position of translator. . . . At a maximum, the nurse is in a position of a research worker. . . . To liberate this crucial subject, nurses must first educate themselves and then the rest of us.'

Professor Patrick D. Wall, 1987

Introduction

Pain is probably the most feared symptom encountered in advanced cancer. To many people pain and cancer are synonymous. It is a common belief that having cancer means pain is unavoidable and must be accepted. Unfortunately poor management of cancer pain continues to perpetuate this myth. However, nothing could be further from the truth. One-third of advanced cancer patients do not experience pain. Of the remaining two-thirds pain relief can be achieved in about nine out of ten patients simply by applying a number of basic principles. Moreover it must be emphasised that this high degree of pain control can be achieved by the non-specialist. For the small minority in whom the pain persists despite the application of this basic approach, the family or hospital doctor should not hesitate to seek consultative assistance. There will be only a very small group in whom complete pain relief is not possible, but even these patients can be helped considerably so that they are able to cope with any residual pain. Thus cancer pain is neither inevitable nor uncontrollable.

Reasons for failure to relieve pain

There are many reasons but they project a single message – the need to educate and train medical students, doctors and nurses in cancer pain management. As part of an endeavour to educate there may be a need to advocate. If a patient is in pain it may be necessary for the informed carer to point out to other medical and nursing colleagues, in a considerate manner, the need to apply certain measures. The reasons for inadequate pain control include the following.

- Lack of factual knowledge about analgesics.

The consequence is the prescribing of analgesics that are inappropriate, insufficient and infrequent. Constant cancer pain requires constant analgesia. This must be adequate and given regularly to stop the pain re-emerging. On demand 'PRN' (as required) prescribing only means 'pain relief now and then'.

- Unfounded fears about addiction, tolerance, respiratory depression.

Too commonly these unnecessary fears mean morphine administration is delayed until the patient is 'really terminal' i.e. moribund. Moreover often it is unappreciated that in cancer pain, morphine doses have no 'ceiling' but must be titrated against the individual's pain.

- Inaccurate assessment and reassessment.

Accurate assessment and reassessment of cancer pain are central to effective symptom control. Inaccurate diagnosis means inappropriate treatment. Inadequate review can mean inadequate control or unheeded resurgence. In other words, advanced cancer demands the logical approach of careful appraisal and repeated reappraisal.

- Inadequate use of co-analgesics.

Often it is unappreciated that pains may be only partially responsive or unresponsive to morphine and a patient may need the support of other drugs. Such 'complementary' drugs, although usually having no intrinsic analgesic activity, can greatly help or even replace conventional analgesics in achieving pain control.

- Inadequate emotional support and communication.

Such deficiencies towards the patient and family may be important reasons for unrelieved pain.

- Non-use of non-drug measures.

Not all pains are responsive to drug therapy and non-drug interventions have an important role. In particular the use of palliative radiotherapy (see p. 46) and nerve blocks (see p. 47) should be kept in mind.

Assessment – the basis of rational treatment

'Pain' in cancer is a very general term. Most cancer patients have a number of pains. Four out of five cancer patients have at least two or more different pains, while one in three patients have four or more pains. Also, every pain is not a cancer pain. Patients often have pains not directly caused by the malignancy (e.g. dyspepsia, constipation, musculo-fascial pains, osteo-arthritis, haemorrhoids, infections, etc.). As already emphasised, unless a considered judgement as to the most likely cause of each pain can be made, then rational treatment cannot be given. It behoves the nurse as much as the doctor to try and differentiate the various pains and to consider the most probable cause of each pain. Thus careful assessment of a patient's 'pain' is a vital part of management. Assessment has four major components.

- A detailed history.
- Accurate measurement.

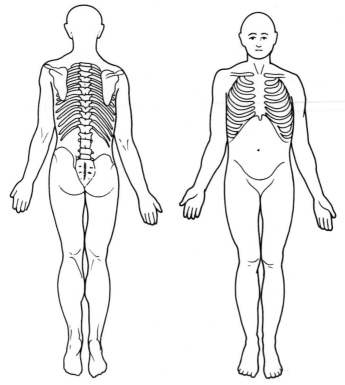

Fig. 3.1   The body diagram (one-third scale).

- Consideration of the patient's 'total pain'.
- Repeated review.

A detailed history

Time spent taking a detailed history is never wasted. The following information should be obtained.

- The sites of the various pains and their radiation.
These are best recorded on a body diagram. (Fig. 3.1). This is especially helpful where there are a number of pains. Completing the body outline in conjunction with the patient can be very rewarding. Its accuracy is affirmed and it is comforting to the patient to see the obvious interest and concern about his or her pains.

- Duration and frequency.
How long has the pain been present, whether it is constant. If it is intermittent, the frequency and length of each episode.

- Quality.
Record the patients description of the pain i.e. whether dull, stabbing, aching, burning, etc.

- Severity.

How severe is the pain? It should be noted that the demeanour of patient and the description of the severity of the pain may not be a reliable guide for a number of reasons. The patient may feel pain is inevitable or may wish to put on a stoic front. He or she may not wish to acknowledge the pain because of its significance (i.e. it indicates the cancer is still present and is progressing) or may fear possible adverse effects if analgestic drugs are prescribed. To obtain a realistic idea the carer should always enquire

– whether sleep is disturbed

– whether daily routines or activities have become restricted

– what drugs have relieved or failed to relieve the pain.

Wherever possible relatives should be interviewed, for their comments may indicate the true level of suffering.

Accurate measurement

The severity of the patient's pain can be measured in a number of ways.

- A popular method is the use of the Visual Analogue Scale (Fig. 3.2)

The patient is asked to put a mark (or says where a mark should be placed) on a 10 cm line according to the severity of the pain, where 0 cm is 'no pain' and 10 cm is 'the worst pain imaginable'. A simple variant of this approach, which most patients have no difficulty in appreciating, is for the carer to draw an imaginary, vertical visual analogue scale in the air with their finger and to ask where, between the imaginary 0 and 10, would the patients put their present pain. Some patients become so adept at this that in subsequent assessments they will quote a figure as the carer approaches, without waiting for a prompt!

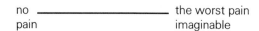

no ———————————— the worst pain
pain   imaginable

Fig. 3.2   The visual analogue scale (not to scale).

- Another method is to grade the pain 0–5 according to the description of the pain's intensity i.e. McGill Melzack Present Pain Intensity (PPI) (Fig. 3.3).

0   No pain
1   Mild
2   Discomforting
3   Distressing
4   Horrible
5   Excruciating

Fig. 3.3   The McGill Melzack Present Pain Intensity (PPI).

- A method that can give patients at home a very real sense of contributing to their management and having some control of the situation is to ask them to keep a pain diary. A set framework can be followed, for example The London Hospital Home Diary (Raiman, 1988), or the format can be personalised according to the individual.

Aspects needing evaluation are pain at or over regular intervals; changes in analgesic requirements; sleep disturbances due to pain; and the development of new pains and other symptoms.

All the above methods can be helpful in monitoring the efficacy of any form of treatment but especially drug therapy.

Consideration of the patient's 'total pain'

Pain is an interweaving of physical and psychological elements and it is essential that an assessment is made of the patient's 'total pain', i.e. not only the physical but the emotional, social and spiritual pain. The intensity of such emotional aspects as anxiety, depression, anger, hostility, should be assessed and note taken of the presence of family, financial or spiritual problems. Any such features can lower the pain threshold and intensify the patient's physical pain. It is so important for the carer to stand back and look at 'the whole person' and consider the various components of the patient's total pain.

Repeated review

Almost invariably the cancer will progress and the clinical situation will change. Thus new pains are likely to develop and old ones re-emerge. It is essential therefore that the patient is repeatedly reviewed.

In addition to the above assessment the overall picture should be completed by taking a detailed history of all drugs administered and making a careful note of the physical findings recorded by medical colleagues.

Setting realistic goals

It is always helpful to delineate in one's mind what one wants to achieve. In pain relief it is useful to have a sequence of realistic goals, such as:
- initially to give the patient a pain-free night's sleep;
- then to relieve the pain at rest during the day;
- then to relieve the pain on standing or moving. This form of pain can be a particular problem.

The need for a personal 'mosaic of therapies'

Although drug therapy is the mainstay of cancer pain management, alleviation of a patient's pain requires more than just the prescribing of analgesics or co-analgesics. Drugs can never be more that one of a number of approaches needed for pain control. Having stood back and looked at the whole person the carer should choose a combination of measures appropriate for the individual. Almost invariably the principle 'pieces' of this personal mosaic of therapies will comprise some or all of the following (Fig. 3.4).

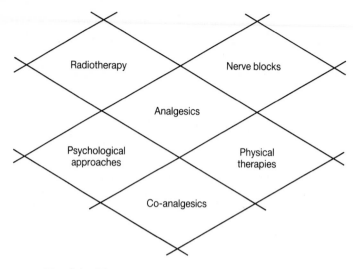

Fig. 3.4   The principal 'pieces' of any personal mosaic.

- Analgesics
- Co-analgesics
- Psychological approaches
- Physical therapies
- Radiotherapy
- Nerve blocks

Analgesics

Analgesics are at the centre of any personal group of therapies. The key to effective pain control is to use a few well known analgesics in a simple sequence of prescribing steps i.e. an 'analgesic staircase' (Fig. 3.5).

The analgesic staircase

For mild to moderate pain   Start at the bottom of the staircase and prescribe a mild 'non-opioid' analgesic such as regular aspirin or paracetamol. If one of these is ineffective it should not be replaced by the other but by regular administration of a drug from the next 'weak opioid' or 'mild analgesic' step, i.e. codeine, dihydrocodeine or dextropropoxyphene, with or without paracetamol or aspirin. If pain relief is still not achieved with the recommended maximum dose of one of these agents then movement should be upwards to the top 'strong opioid' step and regular morphine commenced. There is no particular advantage in using oral diamorphine rather than oral morphine. Both have similar actions and unwanted effects and diamorphine is rapidly converted into morphine following ingestion.

If the pain is severe   Go straight to the top step and administer a strong opioid from the start.

Duration of the effect of oral morphine solution

Morphine is commonly administered as morphine aqueous solution. The doctor can prescribe it as such or as 'morphine aqueous mixture'. Morphine given orally in this form is relatively well absorbed and peak blood levels are reached after one and a half to two hours. The clinical effect of a single dose lasts for about four hours. In general therefore it is illogical to prescribe morphine solution other than every four hours. Despite this, it is not unusual to see it prescribed six or eight hourly. This means for two or four hours the pain will be back, but worse, for it becomes fuelled by spiralling anxiety. Seldom is less frequent administration indicated, although it may be necessary with impaired renal function or if the patient is very old and frail.

Individualisation of morphine dose

Morphine is pre-eminent as an oral analgesic in advanced cancer and, given regularly, will achieve relief in eight or nine out of every ten patients. However, the dose required by any one patient is very variable and the morphine requirements must be individualised. As has been pointed out, there is no 'ceiling dose'. The dose ultimately required must be attained by titration of the dose against the intensity of the individual's pain. Thus there will be a wide range of doses.

Irrespective of its size each four-hourly dose can be dispensed by a pharmacist as morphine sulphate or hydrochloride aqueous solution in a volume of 10 ml. This is preferable and safer for most patients at home. It can be very difficult for some patients and relatives to draw up varying volumes of a concentrated morphine sulphate solution into a calibrated dropper.

NON-OPIOIDS		WEAK OPIOIDS		STRONG OPIOIDS
				Morphine Hydrochloride or Sulphate
		Codeine Phosphate	15–60 mg	
		Tablets	4 hrly	Diamorphine Hydrochloride
		Syrup		
Aspirin	300–600 mg	Dihydrocodeine	30–60 mg	
Tablets	4–6 hrly	Tablets	4 hrly	
(Soluble form available)		Elixir		
Paracetamol	0.5–1 G.	Dextropropoxyphene	2 tablets	
Tablets	4–6 hrly	and Paracetamol	4–8 hrly	
(Soluble form available)		(Co-proxamol)		

Fig. 3.5   The analgesic staircase. See text for details.

Dose titration and increment range

Dose titration is central to successful pain control. About seven out of every ten patients will require no more than 30 mg morphine solution four-hourly. Of the remainder a few will need more than 100 mg four-hourly. More rarely some individuals will need very high doses. By how much should an individual dose of morphine be increased? There are a number of possible sequences. A commonly used sequence is that suggested by Twycross and Lack (1984) i.e. 5–10–15–20–30–40–60–80–100–120–160–200–240 mg/four-hourly etc.

The initial dose of morphine solution

The initial dose of oral morphine solution also must be individualised. It will depend on the patient's previous analgesic requirements, the severity of the pain and the patient's age. If the 'analgesic staircase' has been ascended many will require an initial dose of 10 mg four-hourly: for others 5 mg four-hourly may be more appropriate. If the patient is elderly, frail impaired renal function is suspected, an initial dose of 2.5 mg four-hourly may be adequate. If there is doubt about the magnitude of the initial dose, prescribe a smaller dose and increase this rapidly if it is obvious the pain is not being mitigated. If the pain is controlled by the first dose but the patient is extremely sleepy the next dose should be reduced by 50%.

The bedtime and 'middle-of-the-night' dose

When dose requirements of oral morphine solution have become stabilised often a patient will not need a 'middle-of-the-night' dose i.e. 2.00 am dose. However, should the patient wake with pain this can be negated by doubling the bedtime (10.00 pm) dose (for those having a dose of 40 mg every four hours during the day) or increasing it by 50% (for those having a dose of 60 mg or more every four hours during the day). In some units the augmentation of the bedtime dose is a standard practice. If nightmares or hallucinations should occur with this bedtime increase then routine four-hourly administrations should be adopted throughout the 24 hours.

Controlled – release morphine and mild/moderate pain

Morphine solution can be administered regularly every four hours without difficulty in the hospice or hospital. In the less well controlled environment of home the taking of frequent medication on-time cannot be guaranteed. For this reason, when analgesia requirements for mild to moderate pain have reached the top step of the staircase, many doctors prefer to prescribe twice daily controlled-release morphine (MST Continus).

Controlled-release morphine is a most valuable agent which was developed to reduce dose frequency. The formulation allows the release of morphine over a period of 12 hours. Following the taking of an MST Continus tablet peak plasma concentrations of morphine are achieved after about four hours.

Another great advantage of MST Continus is its various strengths – 10, 30, 60 and 100 mg tablets are readily available and 200 mg tablets will soon be obtainable on a 'named patient' basis. Thus patient and carer are not faced with an inordinate number of single strength tablets as increasing dosage becomes necessary.

When the analgesic staircase has been ascended the starting dose of MST Continus is usually 30 mg 12-hourly. However, as in the case of morphine solution, if the patient is old or frail, or impaired renal function is known or suspected, lower doses may be needed, for example 20 mg 12-hourly or even, very occasionally, 10 mg 12-hourly.

If the pain is not completely allayed MST Continus dosage should be increased keeping the intervals 12-hourly. At high doses, with many tablets to take, some patients may be given MST Continus eight-hourly, but this agent should never be given more frequently, otherwise potentially dangerous cumulation may occur.

Controlled-release morphine and severe pain

The slow absorption of controlled-release morphine and its prolonged action makes this form of morphine unsuitable for the initial treatment of severe pain. The flexibility of morphine solution, given four hourly, is needed to be able to rapidly increase the dose to an effective level. However, once the dosage of morphine solution has been stabilised it is usually possible to revert to 12-hourly MST Continus therapy.

Controlled-release morphine and breakthrough pain

Similarly, controlled-release morphine is too slowly absorbed to be suitable for treating 'breakthrough' pain. Where pain has been well controlled with MST Continus twice daily, 'moderate' breakthrough pain on one or two occasions may be treated with dextromoramide given sublingually or orally, or with a single dose of morphine solution. The additional dose of either of these agents may be half or the whole of a single 4-hourly dose of morphine, depending on the intensity of the pain and the magnitude of the regular dose of morphine currently being given. Very severe breakthrough pain will require immediate review of the clinical situation and usually the administration of subcutaneous diamorphine.

If frequent exacerbations occur and repeated 'top-up' dose of analgesics are needed to achieve pain control, a new adequate level of regular analgesia must be re-established. This may be accomplished by changing the MST Continus therapy to four-hourly aqueous morphine solution and reverting back to MST Continus later at a different dose when a new effective dose level of morphine solution has been achieved. If the breakthrough pain does not respond to additional opioid the patient's condition needs careful reassessment with consideration of other methods of pain control.

Conversion to controlled-release morphine

When transferring from 4-hourly morphine solution, the first dose of MST Continus should be given simultaneously with the last dose of the solution. Giving both at the bedtime dose effects a smooth transfer. Some studies have suggested that MST morphine is equianalgesic mg for mg with diamorphine, others that it is equianalgesic mg for mg with morphine solution.

Although MST morphine is considered to be better absorbed than morphine solution (up to about a fifth) in practice seemingly this has little or no effect. Patients can be transferred from either oral morphine or diamorphine with little or no adjustment of MST needed (Regnard and Davies, 1986). Thus usually the total daily MST dosage is equated with the total daily dose of morphine solution being taken. The strength of each 12-hourly MST dose is obtained by dividing the total daily morphine requirement by a factor of 2; for example

20 mg morphine 4-hourly = 120 mg in 24 hours
= 1 × 60 mg MST Continus tablet 12 hourly

Titrating morphine solution at home

How dose increases of aqueous morphine solution are to be achieved at home needs to be considered, for usually only one bottle of a set strength of morphine will be available at any one time. As suggested by Twycross and Lack (1984), almost all increments in the home will initially be 50% with possibly a second increase of 33% before a new supply of morphine may be prescribed, i.e. an initial dose of 10 ml may be increased to 15 ml (50%) and then to 20 ml (33%). To avoid anxiety it should be explained to the patient and relatives that a dose 'range' may be necessary from a particular bottle, should a fixed initial dose be stated on its label. Clear written instructions should always be given to the patient and family.

Side-effects of morphine and diamorphine

The most common side-effects are drowsiness, constipation, nausea and vomiting.

Drowsiness
Drowsiness when it occurs, is usually transient over two or three days and this will need to be explained to the patient and family.

Constipation
Constipation almost always occurs in patients taking weak or strong opioids and it is imperative that prophylactic laxatives are prescribed. The preferred approach is the administration of a bowel stimulant with a faecal softener. Such a combination can be prescribed together most conveniently in the form of Co-danthrusate capsules (danthron and docusate) or Co-danthramer plain or forte liquid (danthron + poloxamer). Alternatively the combination can be given as two separate products, for example Senna + Lactulose. The latter softens the faecal contents and stimulates peristalsis but often with opiates an additional stronger peristaltic stimulant such as Senna is required. Sodium picosulphate (Laxoberal) is another stimulant that can be used.

Whether given as a combination or two separate agents, conventional doses often are ineffective in the presence of opiates and the laxative dose must be titrated against the patient's response. Constipation due to the failure to give laxatives prophylactically with opiates is a needless, major problem. It causes so much unnecessary trouble, for example nausea and vomiting, anorexia, abdominal pain confusion.

Nausea and vomiting
Nausea and vomiting due to morphine therapy is not inevitable. It occurs in about one in three patients. It is more common in the ambulant. Tolerance develops to

nausea and vomiting and usually it disappears after seven to ten days. In hospice units anti-emetics are no longer given prophylactically but, in the home, practitioners may feel more comfortable to continue this practice for the first week or ten days. An anti-emetic acting against the chemo-trigger zone (the subsidiary CNS emetic centre sensitive to chemical changes) is preferable, for example haloperidol, domperidone, metoclopramide, prochlorperazine.

Confusion and hallucinations
In respect of other side-effects, confusion occurs in about 2% and nightmares and hallucinations in about 1% of patients. If such side-effects do not respond to dose reduction (if feasible) or to an adequate dose of haloperidol, another opioid should be substituted.

Rectal and parenteral administration

Rectal or parental administration will be required when oral administration or morphine is impracticable due to the following.

- Vomiting
- Dysphagia
- Coma
- Profound weakness

Analgesic suppositories
Morphine suppositories may be a useful alternative to injections: 15 mg and 30 mg strength suppositories are readily available but other strengths will be made by the pharmacist. The suppositories may be directly substituted for ordinary oral morphine, i.e. the same dose and same time interval should be used.

Another morphine-like agonist, Oxycodone, is available in suppository form. Oxycodone pectinate (Proladone) suppositories can be used at six to eight hourly intervals. Each suppository is of 30 mg strength and in practice can be considered to be equivalent to about 30 mg oral morphine (i.e. 15 mg morphine solution four-hourly for two doses). The suppository form now available is not easily divided.

Dextromoramide (Palfium) suppositories in 10 mg strengh are also available. These have only a two to three hour duration of action and are best reserved for breakthrough pain.

Parenteral diamorphine
When parenteral medication is required, diamorphine is preferred to morphine. Because of its much greater solubility only impressively small volumes of diamorphine are needed for injection. Generally the oral dose or morphine should be divided by three to obtain the equivalent dose of parenteral diamorphine. The oral dose of diamorphine should be divided by a factor of two. Thus the general rule is 3 mg oral morphine = 2 mg oral diamorphine = 1 mg parenteral diamorphine (Fig. 3.6). For morphine alone 2 mg oral morphine = 1 mg parenteral morphine.

The syringe driver

Subcutaneous diamorphine may be given intermittently at regular intervals. If this is favoured, regular adminstration via a butterfly needle placed in situ will obviate

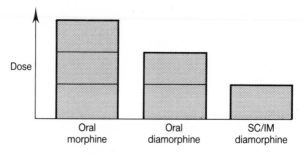

Fig. 3.6   Morphine-Diamorphine equivalents.

repeated piercing of the skin. However the method of choice for this route is to administer the drug continuously via a subcutaneous butterfly needle from a battery operated 'syringe driver'. Some care-givers will only use diamorphine alone in the syringe driver; most will use a mixture of diamorphine and other agents as required.

Advice about syringe drivers
Macmillan nurses and colleagues in Palliative Care Units or in Pain Clinics are always ready to advise about the use of this method. Published information is also readily available (Doyle, 1987; Regnard and Davies, 1986).

Availability of syringe drivers
More and more general practices and hospital units are obtaining syringe drivers but they should never be used as a means of convenience but used only when the above indications are present. The Lisa Sainsbury Organisation kindly loan syringe drivers throughout the United Kingdom, free of charge, for the use of specific patients. Some Macmillan Nurse Home Support Teams, Palliative Care Units and Hospital Support Teams also loan syringe drivers for specific patients.

Diamorphine and other drugs in the syringe driver
Diamorphine used in a syringe driver can be mixed safely with Hyoscine hydro-bromide (Scopolamine), Hyoscine butylbromide (Buscopan), Metoclopramide (Maxolon), Haloperidol, Methotrimeprazine (Nozinan), Midazolam. Cyclizine lactate can react with diamorphine hydrochloride to form an insoluble precipitate. The concentration of each drug has a bearing on the reaction. It is likely to occur if either the concentration of cyclizine or the diamorphine is greater than 25 mg/ml. However, if the concentration of one of these drugs is not greater than 10 mg/ml then the other concentration can be higher than 25 mg/ml.

Sublingual administration

Sublingual administration can be an effective route where doses are relatively low and increases of analgesia are infrequent. On other occasions it can be a dis-appointing approach. Difficulties may arise due to the following.
- Frequent increases mean an increasing number of tablets to be put under the tongue.

- The increasing taste of the drug in the mouth becomes unacceptable.
- The patient has a persistently dry mouth (so common in many patients) so that tablets do not dissolve easily with consequent poor absorption.

Analgesics given sublingually are dextromoramide, phenazocine and buprenorphine. The former two are active if swallowed.

Alternative strong analgesics (Table 3.1)

In the majority of patients morphine sulphate or hydrochloride is effective and acceptable. Occasionally, however, the patient may show an intolerance that necessitates a change to an alternative strong analgesic. Carers who treat advanced cancer patients will need to consider the other strong analgesics available. Some are more potent than morphine and conversion doses will need to be estimated with care. Some features of the principal alternatives are as follows.

- Phenazocine (Narphen) can be a useful alternative on occasions. A 5 mg tablet is equivalent to about 20 mg of oral morphine. Although it can be swallowed the tablet dissolves readily in the mouth and therefore the drug is often used sublingually. A single dose lasts six to eight hours and thus it does not need to be taken as often as morphine solution. Patients may need to be helped to break the small scored tablets when the drug is replacing lower doses of morphine. Sucking a sweet at the same time as the sublingual tablet is under the tongue can mask the bitter taste if this is a problem.

- Dextromoramide (Palfium). This is a valuable agent for breakthrough pain or to cover short interval pain associated with a practical procedure. Although active

Table 3.1 Approximate oral morphine equivalents.

Drug	Tablet strength	Duration of action	Four hourly oral morphine equivalents
Buprenorphine (Temgesic)	0.2 mg	(sublingually) 8 hourly	10 mg
Dextromoramide (Palfium)	5 mg	2–3 hourly	10 mg
Dipipanone + Cyclizine (Diconal)	10 mg (+30 mg Cyclizine)	3–5 hourly	5 mg
Levorphanol (Dromoran)	1.5 mg	4–6 hourly	7.5 mg
Oxycodone pectinate (Proladone)	30 mg (Suppository)	6–8 hourly	15 mg (×2)
Papaveretum	10 mg	3–5 hourly	5 mg
Pethidine	50 mg	2–3 hourly	6 mg
Phenazocine (Narphen)	5 mg	(sublingually) 4–6 hourly	20 mg

orally it is frequently used sublingually. It is rapidly absorbed from under the tongue and as it is not ingested it does not have to pass across the intestinal mucosa or pass through the liver. Both these sites normally metabolise part of the drug (known as the 'first-pass' effect) so by-passing them and this effect will result in higher blood levels. This drug acts for only two to three hours so it should not be used for routine treatment of cancer pain.

● Buprenorphine (Temgesic). This analgesic is a 'partial agonist', i.e. it has a stronger affinity for opioid receptors than a 'pure agonist' such as morphine but evokes less response. The place of the partial agonist in cancer pain management is not fully established (Atkinson *et al.*, 1989). There has been a debate about the use of buprenorphine for a number of years. In the past, authorities have been concerned that because buprenorphine is a partial agonist, it would block or displace morphine from the opioid receptors with impairment of pain control, if they were used together. There is no advantage in using them both simultaneously and no interference has been noted when morphine has been given directly after a patient has been taking buprenorphine (Atkinson *et al.*, 1989).

There has also been concern about buprenorphine's 'analgesic ceiling', i.e. a dose level beyond which no increased benefit occurs. The analgesic ceiling has been stated to occur at a daily dose of about 5 mg i.e. equivalent to about 50 mg of aqueous morphine 4-hourly (Zenz, 1988). Seemingly the position now is that, if a practitioner felt it necessary to add buprenorphine to the analgesic staircase (see Fig. 3.5), its position is between step two and early step three (Atkinson *et al.*, 1989).

● Methadone. This is cumulative and should not be used in the elderly or debilitated. Use in others is best carried out with expert help.

● Levorphanol (Dromoran) should be avoided in the elderly. It has been used successfully in younger patients. It is five times more potent than morphine and the duration of action is about six hours.

● Dipanone (as Diconal) has very limited use owing to its combination with cyclizine.

● Pethidine. This drug has no role in protracted cancer pain. It has too short an action. Cumulation of the toxic metabolite norpethidine and the number of tablets needed when substituted for morphine also negate its use.

● Pentazocine (Fortral). This is another analgesic agent that has no place in the management of chronic cancer pain. The drug should not be given concurrently with morphine. It has partial antagonistic activity that will reduce the effectiveness of morphine and can intensify the pain.

The Brompton cocktail or mixture

This is the name given to mixtures containing morphine or diamorphine in fixed amounts with cocaine, chlorpromazine and alcohol. There is no longer a place for such mixtures in modern therapeutics. They have no advantages over simple morphine solutions and have decided disadvantages. Increasing the opiate means increasing the chlorpromazine (which does not potentiate the analgesic effect of the opiate) and results in unnecessary sedation. Moreover the cocaine can cause unpleasant hallucinations, especially in the elderly.

Co-analgesia

Co-analgesia is an important part of any therapeutic approach and the co-analgesics are a most varied and interesting group of compounds. Almost all have no conventional analgesic activity but nevertheless their actions may complement or supplant accepted analgesics.

Morphine is an excellent drug but it is not a panacea and there are cancer pains that may be only partially responsive or unresponsive to opiates. Co-analgesics often help allay these pains or support more active procedures such as radiotherapy, nerve blocks, surgery, etc.

The two most widely used co-analgesics are corticosteroids and non-steroidal anti-inflammatory drugs.

Corticosteroids

Corticosteroids act as co-analgesics by reducing the overall mass of a malignant tumour. Pain from tumour pressure on nerves, brain or hollow organs is thereby relieved. A malignant tumour comprises a central mass of cancer cells surrounded by a non-cancerous zone of chronically inflamed, oedematous tissue. The latter contributes significantly to the total tumour mass. High dose steroids do not affect the cancer cells but they frequently produce a marked shrinkage of the outer inflammatory zone.

Corticosteroids assist in pain relief in the following situations.

- Raised intracranial pressure
- Nerve compression
- Hepatomegaly
- Head and neck tumour
- Spinal cord compression (as an emergency 'holding' effect)
- Intrapelvic tumour
- Abdominal tumour

There are two principal corticosteroids – Dexamethasone and Prednisolone. Dexamethasone is normally the steroid of choice. It is more potent than prednisolone (2 mg of Dexamethasone = 15 mg Prednisolone) and hence far fewer tablets have to be taken by the patient. There are 2 mg and 0.5 mg dexamethasone tablets available. It is not always appreciated that these tablets can be dissolved easily in water if desired.

When prescribing corticosteroids as a co-analgesic an initial high dose needs to be given to effect reduction of the chronic inflammatory zone. Thereafter the dosage needs to be reduced progressively to the lowest maintenance dose that controls symptoms, otherwise serious side-effects may occur.

There are various patterns of prescribing corticosteroids, as described below.

• Generally the traditional dose to relieve the headache and other effects of raised intracranial pressure from a brain tumour is 16 mg per day. However, on some occasions, 20–24 mg per day may be considered more appropriate.

• Usually smaller doses, for example 8–12 mg per day, may be given to relieve hepatomegaly, nerve compression, bowel or bronchus compression, etc.

• There are various approaches to reducing the dose of steroids. To obviate serious side-effects most practitioners now favour a relatively rapid reduction over 10–14 days once an initial response has been obtained, for example one method is to maintain the high initial dose for 4–5 days and reduce the dosage thereafter by 2 mg per day every third day to a maintenance dose of 2–4 mg per day. Others may favour a more gradual reduction.

• Response to high dose steroids usually occurs within 24–48 hours. If this does not occur generally it is advocated that high doses should be continued for at least a week before it can be said that there has been no response. If there is no improvement after that time the drug can be discontinued.

• The dexamethasone may be given as one or two doses, i.e. in the morning and early afternoon. Sometimes the drug is given four times a day but corticosteroids enhance brain activity and, for some people, later doses may result in insomnia. (Corticosteroids may also stimulate appetite and elevate mood and are often given in small doses to try and produce this effect.)

The nurse will need to become familiar with the patterns of prescribing corticosteroids in his or her own area.

The tumour shrinkage from corticosteroids is temporary. It may last weeks or months. As they have no effect on the actual cancer cells pressure effects will recur as the true tumour mass grows.

Adverse effects of corticosteroids
Corticosteroids are powerful drugs and can give rise to a number of side-effects depending on dosage, duration of therapy and individual response. The adverse effects include the following.

• Oral candidiasis
• Fluid retention – leg oedema
• Moon face (cushingoid)
• Obese abdomen
• Gastritis, peptic ulceration, with possible perforation or haemorrhage
• Muscle weakness and wasting (myopathy); especially of anterior thigh muscles
• Steroid psychosis
• Steroid diabetes
• Osteoporosis

Patients on corticosteroids are very prone to develop oral thrush and, whatever the dose being taken, the mouth needs to be inspected regularly and frequently. In respect of steroid diabetes, beware of the patient on corticosteroids who develops

Table 3.2 Principal NSAIDs used for painful bone secondaries (grouped into separate chemical classes).

Aspirin	600 mg 4 hourly Aspirin–paracetamol ester (Benorylate) 4–8 G of ester daily (5–10 ml bd)
Ibuprofen Flurbiprofen	1.2–1.8 G daily in 3–4 divided doses 150–300 mg daily in 3–4 divided doses
Naproxen	0.5–1 G daily in 2 divided doses
Diclofenac	75–150 mg daily in 2–3 divided doses
Sulindac Indomethacin	200 mg twice daily 25–50 mg 2–3 times daily. Max. 200 mg daily
Piroxicam	20 mg daily initially 10–30 mg maintenance in single or divided doses

polyuria and increasing thirst. Keep the possibility of steroid psychosis in mind if a patient on corticosteroids, especially a high dose, becomes increasingly euphoric, is not sleeping, is paranoid, or is verbose with grandiose ideas.

Non-steroidal anti-inflammatory drugs (NSAIDs)

Non-steroidal anti-inflammatory drugs (NSAIDs) are used as co-analgesics particularly to help allay the pain of bone secondaries. NSAIDs have analgesic, antipyretic and anti-inflammatory properties. They probably exert most of these effects by impairing the synthesis of prostaglandins. They inhibit an enzyme called cyclo-oxygenase which is needed for the completion of one of the final steps leading to the formation of prostaglandins.

In many of the bone metastases which are 'osteolytic' (i.e. destroy bone), prostaglandins appear to play an important role in causing the bone destruction and therefore the associated pain. Prostaglandins also sensitise nerve endings making them respond more easily to painful stimuli. Thus the basis for giving NSAIDs to patients with painful bone secondaries is to inhibit the production of prostaglandins by the bone cancer cells.

There are many different NSAIDs available belonging to different chemical categories. Different medical practitioners favour different agents. There is variability in their effectiveness and if one NSAID does not help it is well worth trying another, preferably from a different chemical class. A helpful scheme has been proposed (Mannix and Rawlins, 1987). The principal NSAIDs used for painful bone secondaries are listed in Table 3.2.

Adverse effects
Like corticosteroids, NSAIDs are powerful drugs and adverse effects are frequently seen. These include the following.

- Dyspepsia: this is common
- Fluid retention with leg oedema: this is common
- Gastro-intestinal bleeding (with melaena or frank blood per rectum), gastro-intestinal ulceration and perforation

- Hypersensitivity reactions (asthma, urticaria and other skin rashes)
- Blood dyscrasias: rarely

NSAIDs are to be used with caution in peptic ulceration, allergic disorders (particularly asthma and hypersensitivity to aspirin) and renal and hepatic impairment.

Fluid retention with NSAIDs
The fluid retention associated with NSAIDs is of interest because it is often resistant to ordinary doses of diuretics. Far higher doses than usual may be needed to achieve an effect. The reason is that prostaglandins are necessary within the tubules of the kidney to facilitate excretion of fluid and often this will remain reduced despite conventional doses of diuretics.

Other co-analgesics

Important other components include muscle relaxants, antidepressants, other deafferentation pain co-analgesics, anticonvulsive drugs and antimicrobial agents.

Muscle relaxants

The pain of skeletal muscle spasm has a variable response to opioids and is best treated by measures directed to relax the muscle. Muscle spasm may arise from irritation from an underlying bone secondary or be due to nerve involvement. The spasm may be relieved by massage, relaxation and the use of drugs. Useful agents are diazepam and baclofen (Lioresol).

- Diazepam. Because this drug and one of its active metabolites exert a prolonged effect a single bedtime dose is usually sufficient, i.e. 5–15 mg. Response is often at the expense of drowsiness.

- Baclofen (Lioresol). The dose of this drug should be gradually increased from 5 mg 8-hourly to 15 mg 8-hourly. Again drowsiness often occurs. Nausea and vomiting and confusion are other side-effects.

Muscle pain may not always be due to generalised spasm. The pain can arise from an area of excessive irritability in the muscle or its covering (fascia) caused by strain. This area is called a 'trigger point'. It is a tender, palpable band of muscle fibres. The pain tends to be referred away from the trigger point with a distinctive pattern specific for the muscle involved. The painful condition is called an acute myofascial pain syndrome. The pain can be relieved by application of Transcutaneous Electrical Nerve Stimulation (TENS; see p. 45–6), acupuncture or an injection of local anaesthetic and a corticosteroid (e.g. bupivacaine and depomedrone) to the trigger point area.

Antidepressants

Antidepressants can be effective in relieving pain resulting from the nerve being destroyed by malignant infiltration. This disturbing type of pain, which does not respond to opioids, is called deafferentiation pain. Characteristically it is felt in areas of the body supplied by particular spinal nerves, i.e. in the distribution of dermatomes. The pain is felt as a superficial burning or scalding. In many, the lightest of touch can arouse an intense exacerbation of the pain (a phenomenon called allodynia). Stabbing pain is also felt and may be the predominant feature.

Amitriptyline or dothiepin are popular choices of antidepressant. The starting dose of amitriptyline varies from 10–25 mg daily with a slow increase to 50–70 mg daily. Dothiepin is commenced at 50–75 mg daily increasing slowly to 150 mg daily. The drugs can be given as single doses at bedtime. Such drugs produce analgesic effects at doses lower than those used to treat depression. Side-effects are common including sedation, dry mouth, constipation, urinary retention, dizziness and confusion. These drugs are contra-indicated in patients with glaucoma.

Other deafferentiation pain co-analgesics

Other interesting drugs used to try and mitigate this non-opioid responsive pain include mexiletine hydrochloride and clonidine hydrochloride.

- Mexiletine hydrochloride: This is an anti-arrhythmic agent. It is normally used to treat abnormal rhythms after myocardial infarction or with ischaemic heart disease. Essentially it 'stabilises' nerve cells so they are not so easily stimulated. For this reason it is used to try and inhibit the nerve cells in the spinal cord concerned with pain transmission.

- Clonidine hydrochloride: This drug is normally used against migraine in lower doses and as an antihypertensive agent at higher doses occasionally it is also used to try and inhibit the nerve cells in the spinal cord involved in pain transmission.

These agents are best avoided for pain therapy if a patient has heart trouble or is hypertensive. The advice of a Palliative Care specialist or an anaesthetist should always be sought before using these drugs for cancer pain.

Anticonvulsive drugs

Such drugs are used to dampen down the erratic firing of nerve cells. In cancer patients they can be useful in relieving the stabbing pain of nerve compression (which often does not respond to morphine alone) or the lancinating component of deafferentation pain.

Carbamazepine (Tegretol) is a popular choice. A small starting dose is best, for example 100 mg twice daily with a gradual increase. The average dose is 200 mg 8-hourly. Occasionally doses of 400 mg 8-hourly or 6-hourly may be reached. Drowsiness and dizziness may occur, also nausea and vomiting. Rashes may appear after some weeks on therapy. Hepatitis and bone marrow depression are rare adverse effects.

Other anticonvulsants such as sodium valproate or phenytoin may be favoured.

Antimicrobial agents

The pain from cellulitis associated with ulcerating or fungating cancers, or complicating lymphoedema, can be allayed by an appropriate antibiotic, for example Phenoxymethylpenicillin (Penicillin V) 500 mg orally 6-hourly, Flucloxacillin 250 mg orally 6-hourly, Erythromycin 500 mg orally 6-hourly. Metronidazole 400 mg orally 8-hourly can be added when an anaerobic infection is also suspected.

Psychological approaches

This piece of the mosaic has many components and these include the following.

- Sensitive listening
- Relaxation therapy
- Hypnosis
- Distraction
- Imagery

Sensitive listening

All carers should aim to be 'good' or sensitive, empathic listeners. Such listening is a disciplined skill. It does not come naturally as one might think and the carer should read and practise appropriate approaches (Nelson-Jones, 1988). Sensitive listening is an essential adjunct to any form of pain therapy. Such listening involves the characteristics given below.

- Not just hearing words, but listening for cues, for example the way the words are said and the implications behind their content.
- Seeing as well as hearing, i.e. perceiving 'body messages'.
- Conveying one's attention, interest and availability ('attending' the patient). This is a powerful way of affirming a patient's worth and reducing isolation.
- Encouraging the patient to talk, so that pent up frustration and anger are released and anxieties are expressed.

Communication skills are discussed further in Chapter 14.

Relaxation therapy

Although there is widespread belief that relaxation helps to relieve pain there is little research to demonstrate its effectiveness, especially in cancer pain. Nevertheless, the benefit to individuals and the knowledge of how pain, anxiety and muscle tension tend to intensify each other, form a reasonable basis for its use. It seems that even if it does not have an effect on the pain, relaxation therapy improves the person's mood and attitude so that he or she can cope better with the pain.

There are many relaxation techniques available and they need to be matched to specific patients and specific situations. Some have an inward focus on the body (e.g. rhythmic breathing, jaw relaxation) and these may not be the best for a patient distressed about body changes. Others have an outward focus, for example pleasant imagery, when one imagines oneself back in a secure and peaceful environment. For those with pent up emotions 'progressive relaxation' may be beneficial, i.e. various muscle groups are tensed, held and then relaxed. For others with prolonged pain a meditation technique may be preferable.

Relaxation is a skill that has to be learnt by patients. It is not simply resting or reading a book or watching television. Relaxation therapy for a cancer patient is a helpful adjunct. It can never be a substitute for other therapies such as analgesics. Nurses who are interested may wish to seek suitable education and experience and read appropriate accounts, for example McCaffery and Beebe (1989).

Hypnosis

There are numerous reports about the successful use of hypnosis in reducing cancer pain. The problem again is that much of the published evidence is inadequate, i.e. reports are either on single cases or on small numbers of patients, there are no appropriate controls and pain measurements are variable. Doubters question whether hypnosis is any more beneficial than just the emotional support given by the carer. Nevertheless, there have been impressive responses in certain individuals and these, allied to the other many anecdotal reports, suggest that hypnosis can be of great help to some patients (Wood, 1989).

Once the hypnotic stage has been entered various approaches may be used. These include such highly interesting strategies as outlined below.

• Dissociation of the patient from the pain and from his or her current body state, back to a pain free, enjoyable period. Patients can be taught simple techniques to enter this dissociation state themselves i.e. auto-hypnosis.

• Suggestion of anaesthesia being generated in the hand and transferring this to the part of the body in pain by touching that area with the hand.

• Suggesting that the pain is a pulsating light which decreases in frequency and intensity and as the light diminishes so does the pain. A train disappearing into the distance taking the pain with it is another imagery form.

• Substituting the pain with a less disturbing sensation, i.e. a tingling sensation or a pressure.

• Displacing the focus of the pain to a less important part of the body, i.e. to a toe or to a thumb with the pain leaking away from its tip.

Distraction

Distraction is drawing the patient's attention away from pain onto other stimuli. All sensory approaches can be used, i.e. hearing, seeing, touching, moving. Distraction strategies may be used against both short episodes of pain (less than an hour) and chronic pain (McCaffery and Beeb, 1989). In all instances the content of the techniques must be individualised.

For brief episodes of pain, i.e. from short practical procedures or for pain on movement, a number of techniques can be used. These include focusing on an object (e.g. a flower or picture in a magazine) and describing it mentally or verbally, listening to music through a headset or singing a tune mentally, tapping out a rhythm with the fingers or feet, holding onto or rubbing an object.

For ongoing cancer pain the strategy is to improve the level of sensory input so that the patient does not lie in bed or sit in a chair thinking only of his or her pain and impending death. Commitment and consideration are needed by the carer so that a structured programme is elaborated for the patient, including adequate periods of rest. The programme may include such inputs as listening to music or a talking book, craftwork, exercise, conversation with individuals, selected television and video viewing, being taken out for visits, etc. In the home simply putting the bed by a window so a patient can look out and watch the world go by can be a great help. There is a great need for well planned, individualised programmes for patients. An occasional, single distraction episode is of minimal use.

Imagery

This is another well known supportive technique which is gaining popularity. Again there is no definitive research data available but individual reports support the benefit of this approach. In this technique the patient is helped to use his or her imagination to develop sensory images to help reduce the pain intensity. If the pain is brief the carer may suggest that the patient imagines the pain is becoming stinging rather than lancinating or a pleasant warmness rather than an ache.

If the pain is prolonged then a more lengthy, systematic approach is needed. The patient may benefit from 'guided imagery'. Two examples of the latter approach are given below.

● The patient is helped to imagine the body to be a bag which becomes slowly filled with sand. When full a slit in the bag is imagined and as the sand slowly trickles away so does the pain.

● After an appropriate preamble the patient is helped to imagine that there is a hole in the body close to the painful area. Each time the patient breathes out it is imagined that more and more of the pain leaks out through the hole.

Helpful accounts on the use of imagery are readily available (McCaffery and Beebe, 1989).

Physical therapies

In physical therapies some form of stimulation is applied to the skin and superficial tissues. Stimulating the skin to relieve pain is probably as old as the human race. It is seen in its simplest form in everyday life with the mother rubbing the painful area of the child's arm or leg hurt by a fall.

The physical therapies commonly used in practice include the following.

- Superficial application of heat or cold
- Superficial body massage
- Transcutaneous Electrical Nerve Stimulation (TENS)
- Acupuncture

Superficial heat or cold

Provided they are applied at a comfortable intensity, the application of heat or cold may help bring relief when there is localised pain. Heat may be applied in a variety of forms including via an electrical heat pad, a hot water bottle (wrapped in cloth to prevent burns), radiant heat, immersion in a warm bath or jacuzzi. Cold may be applied in various containers wrapped in cloth to prevent tissue damage, for example cold gel pack, plastic bag containing ice and water, a bag of frozen peas (hit gently to separate the constituents).

Application of heat and cold is suitable for the non-cancer types of pain occurring in the cancer patient, for example musculo-fascial strain, muscle spasm, joint stiffness. It is generally suggested that application of heat directly over an area of malignant infiltration should be avoided in case this favours an acceleration of the growth. Cold has a more prolonged pain relieving effect than heat but usually the latter is preferred by patients.

Superficial body massage

Many carers are becoming proficient in the use of superficial body massage. To many cancer patients this is most pleasurable and the relief of physical and mental tensions can help to decrease the pain.

Physical well being is enhanced, probably by relaxation of muscle tension and by increasing skin circulation. Also a caring touch usually brings comfort and re-assurance. In addition, the degree of intimacy afforded by this procedure may give a patient the confidence to talk about underlying fears and other problems.

Extensive body massage is too tiring for most advanced cancer patients and any areas with underlying cancer infiltration need to be treated with caution. However, limited massage of the hands or feet, or a back and shoulder rub, can be most pleasant and comforting. Some nurses may wish to gain the knowledge and skill of superficial body massage and there are appropriate courses available.

A growing interest is developing within palliative care in the use of essential oils and massage (aromatherapy, see p. 112) and in a particular form of massage involving reflex areas in the feet and hands (reflexology).

Transcutaneous Electrical Nerve Stimulation (TENS)

In this technique low intensity stimulation of large nerve fibres within a painful area is carried out through electrodes applied to the overlying skin. These large nerve fibres rapidly conduct the stimuli along to the spinal cord where they activate an agent called enkephalin. This agent inhibits, or 'closes the gate' on the painful stimuli being conducted from the area at a slower rate along smaller nerve fibres.

The patient wears a battery-powered stimulator and flexible wires conduct the current to electrodes on the skin. The electrodes are applied with a conductive gel and held in place with adhesive tape. The aim is to induce a tolerable tingling sensation. The technique is taught to patients so that it can be self-administered. The patient may need to use the stimulator for a few hours or for the entire day.

It is uncommon for the technique to be useful in severe cancer pain. Beneficial effects have been found in moderate pain in cancer patients, especially for benign musculo-fascial pains, scar pain, post herpatic neuralgia and phantom limb pains.

A significant limitation of the usefulness of TENS in cancer pain is that its efficacy rapidly declines with time. In some studies (Ventafridda *et al.*, 1979) only 10% to 30% of patients who obtained initial relief were still using the technique after a month. Another problem is that the positioning of the electrodes in relation to the painful area and the finding of the optimum electrical stimulus can be very time consuming. TENS should be performed by trained personnel, for example physio-therapists, who can explain the technique to the patient in simple terms and who have the skills and patience to correctly position the electrodes and find the optimum electrical stimulus.

TENS should not be used in patients with a pacemaker and the electrodes should not be placed over the carotid sinus.

Although only a few patients with cancer pain have long term benefit this procedure is simple and safe and it may be worth considering before embarking on more involved therapies.

Acupuncture

Generally acupuncture is not sufficient to relieve severe malignant pain. It is useful for non cancer pain such as musculo-fascial pain and muscle spasms. Different intensities of acupuncture therapy may be applied varying from passive needle insertion to electrical stimulation.

Palliative radiotherapy

Palliative radiotherapy can be very effective in relieving cancer pain in selected patients. Doctors and nurses should appreciate that radiotherapy is the treatment of choice for metastatic bone pain. Painful bone secondaries should be discussed with the local radiotherapy and oncology service irrespective of whether the patient is at home or in hospital.

For localised bone secondaries usually a single treatment as a day patient can be given and if pain is not relieved, or if it re-emerges, retreatment is possible. For a larger 'field', for example secondaries throughout the bony pelvis, five to ten treatments may be necessary. For painful, more widespread bone metastases 'half body' irradiation may be indicated. An appropriate single treatment is to the upper or lower half of the body. If necessary, irradiation to the other half of the body can be carried out six weeks later. Admission to hospital for a short period is required to alleviate possible nausea and vomiting.

Treatment with morphine and non-steroidal anti-inflammatory drugs should be commenced while radiotherapy is being arranged and continued until the radiotherapy has taken effect. Pain relief commences about seven to ten days after radiotherpay in many patients: in others it may take three to four weeks. As increasing alleviation of the pain occurs so it may be possible to reduce drug therapy or even stop it eventually.

Other painful conditions where radiotherapy may be of help include the following.

- Painful ulcerating or fungating superficial lesions
- Painful solid growths on the surface of the body
- Severe perineal pain from an unresectable rectal carcinoma left in situ
- Painful metastatic liver enlargement not allayed by drugs

Nerve blocks

It is possible to relieve cancer pain by blocking the nerve pathways along which the pain stimuli are conducted to the central nervous system. Nerve blocks are a valuable approach but patients and procedures need to be selected with care if pain relief without adverse sequelae is to be achieved. Nerves can be interrupted either temporarily or for a long period.

- Temporarily by injecting a local anaesthetic (such as bupivacaine or lignocaine) around the nerve.

- For a prolonged period, by destroying a portion of the nerve by one of several techniques, i.e. local infiltration of chemicals such as alcohol, phenol, chlorocresol, or by the application of cold (cryotherapy) or heat (thermo-coagulation).

These techniques are usually carried out by specially trained anaesthetists. The anaesthetist will always be pleased to see the patient initially in the hospital ward, or at home as a domiciliary consultation. Alternatively, it may be possible for the patient to attend a local Centre for Pain Relief.

Nerve blocks can be carried out at a variety of sites and can be directed at:

- the spinal nerves; and
- the sensory fibres which transmit pain from the organs (viscera) within the body. These accompany the autonomic nerves.

The spinal nerves

Spinal nerves may be interrupted outside or inside the vertebral column.

Outside the vertebral column, the principal sites are as given below.

- As the nerve emerges from the vertebral column, i.e. a paravertebral block. This may be indicated, for instance, in the thoracic region for pain in the thoracic spine or posterior ribs or upper abdominal wall.

- As a single nerve coursing across the body, for example an intercostal block, where a thoracic nerve is interrupted as it runs beneath a rib, to treat rib pain at the side or front of the chest.

- When joined with others as a nerve plexus, for example a brachial plexus block, for pain down the arm from malignant infiltration of the plexus not responding to morphine and cortico-steroids. In this situation such a procedure has to be considered very carefully as the nerve destruction (neurolytic) agent will affect motor function leaving the patient with a useless arm. Generally when neurolytic agents are to be injected at any site, initially a block with a local anaesthetic is performed to allow the patient to observe the effects. Only if these are acceptable to the patient is the neurolytic block then performed.

Within the vertebral column the block is directed at the sensory roots of the spinal nerves as they traverse the vertebral canal to join the posterior aspect of the cord. The most common sites for the block are given below.

● In the space between the inner surface of the vertebrae and the outermost layers of the meninges (the dura mater), i.e. the intradural or epidural space. Thus the procedure is termed an epidural block.

● In the space filled with cerebrospinal fluid, between the inner covering of the spinal cord (the pia mater) and the middle layer of the meninges (the arachnoid mater), i.e. the subarachnoid space. This is termed an intrathecal block.

Epidural block

A common indication for an epidural block in the cancer patient is back pain with nerve root pain, due to malignant bone disease of the spine. Usually an epidural catheter is inserted to administer a regular top up of local anaesthetic solution alone or to complement an infusion of epidural opiates (see below). Single injections of the cortico-steriod depomedrone mixed with a local anaesthetic, also may be given epidurally to reduce local chronic inflammatory changes around a malignant focus and nerve-root compression.

Epidural opiates

This is a route which has been controversial but is becoming more widely used. By this method opiates are deposited through a fine catheter into the epidural space. In the UK diamorphine is favoured because of its greater safety and is usually given as a continuous infusion over 24 hours via a syringe driver. The opiate is absorbed across the meninges and cerebrospinal fluid (CSF), into the posterior horn of the spinal cord where it stimulates opioid receptors on neurones there and inhibits the onward transmission of pain stimuli. The opiate also diffuses upwards through the CSF to gain access to the brain itself.

Increasingly epidural opiates are being used where hitherto a neurolytic block would have been the next approach, for example they are being used in difficult cancer pain problems such as intractable back pain and intrapelvic pain with or without nerve root involvement, and for the pain from intra-abdominal infiltration.

Epidural opiates are especially useful if the patient seems to have a morphine responsive pain but the overall amount of oral or subcutaneous opiate is causing excessive drowsiness or confusion or hallucinations. Only about an eighth to a tenth of the total 24 hour oral dose may be needed epidurally.

Intraspinal morphine

Morphine is used in centres where diamorphine is not available (the UK is one of the few countries where diamorphine can be legally administered in routine practice). It is given directly into the CSF (i.e. intrathecally) as well as epidurally.

A number of side effects can occur with intraspinal opiates but delayed respiratory depression has to be especially considered when morphine is given. Such an effect can occur hours after the initial administration. This seemingly represents the time taken for the morphine to diffuse upwards within the circulating CSF to be absorbed by the brain tissues, including the respiratory centre. Such delayed respiratory depression is infrequent with epidural diamorphine.

Closed systems

For prolonged epidural or intrathecal administration the epidural catheter may be implanted beneath the skin. Using a tunnelling technique the catheter is 'threaded' subcutaneously around to the anterior chest wall where its free end is attached to a reservoir also buried beneath the skin. The reservoir can be filled daily by the percutaneous injection of the appropriate amount of opiate. Alternatively the free end can be brought out and attached to some form of pump and the opiate administered continuously. These closed systems are expensive.

Intrathecal block

A common indication for an intrathecal block is pain in the perineum, usually from cancer of the rectum. A small amount of phenol in glycerine is injected via a needle inserted between the 5th lumbar vertebra and the sacrum. The patient is tilted backwards (at an angle of 30° and maintained like that for half an hour so that the solution drops down to pool around the lower sacral roots). This indication is a good example of the need for careful consideration and careful selection of patients when neurolytic solutions are to be used. With this procedure there is a real risk of bladder and rectal dysfunction, because among the sacral nerve roots affected by the chemical lesion are those which supply the rectal and bladder sphincters.

The sensory fibres carrying visceral pain

These fibres accompany the autonomic nerves and are usually interrupted at the sympathetic ganglia.

Coeliac plexus block

One of the most useful techniques is the coeliac plexus block. This is especially helpful for intractable pain in the upper abdomen and back, associated with carcinoma of the pancreas or stomach. The plexus also receives pain fibres from the gall bladder, liver, kidney, adrenal and ureter. The block is carried out under local anaesthesia with the patient lying face downwards. The needle is inserted through the skin to either side of the vertebral column just under the 12th rib. Using X-ray image intensification the needles are advanced upwards and inwards to the front of the aorta. If a 'prognostic block' is being carried out, i.e. to observe if the procedure will relieve the pain, local anaesthetic solution is injected through each needle. If destruction of the nerve plexus has been decided upon an equal volume of absolute alcohol and local anaesthetic is injected. A coeliac plexus block requires admission to hospital for about three days. Its effect may last for about six months and often complete abolition of the pain is achieved.

Lumbar sympathetic block

A block of the lumbar sympathetic ganglia is another very useful procedure for bladder and rectal pain, especially tenesmus. The ganglia also receive pain fibres from the uterus, ovary and testis. The block is carried out in much the same way as the coeliac plexus block but at a slightly lower level. The neurolytic solution usually used is phenol in water. This procedure also will require the patient to be admitted to hospital for about three days.

When to refer to the anaesthetist or pain clinic

The possibility of some form of nerve block should be considered for any cancer pain not responding to drug therapy. The anaesthetist will be only too willing to discuss whether or not a nerve block is appropriate for a particular problem.

The possibility of a nerve block should be considered when the following types of pain cannot be controlled with drug measures.

- Pain that is 'anatomically suitable', that is unilateral pain, on one side of chest, upper abdomen or trunk, or in a leg or arm
- Pain across the upper abdomen or radiating through to the back from cancer affecting the stomach, liver, gall bladder or adrenal
- Pelvic pain
- Rectal/bladder tenesmus
- Lower back pain, alone or with nerve root pain radiating down one or both legs
- Pain controlled at rest but not on movement.

Other 'special therapeutic pieces'

Expert assistance from a variety of specialties may be needed if the pain remains difficult to control or certain pathological conditions develop. Certain 'special therapeutic pieces' may need to become incorporated into the mosaic of pain management. These include hormone therapy and chemotherapy, general surgery, orthopaedic surgery, neurosurgery.

Hormone therapy and chemotherapy

Modification of the cancer by either of these methods alleviate pain and they may be considered even in an advanced malignancy. Examples of hormone therapy include progestogens for metastatic breast and renal carcinoma and anti-androgen therapy for advanced prostatic carcinoma. Chemotherapy may be used occasionally, for example for pain relief in advanced breast and head and neck cancer, but the benefits need to be weighed very carefully against the side effects.

General surgery

The general surgeon may be able to help alleviate pain due to advanced cancer in certain circumstances. Surgical intervention may relieve pain by such procedures as laying open painful intestinal-cutaneous fistulae, draining superficial abscesses, relieving intestinal obstruction by a colostomy or a by-pass operation.

Orthopaedic surgery

Orthopaedic management of skeletal metastases may achieve considerable pain relief. Treatment may be required for a pathological fracture, impending fracture or spinal instability.

Pathological fracture   For a pathological fracture some form of internal fixation is commonly carried out, followed by radiotherapy. Local irradiation is an essential part of treatment in order to inhibit further tumour growth.

Impending fracture   There is a high risk of fracture of a long bone if a large bone destroying (lytic) metastasis is present. (Such metastases are not seen on X-ray until at least 50% of the bone has been destroyed.) Some form of internal stabilisation of the weakened bone is then necessary, followed by radiotherapy.

The unstable spine   The spine may become unstable as a result of bone destruction of the vertebrae and any movement is associated with severe pain. X-rays show various degrees of vertebral collapse. Various methods of stabilisation are used and fixing the vertebrae at and around the level of the bone metastases to a rod or rectangle can bring immense relief of pain. Post-operative irradiation is essential.

Neurosurgery

Recourse to neurosurgical techniques to relieve advanced cancer pain varies from centre to centre. In general it is an infrequent approach.

Cordotomy
When pain remains intractable a procedure such as cordotomy may be indicated. This involves sectioning the tracts which convey pain stimuli from the spinal cord to the brain in the antero-lateral quadrant of the spinal cord. Such a procedure is used mainly for pain on one side of the body below the mid-chest.

Percutaneous and surgical cordotomy
Cordotomy is achieved in two ways; percutaneous or surgical. In the former a needle is inserted between the first and second cervical vertebrae under X-ray control. The patient is not anaesthetised but sedated with premedication. Using an electrode a heat lesion is produced in the antero-lateral quadrant of the spinal cord. Surgical cordotomy is an operative procedure under anaesthesia and is usually carried out in the upper thoracic region. The antero-lateral quadrant of the spinal cord is cut under direct vision.

A decreasing demand

The increasing use of other techniques, especially implanted drug delivery systems for the chronic administration of epidural or intrathecal opiates, has greatly reduced the need for cordotomy. Similarly there is a decreasing demand for other approaches such as the ablation of the pituitary gland, section of dorsal roots of spinal nerves, or the use of stereotactic surgery. In the latter, various nerve tracts or collections of nerve cells are destroyed by means of a probe or energy beam directed through the brain.

Conclusions

The nurse has a unique, privileged position having trusted, close contact with patients. Such a relationship should be used to the full to help relieve the pains of advanced cancer. The nurse should consistently keep in mind the following considerations.

- Cancer pain is not inevitable. It is treatable and controllable.

- The majority of cancer patients have more than one pain.

- Assessment of a patient's 'pain' is essential. Repeated review is equally important – new pains develop, old ones recur.

- It is essential to stand back and look at the person's 'total pain'.

- Analgesics are the mainstay of pain relief. For persistent pain they should be taken 'by mouth', 'by the clock' and 'by the ladder' (WHO , 1986).

- Morphine is the opioid of choice. Addiction, tolerance and respiratory depression are myths.

- Analgesics are only one of a number of measures and each patient should have a personal 'mosaic of therapies'.

- If pain persists ask questions. Is the pain Morphine responsive? Has the 'whole person' been addressed? Is the patient frightened, angry, depressed or lonely? Have co-analgesic drugs been considered? Is there any indication for radiotherapy or nerve blocks? Has some basic principle been overlooked?

- Pain is only one of many distressing symptoms of advanced cancer. Pain control should be but one part of a comprehensive approach to the care of the patient and family.

References

ATKINSON, R. E., SCHOFIELD, P. A. and MELLOR, P. (1989). *Buprenorphine Morphine Transfer Trial in Cancer Pain.* Meeting of Intractable Pain Society of Great Britain and Ireland, Nottingham.

DOYLE, D. (1987). *Domiciliary Terminal Care.* Churchill Livingstone, Edinburgh.

MCCAFFERY, M. and BEEB, A. (1989). *Pain. Clinical Manual for Nursing Practice.* The C. V. Mosby Company.

MANNIX, K. A. and RAWLINS, M. D. (1987). The management of bone metastases: non-steroidal anti-inflammatory drugs. *Palliative Medicine,* 1, 128–31.

NELSON-JONES, R. (1988). *Practical Counselling and Helping Skills,* second edition. Cassell Education Limited, London.

RAIMAN, J. (1988). *Nursing Issues and Research in Terminal Care.* John Wiley & Sons Ltd, Chichester.

REGNARD, C. F. B. and DAVIES, A. (1986). *A Guide to Symptom Relief in Advanced Cancer.* Haigh and Hochland Ltd.

TWYCROSS, R. G. and LACK, A. (1984). *Symptom Control in Far Advanced Cancer.* Pitman Publishing Limited, London.

VENTAFRIDDA, V., SGANZERLA, E. P., FORCHI, C., POZZI, G., CORDINI, G. (1979). *Transcutaneous Nerve Stimulation in Cancer Pain. Advances in Pain Research and Therapy, Vol. 2.* Raven Press, New York.

WALL, P. D. (1987). Foreword in *Pain Control,* Jane Latham. Austen Cornish Publishers with The Lisa Sainsbury Foundation.

WOOD, M. (1989). Pain control and hypnosis. *Nursing Times,* 85, 38–40.

WORLD HEALTH ORGANIZATION (1986). *Cancer Pain Relief.*

ZENZ, M. (1988). Personal communication in R. G. Twycross, Opioid analgesics in cancer pain: current practice and controversies. *Cancer Surveys,* 7, 29–53.

Further reading

MCCAFFERY, M. and BEEB, A. (1989). *Pain. Clinical Manual for Nursing Practice.* The C. V. Mosby Company.

REGNARD, C. F. B. and DAVIES, A. (1986). *A Guide to Symptom Relief in Advanced Cancer.* Haigh and Hochland.

WORLD HEALTH ORGANIZATION (1986). *Cancer Pain Relief.*

4

The management of other frequently encountered symptoms

Ilora Finlay

'I do not want two diseases, one God made and one the doctor made'
Napoleon Bonaparte

Symptom analysis

The only way that a symptom can be brought under control is to understand the cause and then provide the appropriate therapy. Knowledge of the cause of a symptom is the guide to therapy. When a patient is beyond curative treatment, it is not permissible to blame everything on the underlying disease; fear, depression and intercurrent infections will aggravate disorders already present or give new symptoms of their own. A dry mouth becomes drier with fear; cystitis can cause vomiting; candida infection can give dysphagia and oesophagitis; insomnia may be a side-effect of corticosteroids – the list is almost endless.

The interplay between the psyche (mental, social and spiritual state) and pain has been described; it applies equally to all the symptoms the patient presents with (Fig. 4.1). Thus the patient's experience of the symptom and the consequent distress is aggravated if all aspects of the patient's care are not attended to (Baines, 1981).

Patients deserve the best of care and that depends on the best of medical diagnostic skills and nursing observations. The challenge to the professions is to continually review the clinical situation in the face of constant change. Patients with cancer have a disease that is progressing; no sooner is a symptom under control than another emerges. Some problems can be anticipated, enabling the patient at risk of bowel obstruction to be treated with stool softeners early or prophylactic antiemetics to be left in the house when starting a patient on opiates. But when the unexpected occurs the carer is left like the sleuth in a detective story asking the question 'WHY?' – there must be a cause for the symptom and that cause must be sought to guide appropriate therapy.

Pain has had much publicity and so patients are more willing to complain of pain, partly as they have the hope and the expectation that something can be done. For some symptoms, such as nausea, that expectation does not exist and many patients submit to distressing symptoms feeling they cannot complain about too many. Actively questioning about different symptoms is important to obtain a full picture of the various sources of distress to the patient. In many patients the problem list then obtained will contain over five, sometimes over fifteen problems. Each of these

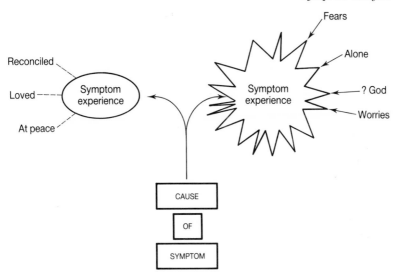

Fig. 4.1 The interplay between the psyche and pain. The same symptom will be perceived as terrible by the frightened patient and less distressingly when the patient is calm.

symptoms interplays with the others so that therapy must be aimed to hit several targets at once.

There are so many symptoms that cancer patients can have. The presenting complaint may be, for example, dyspnoea; on direct questioning these patients often have weakness, weight loss, loss of appetite, constipation, nausea and pain to name but a few symptoms. The dyspnoea and pain will cause insomnia so that chronic fatigue lowers the patient's ability to cope with persistent pain. The constant effort to breathe combined with a low dietary intake aggravates weakness already caused by the tumour and breathing through an open mouth further dries mucous membranes already dry from the anticholinergic effect of analgesic and antiemetic drugs. Thus, the picture is always complex in these patients.

Swollen ankles, nausea, anorexia, abdominal discomfort, hallitosis and diaphragmatic pleuritic pain can all be caused by liver involvement with cancer. Metastases can occur at multiple sites, hence a patient with lung metastases can also have dyspnoea, haemoptyses and chest pain on their problem list. Bone metastases will cause pain and risk of pathological fracture or hypercalcaemia; all can confound the professionals by the sheer complexity of the symptoms presented. There is no substitute for taking a good history. Each symptom must be differentiated from another to evolve a problem list (often long) specifying the symptoms individually. For example: Is the patient nauseated all the time; only after eating; only at the smell of food; or does the patient vomit with no preceding nausea? Such attention to detail is imperative to provide an adequate guide to management.

When drugs are used their dose and route of administration must be appropriate. Intramuscular injections are painful and should not be given; the same clinical effect can be obtained by giving drugs subcutaneously through a small gauge needle. Intravenous administration is the route of choice when a rapid effect is needed.

Rectal administration of drugs is very useful at home when drugs cannot be taken by mouth (e.g. rectal antiemetics in nausea and vomiting).

The following problems are considered below.

Nausea and vomiting
Eating and feeding
Anorexia
Mouth care
Ascites
Constipation
Intestinal obstruction
Diarrhoea
Rectovaginal fistula
Bladder pain
Dyspnoea
Itch
Fungating lesions
Weakness
Hypercalcaemia
Cerebral tumours
Corticosteroids
Lymphoedema
Depression
Fear and anxiety
Insomnia

The incidence of some of these problems is indicated in Table 4.1.

Nausea and vomiting

Nausea and vomiting is experienced by over one third of patients admitted to a Palliative Care Unit, which is about half the incidence of pain in patients on admission. It is therefore evident that the problem of nausea and vomiting would be a commonly occurring symptom in any area of clinical practice (see Table 4.1). Nausea makes a person listless, 'off food', withdrawn and disinterested in surroundings, sweaty and pale. Patients are often reluctant to complain of nausea, attributing it to 'something I ate', 'the car ride' or 'the tablets'. The mechanisms of nausea and vomiting are complex and the causes are many. There are many different centres in the brain involved but, for practical purposes, they can be considered under two main areas: the chemoreceptor trigger zone which detects blood borne chemicals and the integrated vomiting centres of the lateral medulla of the brain. The latter co-ordinates all impulses coming in and results in the vomiting process. Impulses come to the lateral medulla from the gut, from the higher centres such as memories and the sights and smells experienced in the conscious state, and also from the balance organs of the inner ear (Fig. 4.2).

Table 4.1 Results of the survey of 200 consecutive admissions to Holme Tower Marie Curie Home, Penarth, Wales in 1989. Published on Interactive Video Disc, produced by Marie Curie Education Department.

Symptoms on admission	% incidence of symptoms (i.e. % of patients with this symptom)
Pain	62
Weakness	39
Constipation	34
Nausea and vomiting	30
Dypsnoea	26
Fear	20
Confusion	16
Anorexia	14
Depression	8
Incontinence	8
Lymphoedema	7
Skin problems	5
Fungating lesions	5
Sore mouth	4
Ascites	3
Dysphagia	2
Cough	0

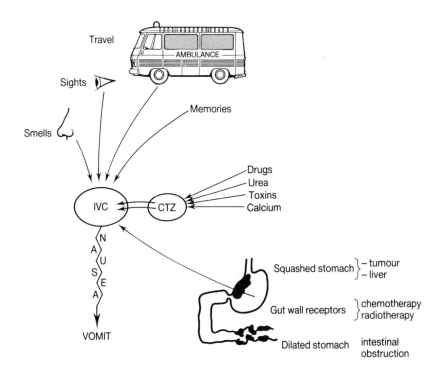

Fig. 4.2 Causes of nausea and vomiting. The cause of the nausea and vomiting must be understood before an appropriate antiemetic (see Fig. 4.3) can be chosen.

Drugs such as opiates cause vomiting by stimulating the receptor cells in the chemoreceptor trigger zone. Other drugs such as cytotoxic drugs and antibiotics stimulate receptors in the gut wall to cause vomiting. Toxins are released from bacterial breakdown in infection, and are re-absorbed from the gut wall in severe constipation or circulate following tissue damage breakdown in the patient who has had radiotherapy to tumour. Uraemia and liver failure are other sources of toxin; all these toxins are detected by gut, liver or brain chemoreceptors and impulses pass into the integrated vomiting centres. Some causes of vomiting are easier to control with antiemetics than others; hypercalcaemia can cause very severe vomiting, particularly resistant to antiemetics, but coming rapidly under control when the serum calcium is brought down by intravenous rehydration and treatment (Heath, 1989).

Different antiemetics act at different points in the vomiting mechanism. There is no place at all for plucking the name of an antiemetic out of the air and expecting it to work; the drug used must be appropriate to the cause of the nausea and vomiting (Sykes, 1990) (Fig. 4.3). When there is no obvious cause, then the most appropriate drug to try is cyclizine as it acts on the histamine transmitters in the integrated vomiting centres and is better at stopping vomiting than stopping nausea. Haloperidol which acts on dopamine receptors is the drug of choice in opiate induced vomiting; it can be given in conjunction with cyclizine. Metoclopramide has a weak central action but acts on the gut wall making it useful in chemotherapy or radiotherapy induced vomiting. It is associated with extrapyramidal reactions when given in large doses, especially in younger female patients. Domperidone acts more selectively on the gut and does not cross the blood/brain barrier. The newer drug, cisapride, acts by improving motility of the stomach, making it possibly the drug of

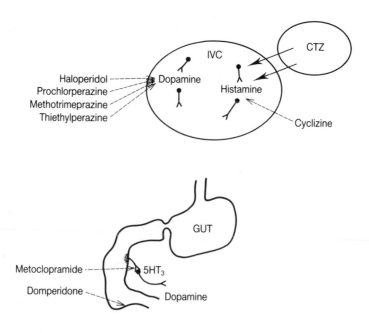

Fig. 4.3   Sites of action of antiemetics.

Table 4.2 Antiemetics in nausea and vomiting.

Drug	Dose	Timing	Indication	Disadvantages
Cyclizine	50 mg s/c	4 hrly	Good for established vomiting	Painful injection; causes dry mouth
Haloperidol	5 mg s/c oral	once daily	Opiate induced vomiting	Sedative; risk of extrapyramidal side effects*
Methotrimeprazine (Oliver, 1985)	25 mg s/c oral	25 mg 8 hrly	Opiate induced vomiting	Very sedative; risk of extrapyramidal side effects*
Metoclopramide	1–2 mg/Kg body per day in divided doses		Chemotherapy; radiotherapy; gut damage	Risk of extrapyramidal side effects*
Domperidone	30 mg pr	6 hrly	Action on rectal route	Ineffective in opiate induced and other central causes of vomiting
Hyoscine	0.4 mg	4 hrly	Weak antiemetic; action centrally	Very dry mouth; slows gut peristalsis
Thiethylperazine	6.5 mg pr	8 hrly	Central effective antiemetic	Risk of extrapyramidal side effects*

*Extrapyramidal side effects

(1) Occulogyric crisis, seen in the young, especially women
(2) Parkinsonian rigidity, usually of gradual onset over a few days

Reversal of the extrapyramidal side effects is by procyclidine injection. This is a medical emergency.

choice in squashed stomach syndromes where there is a need to hasten gastric emptying into the duodenum as the intragastric volume is small (Table 4.2).

When the patient is vomiting, drugs cannot be given orally. Rectal or subcutaneous routes become important. Antiemetics such as thiethylperazine can be given as a suppository eight hourly; it is effective for most causes of vomiting since it acts centrally. When a syringe driver is available the antiemetics can be put in to run over 24 hours and can often give good control of vomiting (Dover, 1987; Oliver, 1988). Cyclizine, 200 mg in 24 hrs, can be given as a subcutaneous infusion. If this fails to control vomiting, then haloperidol 5 mg can be added. An alternative infusion is methotrimeprazine in doses of 50–75 mg in 24 hrs. When a syringe driver is not available, metoclopramide at 10 mg IV may gain control of vomiting and can be followed up by cyclizine 50 mg subcutaneously. Once control has been gained over the vomiting, the maintenance dose of antiemetic is often much smaller and so the dose can be reduced fairly rapidly when the patient has control of nausea.

The nauseated patient will tolerate cool fizzy drinks better than tea, coffee or still drinks; and low fat foods, for example white bread, mashed potatoes and savoury foods can be eaten when other sweet foods are nauseating (see Chapter 6 on Nutrition).

Eating and feeding

Patients with a small stomach, for whatever reason, need good dietary advice. Small meals taken often are the order of the day; this is easily done if savoury snacks are provided and the courses of a meal given with a time gap between. For those at home, this can mean that the family meal pattern needs to be altered; this is most easily done by courses being prepared and eaten separately so that soup is prepared and eaten and then the main course prepared. These seemingly small modifications can be sensitively suggested to the family and will allow the important social function of the family eating together to be maintained. It is disheartening for all to sit at table with the patient who can't eat anything, both for the patient and for those with a hearty appetite who feel guilty eating in front of someone who is not eating. Small plates with small helpings for the patient can make meals easier.

The advice of a dietician with specialised skills in dealing with the terminally ill can be invaluable (see Chapter 6 on Nutrition). Much has been written of different diets which claim to 'help the body fight the cancer'. Sadly, the objective evidence is lacking and the tenacity with which patients and their families will try the diets is a mark of their distress at the whole disease process (McKillop *et al.*, 1988). Dismissing the diets on lack of evidence will only make the patient feel isolated, rejected and that the professionals 'don't understand'. The terminally ill, like all patients, need to keep an adequate dietary intake of calories and especially fluids and a dietician can advise on ways to enhance the intake, either with some dietary supplement drinks or with techniques such as cream in coffee, butter on vegetables, gravies and sauces with meats. The food value of fluids should be stressed to relatives, who can otherwise fear the patient is starving. Feeding is a fundamental way of showing love; the importance for the carers should not be underestimated.

Dysphagia

Feeding the patient with a carcinoma of the oesophagus can present an ethical dilemma. Allowing a person to starve to death is terrible, but the question of parenteral feeding is fraught with difficulties. Assessment of a patient with dysphagia begins with examination of the mouth to look for oral candida. Patients with marked oral candida often have an extension of candidal plaques down through the pharynx and the oesophagus. Patients point very accurately to the level at which food sticks; this usually represents the level of obstruction.

Obstruction from tumour of the oesophagus can respond to corticosteroids; they may decrease oedema around the tumour to restore swallowing for days or even weeks. Dexamethasone in high dose (12 to 16 mg) should be given as divided doses through the day; any improvement in swallowing is temporary. If the patient has no benefit in the first five days, there is no point continuing to administer corticosteroids. Dexamethasone tablets can be dispersed by stirring in a small amount of water, making it easier for the patient to swallow than when they are whole. In the patient unable to swallow Dexamethasone at all, the drug can be given as Betamethasone subcutaneously, although this would not normally be done at home.

Where tumour is gradually growing into the lumen of the oesophagus, laser resection can be a simple, safe procedure in expert hands. Over the next ten years this type of therapy should probably become more widely available through regional surgical units. Palliative radiotherapy can be remarkably effective for some tumours and the technique of intra-oesophageal radiotherapy via an endoscope is available in some centres, although it is less pleasant for the patient than external beam radiotherapy. Radiotherapy must always be considered early as dysphagia is often transiently worse in the immediate post-treatment period.

When these measures are not applicable, a fine bore feeding nasogastric tube or even a simple gastrostomy are occasionally indicated where the patient wishes something done; each case must be individually assessed.

Anorexia

Anorexia can be due to tumour effect alone. A few patients will complain only of anorexia, but do have a degree of nausea; for these patients, antiemetics will increase appetite again. Corticosteroids have been advocated and used for increasing appetite. Their effect is unpredictable, they can cause gastric irritation and the systemic effect may in time predispose the patient to oral thrush and to skin fragility, risking pressure sores. Corticosteroids do however provide a sense of well-being in some patients which can almost appear to 'resuscitate' the patient for a time. False hopes in the family can be raised all too easily by implying that the return of appetite means the disease is being conquered; the importance of quality rather than quantity of life is the realistic goal.

Mouth care

Loss of taste and alterations in taste are common in the patient with metastatic malignancy and in many who are dying of metabolic disturbances, such as liver or renal disease. Savoury foods are preferred to sweet and some foods become flavourless. Oral thrush is so common in these patients that it is probably secondary to other mouth problems rather than the cause of the mouth problem (Finlay, 1986). Good oral hygiene is the single most important factor in such care. Debris should be removed with a soft toothbrush and toothpaste, then chlorhexidine mouthwash used as a rinse.

Only after this cleansing can topical agents such as Nystatin or Amphotericin have any effect. In those with severe oral and pharyngeal candida causing sore throat or dysphagia, systemic fungicides such as ketoconazole or fluconazole are indicated as the candidiasis usually extends down the oesophagus.

Dentures often become loose fitting as a patient loses weight and can cause local ulceration of the gums. Quick-set dental relining materials are now available so that dentists can rapidly refit dentures without needing to take new moulds and casts. Mouth ulcers can be extremely sore. Cancer patients are often partially immuno-compromised by their tumour as well as by treatments such as radiotherapy or chemotherapy. Herpes simplex should always be considered as a cause of mouth ulcers in these patients. Bacterial infections of the oral pharynx are likely so a simple throat swab may help. In some patients with a very smooth red tongue, vitamin deficiencies should be considered. Patients who have had a very poor dietary intake for a long time may well be vitamin C deficient; a deficit of B vitamins will also cause sore mouth. Oral supplementation with B or C vitamins is easy.

Ascites

Intra-abdominal tumours, particularly carcinoma of the ovary and colonic carcinoma, are associated with ascites. As girth increases patients feel heavy and uncomfortable. The fluid in the abdomen is usually very high in protein so there is a danger that the patient will become protein depleted when the ascites is tapped. Ascites tends to re-accumulate fairly rapidly after tapping. Diuretics such as spironolactone have been recommended for patients with ascites but often seem very ineffective. Diuretics have to be given in very large doses, usually making the patient dehydrated. The patient can end up with a very dry mouth and feeling very thirsty before any reduction in abdominal girth is seen. The half-hearted administration of diuretics seems to provide the worst of both worlds, leaving the patient dry and thirsty but not affecting the increasing volume of ascites in the abdomen.

Tapping ascites is relatively easy. A small intravenous cannula can be inserted directly through the abdominal wall and the ascites drained off through plastic drip extension tubing via a three way tap using a 50 ml syringe. However the protein depletion that occurs can result in a rapid deterioration in the patient's general condition after the ascites has been tapped, so it is only worth considering in patients who have marked symptoms, such as a patient who has difficulty in sitting because of the pressure of the ascitic fluid. However, to nurse a patient 'who cannot bend in the middle' can be extremely difficult; the simple expedient of withdrawing a litre of ascitic fluid may allow the patient to be comfortable when sitting in bed or a chair.

A few patients accumulate vast quantities of ascites very early in their illness. These patients, who are otherwise relatively fit, can benefit from the insertion of a LeVeen shunt which is usually done by a hepatic surgeon. It is a simple procedure: a shunt is inserted into the abdominal cavity and run subcutaneously to drain into the superior vena cava. Through this system the ascitic fluid drains directly back into the patients circulation, avoiding protein depletion (Morris, 1984).

Constipation

Constipation is so common in ill patients that it is almost accepted as a 'normal occurrence' by some nurses and doctors (Regnard, 1988). Constipation makes a patient uncomfortable, causes colicky abdominal pain, anorexia and in some elderly patients causes confusion.

Many drugs are anticholinergic and cause constipation by a direct action on the gut wall slowing down peristalsis. The opiate drugs are the commonest culprits in these patients, but other analgesics containing codeine in small doses are equally capable of causing severe constipation.

As with other symptoms, the cause must be determined to enable treatment to be appropriate (Fig. 4.4). Where peristalsis has been slowed by drugs, stimulant

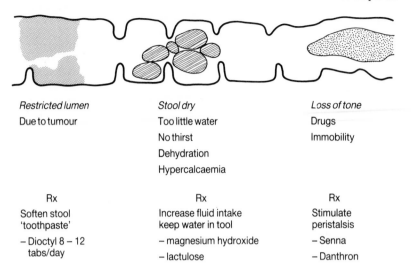

Restricted lumen	Stool dry	Loss of tone
Due to tumour	Too little water	Drugs
	No thirst	Immobility
	Dehydration	
	Hypercalcaemia	

Rx	Rx	Rx
Soften stool 'toothpaste'	Increase fluid intake keep water in tool	Stimulate peristalsis
– Dioctyl 8 – 12 tabs/day	– magnesium hydroxide	– Senna
	– lactulose	– Danthron

Fig. 4.4 Constipation. The cause of constipation must be sought before deciding which laxative to give.

laxatives such as senna should be used to reverse this. The stool can be kept soft by drawing water into the small bowel with a flusher such as magnesium hydroxide mixture. Thus a suitable combination for a patient on morphine is Senna liquid 10 mls and Magnesium hydroxide 10 mls given two to four times a day.

Where the bowel is sluggish from immobility of the patient or a low residue diet, the osmotic laxative lactulose may be used. Water is held in the stool and therefore not reabsorbed in the large bowel, so the patient must have a good fluid intake for it to be effective. Unfortunately, the gut bacteria tend to cause fermentation of lactulose (a non-absorbable sugar) with gas formation; these patients can have uncomfortable and embarrassing flatus. The oily syrup texture of lactulose makes it unpopular with patients who are anorexic.

Patients with tumours of the gut wall risk intestinal obstruction. This can be avoided by keeping the stool as soft as toothpaste with a pure stool softener such as dioctyl (docusate), which needs to be given in high doses of 8–12 tablets a day. Dietary advice is very important as the patients should avoid non-digestible foods; fruit should be peeled and oranges and grapefruit squeezed so the pith is not eaten. It is particularly important for these patients to maintain an adequate fluid intake as a hard dry lump of stool will not pass easily through a narrowed segment of bowel. These measures must be instigated early to assure the constipation is avoided (Table 4.3).

All too often the patient presents with constipation. Both the cause of the constipation and probable site of the stool must be located. A rectal examination must be done to ascertain if the stool is sitting in the rectum and its texture. Large 'rocks' of stool may need to be partly removed manually before any enema can bring stool down from the upper rectum, let alone from the rest of the gut with laxatives. The procedure is very distressing and the patient must be given adequate analgesic

Table 4.3   Constipation and laxatives.

Drug	Effect	Dose	Indication
Senna liquid	Bowel stimulation	10 mls bd/tds	On opiates
Senna tabs	Bowel stimulation	2 tabs tds	On opiates
Magnesium hydroxide	Small bowel flusher	10 mls bd/tds	With senna in patients on opiates
Codanthrusate Codalax	Bowel stimulation with stool softener	10 mls bd/qds	On opiates
Dioctyl	Stool softener	4–12 tabs/day	Avoid bowel obstruction
Lactulose	Stool softener	up to 60 mls a day ⎫	The frail immobile patient on few drugs (not opiates)
Fybogel and other fibres	Bulking agents	1–2 sachet a day ⎭	

cover. Sublingual dextromoramide 10 mg with 1 mg lorazepam is a useful combination for the patient at home and should be given half an hour before commencing the manual removal of faeces.

Where the rectum is full, but not so impacted, an enema can be given. Phosphate and other enemas such as sodium citrate are stimulant whereas the lubricant arachis oil enema will help the stool slip lower into the rectum to then be passed. However, enemas are tolerated as a necessary expedient by those who are severely constipated – they are unpleasant procedures and avoidable with the use of adequate doses of preventive laxatives in most patients. The paraplegic patient is the only one who may benefit from constipation with rectal clearance twice or three times a week – there is no sensation in the rectum and the firm stool avoids the embarrassment of faecal soiling. No enemas should be given without first doing a gentle rectal examination.

Intestinal obstruction

Intestinal obstruction must not be confused with constipation. Patients present with nausea and vomiting often long before the constipation occurs since the gut beyond the site of obstruction continues to empty material as faeces via the anus and often the obstruction is not total. Classically the patient has large volume vomits, often foul smelling and sometimes frankly faeculent. The patients may also have severe abdominal colic. The days of drip and suck regimes are over. The patient with a single site of obstruction should be referred for surgery to bypass this site. Most patients sadly have multiple sites of obstruction and have an abdomen riddled with tumour; for them surgery is not a viable option and they do best kept away from the surgical unit who will be tempted to put down a nasogastric tube and put up an IV line.

Treatment is aimed at the specific symptoms caused by the obstruction. Nausea should be controlled with a continuous subcutaneous infusion of an antiemetic via a syringe driver; for example cyclizine 200 mg with or without haloperidol 5 mg over 24 hours will control nausea and vomiting in many of these patients. If symptoms persist, further antiemetics such as metoclopramide should be added. The colic can be controlled with an antispasmodic, such as loperamide, or with an opiate, such as diamorphine, added into the syringe driver. Diamorphine is a good analgesic and decreases gut motility, making it a suitable drug; doses should be titrated as for any pain. In some patients with severe colic, hyoscine can be helpful.

As outlined in the preceding section, these patients should be managed early with prevention of the intestinal obstruction by keeping the stool as soft as toothpaste. However, this ideal situation often does not occur, the patient presenting with a subacute intestinal obstruction. As well as antiemetics and antispasmodics a stool softener, such as Dioctyl, should be used. Stimulant laxatives must be avoided since these will aggravate colic. I have seen one patient with a bowel perforation because she was given a stimulant enema into an empty rectum. The situation of intestinal obstruction underlines yet again that no aperient drugs should be put in the rectum unless you know that there is stool in there to be passed.

Diarrhoea

The causes of diarrhoea can be considered under simple headings which then guide management.

Gut surgery may leave a blind loop of non-functioning bowel in which bacteria proliferate causing intestinal hurry. The putty coloured floating stool of intestinal malabsorption may also be caused by lack of pancreatic enzyme secretion. Laxative overdosing must not be confused with constipation and overflow – in both states the stool is normal colour. Tumours in the large bowel frequently secrete mucus and act as an irritant focus; these patients risk intestinal obstruction and should be given antidiarrhoeals with caution. When there is a large mucus-secreting tumour on the lower bowel, corticosteroids can be given as predsol retention enema; the direct action of the corticosteroid on the tumour surface will often help greatly (Table 4.4).

Rectovaginal fistula

Passing faeces per vagina is foul for any woman. The vagina should be gently douched with saline to wash out faecal matter and be assessed. In some women a

Table 4.4 Diarrhoea.

Stool type		Cause
Grey, floating	= Malabsorption	Blind loop syndrome, pancreatic duct blocked
Watery, undigested food	= Intestinal hurry	Infection, laxative overdose, shortened bowel
Black	= Melaena	G.I. bleeding
Brown sticky fluid, occasional pellets	= Overflow	Constipation
Mucoid	= Tumour secretions	Tumour in lumen of bowel

small tampon may help absorb vaginal leak and contain the flow. Tampons extending widthways (Lillets and Dr Whites) tend to be more comfortable than those expanding lengthways (Tampax).

A defunctioning colostomy may help where lumps of faeces are being passed, although tumours tend to secrete a lot of mucoid material which continues to be passed per vagina even after the faeces are diverted. Topical corticosteroids can be given either as a vaginal douche (rectal predsol enemas can be used vaginally) or as creams on a tampon; the topical corticosteroid may decrease the rate of discharge from the tumour surface into the vagina.

Bladder pain

Cystitis is common and very painful. Smelly urine, incontinence or dysuria warrant immediate treatment with an antibiotic. The patient should not be left for days

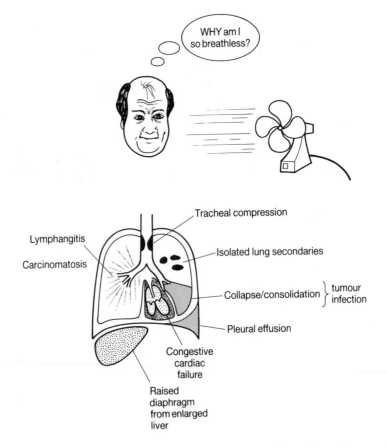

Fig. 4.5   Threat the cause of dyspnoea. Facial cooling with a fan will ease the sensation of dyspnoea, but the cause to be treated will lie in the chest.

Table 4.5 Observations which suggest various causes of dyspnoea.

Causes of dyspnoea	Pointer signs/Symptoms
Tracheal compression	• Stridor/wheeze audible on inspiration and expiration NB: easily mistaken for wheezing • Inspiratory and expiratory effort
Tumour at epiglottis	• Marked inspiratory stridor sometimes partly relieved by sitting forwards
Infection	• Sputum volume increase • Sputum colour change • Pyrexia is not always present early • Tachycardia, sweating
Pulmonary emboli	• Sudden episodes of deterioration (may be multiple and small) • Tachycardia • Apyrexial, no chest signs
Congestive failure	• Tachycardia • Patient sitting up, legs over the side of bed • Frothy white sputum when severe
Lymphangitis } Lung secondaries }	• Steady deterioration • Dyspnoea on exertion progress to dyspnoea at rest
Pleural effusion	• Steady deterioration, may be rapid • No vocal resonance felt when a hand put on the chest wall over the effusion • Stony dull to percussion • Trachea may be deviated towards the unaffected side
Anaemia	• Marked pallor • Marked tachycardia • Wide pulse pressure • Air hunger

awaiting the result of urine culture; a clinical response of symptom relief can be achieved in one to two days with simple antibiotic therapy such as trimethoprim or amoxycillin.

Dyspnoea

Dyspnoea must be one of the worst symptoms a patient can suffer. The sensation of being unable to breathe adequately will generate tremendous fear and panic. The danger is in mistaking the distress of dyspnoea for a panic attack.

As for every symptom, seeking the cause is the challenge (Fig. 4.5). Simple baseline observations give many clues to the cause (Table 4.5): respiratory rate, pulse rate, blood pressure and observing for peripheral or central cyanosis are all simple bedside procedures. The history of the onset, the presence or absence of cough, pleuritic pain and the changes in sputum volume and colour are important clinical clues.

A wheezing chest does not only occur in asthma. Reactive bronchospasm is seen in patients in congestive cardiac failure (cardiac asthma) and with retained secretions or tumour in the main bronchi. Whilst bronchodilators such as nebulised salbutamol help greatly, any patient with recent onset wheezing must be adequately examined to define and treat an underlying cause appropriately. Diuretics and other treatments for heart failure must be given to avoid the distress of a patient drowning in his or her own secretions (Allen, 1985)

Tumour invading the main bronchi may respond well to palliative radiotherapy in the short term, particularly if causing haematemesis; expectorated blood is always frightening for patients and relatives.

A pleural effusion can be drained through a small plastic intravenous cannula almost painlessly – this can be done at home if the patient is too ill and too distressed to be moved.

Cough is remarkably uncommon in these patients even when they may have carcinoma of the lung. This is usually because they are already on opiates and opiates are potent cough suppressants. Simple cough linctus really does nothing for a patient with carcinoma of the lung who has an irritant cough and codeine is usually too mild a cough suppressant. Methadone linctus can be used (2 mg in 5 ml) given once or twice a day to control cough in these patients. Methadone is an opiate and the dose must be titrated just as the dose of morphine must be titrated in pain (see Chapter 3 on Pain).

Infections causing symptoms warrant treatment with the appropriate oral antibiotics. When the patient continues to deteriorate and becomes unable to take medication, then it may be injudicious to resort to parenteral antibiotics in some patients but each individual case must be considered ethically.

When the underlying cause has been treated, the sad reality of tumour in the chest is that the patient often remains dyspnoeic from shunting of blood through a portion of non-ventilated lung. Oxygen by mask does little to relieve this as the arterial oxygen tension remains unaltered because the blood which has passed through collapsed areas of lung dilutes down the remainder returning to the left atrium. Facial cooling has been shown to relieve the sensation of dyspnoea, which is why patients feel 'better sitting by an open draughty window'. A small electric fan can produce the same breeze most effectively.

The patient's respiratory drive can be damped down by the judicious use of opiates. The dose should be titrated up in small (10%) dose increments above the pain threshold until the sensation of severe dyspnoea is eased. The respiratory rate must be monitored and will fall as the dose of opiate rises. The side effect of drowsiness is inevitable but may be the right price to pay to relieve a dying patient from the sensation of having to struggle to get enough breath and allow rest with peace and dignity. For these patients eating and talking will always be an effort but the family should be able to sit with the patient and not have to witness distress.

Itch

Many patients' skin becomes dry and scaly with cancer. This ichthyosis is easily relieved with simple emollients such as the many simple liquid oils and creams available on prescription. Cetomacrogol is particularly good for itchy skin, whereas oilatum emollient is better when the skin is very dry and simple creams such as E45 have not been moisturising enough.

Severe itching is sometimes due to liver failure; the patients are icteric by this stage. Very severe pruritis must raise suspicion of scabies – all too often the simple diagnoses are missed when a patient carries the label of major disease such as carcinoma. Careful examination of the skin will reveal the burrows of the mite which is easily killed by appropriate topical treatment such as gamma benzene hexachloride. The worst cases occur in patients who are partly immunosuppressed either by corticosteroids or by chemotherapy and who get a severe eczematous reaction to the scabies mite, making the diagnosis more difficult.

Fungating lesions

The visible marker of disease that literally eats through to the body surface requires the most sensitive and tactful nursing. It is so important to remember that the patient will be embarrassed by the smell of necrotic tissue, by soiling and oozing from the tumour surface and by the indignity of having a sensitive part of the body destroyed (Lancet, 1990). All too often the breast, the genital area or part of the face become eroded by locally aggressive tumour. Those nursing the patient must set different care goals than for surgical wounds or varicose ulcers – these fungating lesions will not heal and will look worse as the tumour grows. Containment of smell and exudate must become the markers of successful therapy. Palliative radiotherapy (see p. 46) can provide a dramatic shrinkage of tumour and must always be considered.

The smell is caused by anaerobic organisms on the necrotic tissue surface. Dead black and grey sloughing tissue should be cleared away by debridement with a scalpel blade or scissors. Small amounts remaining may be then digested off by aserbine cream or varidase mixed with glycerine or sherisorb gel. Granuflex will help remove slough but the sticky layer tends to damage adjacent skin.

Topical metronidazole as 0.8% gel will decrease smell by killing the anaerobes on the fungating surface (Newman *et al.*, 1989). Continued bacterial colonisation can be decreased with topical 0.5% silver nitrate solution or with Flamazine cream which contains silver nitrate.

However, it is very important to remember that the quality of the patient's life must be preserved at all times. There is no excuse for painful dressing changes, for obsessionally trying to make the lesion look better if pain is caused to the patient in the process. Dressings should be done with adequate analgesic cover such as sublingual dextromoramide 10 mg give half an hour before starting. Bleeding points will stop oozing with topically applied adrenalin or the seaweed alginate dressing Kaltostat.

Light absorbent gauze and gamgee dressings can be prevented from sticking by soaking the layer adjacent to the skin in liquid paraffin before applying. Telfa and melonin non-stick dressings are also useful. Silastic foam can be moulded to provide a comfortable surface dressing over a craggy lesion and held in place by tubigauze or netelast stocking dressings (Fig. 4.6). The nurse doing the dressing needs to be very sensitive throughout; facial expression often gives away far more than ever intended and the patient's sense of dignity can be maintained by gentle conversation.

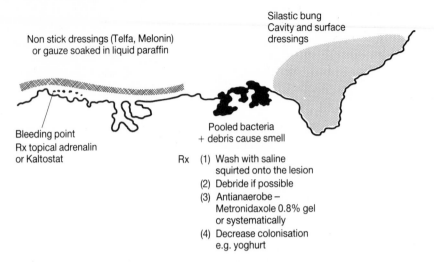

Non stick dressings (Telfa, Melonin)
or gauze soaked in liquid paraffin

Silastic bung
Cavity and surface
dressings

Bleeding point
Rx topical adrenalin
or Kaltostat

Pooled bacteria
+ debris cause smell

Rx   (1) Wash with saline
        squirted onto the lesion
     (2) Debride if possible
     (3) Antianaerobe –
        Metronidaxole 0.8% gel
        or systematically
     (4) Decrease colonisation
        e.g. yoghurt

Fig. 4.6   The fungating tumour surface.

Weakness – 'gone off his legs'

Weakness often accompanies advancing disease and may be most distressing. Physiotherapy has much to offer in teaching patients to move within their new limitations but, more importantly, the physiotherapist's role maintains hope by maximising movement. A hydrotherapy pool may enable the patient to experience some movement in limbs normally too heavy to move out of water, an experience which, psychologically, can be very beneficial.

Hypercalcaemia should be considered in any patient who has become inexplicably drowsy, confused, nauseated and dehydrated. I have seen two patients in whom polyuria from hypercalcaemia was initially mistaken for diabetes insipidus; they both presented with rapidly increasing drowsiness over a week.

Spinal cord compression is a medical emergence that warrants special mention. Tumour compressing the cord will cause a progression of symptoms, often over several days that can be halted by the immediate administration of radiotherapy or by surgery if appropriate. Pain in the thoracic or cervical spine region associated with leg weakness comes first. The arms are only weak if the lesion is very high in the cervical region. There may be parasthesiae and tingling in the lower limbs and skin sensation is decreased at a sensory level corresponding to the level of compression. As motor and sensory loss worsen, the paraplegia develops. This is irreversible and followed by loss of sphincter control. These patients must be actively treated immediately the lesion appears – to wait until the sphincters are lost is negligent. Paraplegia is terrible enough, let alone when compounded by incontinence.

Parkinsonism can be caused as a side effect of drugs that act on dopamine receptors; these include most antiemetics. The patients are less mobile and have an expressionless face, all too often mistaken for depression. The other common causes of weakness include infection and steroid induced muscle wasting (Fig. 4.7).

Hypercalcaemia

Hypercalcaemia is a specific entity which occurs in patients who have cancers, particularly those which metastasise to bone. It is caused by rapid reabsorption of calcium from the bones occurring more quickly than this calcium load can be excreted through the kidney (Heller and Hoskins, 1986). It is a diagnosis that is not made unless you think of it.

The hypercalcaemic patient is drowsy, constipated, nauseated and dehydrated, causing a dry mouth. All of these symptoms are so common in cancer patients that it is very important that when all four occur together the clinician thinks of checking a serum calcium. A serum albumin must be done at the same time because a low serum albumin alters the interpretation of the serum calcium result. Thus the corrected serum calcium is the important figure. The conversion factor is:

Corrected serum calcium = measured serum calcium + 0.02(42 − serum albumin)

Levels above 2.6 mmol/l are raised and levels above 3.4 mmol/l are life-threatening (Iqbal *et al.*, 1988).

Management of hypercalcaemia is a medical emergency and requires admission to an inpatient unit. There are now new intravenous treatments available which cause minimal distress to the patient and can provide an excellent response allowing the sick, dry, drowsy, confused patient to return to activity and lucidity within 48 hours. Patients should not be allowed to die prematurely from a condition that is now easily treated. It is important to remember that a few months of life can be very, very important to a patient, particularly a young parent preparing his or her family for their life after the bereavement.

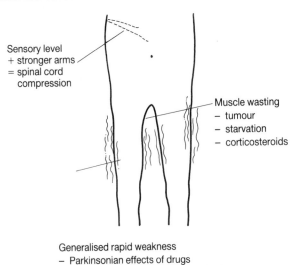

Sensory level
+ stronger arms
= spinal cord
  compression

Muscle wasting
– tumour
– starvation
– corticosteroids

Generalised rapid weakness
– Parkinsonian effects of drugs
– Metabolic disturbance Ca^{++}; Na^+; K^+
– Toxic from infection

Fig. 4.7 Common causes of 'going off his legs'. Leg weakness must not be assumed to be an irreversible or untreatable effect of tumour.

Cerebral tumours

Cerebral tumours can be particularly distressing. Patients with cerebral tumours are often young and can undergo personality changes when the tumours involve the frontal lobe areas although, fortunately, personality changes seem to be relatively rare. Neurosurgery can sometimes be palliative in debulking tumours and will allow radical radiotherapy. In those tumours which are resistant to radiotherapy some control can be gained with corticosteroids. However, these patients are often best left without corticosteroids until symptoms are marked. The long-term use of corticosteroids can create many problems in both the physical and emotional sphere (see below).

The tumour itself is usually surrounded by an area of oedema and hyperaemia; this is the area affected by high dose corticosteroids. Thus the total tumour bulk is not affected, but pressure effects can be temporarily relieved. As the tumour grows the pressure effects recur but, as these are directly from the tumour itself, there is no longer a corticosteroid response. Thus the patients appear to escape from the benefit of corticosteroids.

Corticosteroids can be used to 'buy back' a little bit of time of reasonable mobility (Kirkham, 1988) for patients who have special events ahead of them, such as a family wedding, but there is a danger in corticosteroids being raised and lowered in a yo-yo fashion so the patient appears to be transiently brought back only to deteriorate again. In patients who are on corticosteroids, and in whom deterioration has become marked, the tailing down of corticosteroid therapy may allow the cerebral tumour to swell enough for the patient to become gently comatose and this can take the patient fairly rapidly through the twilight state of awareness of tremendous disability into the comatose state, which at times may be more humane.

Thus, when patients can no longer swallow their corticosteroids due to advancing cerebral tumour, I am inclined to feel that administration of large doses of corticosteroids parentally is not indicated. These are all very difficult ethical decisions and no firm rules can be drawn. It is imperative that the nurses, doctors and other professional carers involved in the care of the patient are able to weigh up the pros and cons and present the family, and sometimes the patient, with a clear sensible and humane rationale which fits in with the goals the patient has set and the desires expressed by the patient him or herself. Even when patients are extremely ill, they have a right to their autonomy. This does not mean that the carer leaves the decision taking to the patient; it means that they do not exclude the patient. The carers' aim must be to obtain the best possible outcome for each patient at each time in their illness, given the realistic goals available within the limitations of the disease present.

Corticosteroids

Corticosteroids are not without their problems. Although used fairly widely in palliative care for the relief of raised intracranial pressure, the indiscriminate use of corticosteroids can give more problems than they can help. Corticosteroids should not be given late at night as they will prevent the patient sleeping. After a few weeks on high doses of corticosteroids patients can become Cushingoid and the facial puffiness and plethora can be particularly distressing. Muscle wasting is a specific side effect of corticosteroids.

Skin changes induced by steroids will make the patient at greater risk of pressure sores when immobile. Their immunosuppressant effect makes the patient more prone to infections and the symptoms of infection tend to be masked, making diagnosis harder. Some degree of emotional lability is common in patients on corticosteroids, even though only a few exhibit a full-blown steroid psychosis. Patients can feel anxious, weepy, frightened, insecure. These distressing psychological alterations are damaging for the patient to experience and the family to witness.

Lymphoedema

Lymphoedema occurs commonly at two main sites. Lymphoedema of the arm is frequently seen in women who have undergone mastectomy. Gross lymphoedema from the waist down is frequently present in patients who have tumour in the abdomen involving the para-aortic nodes.

Arm lymphoedema requires two main strategies. Firstly, the collapsed lymphatics beyond the site of obstruction need encouragement to open again with gentle massage or efflurage. This can be done by a physiotherapist or other masseuse. Rhythmic, gentle massage should be undertaken working furthest away from the affected site and gradually massaging the area to include the zones nearer and nearer the affected site. The second strategy involves compression bandaging. Firm compression bandaging which becomes tight or wrinkled should be re-applied immediately.

Mechanical lymphoedema compression devices are useful; the most useful are graduated sleeves which compress serially working from the fingers up through the hand, the lower then upper forearm, on up through the upper arm towards the shoulder. These machines are usually available only at a lymphoedema clinic.

Diuretics have no place at all in the management of lymphoedema. The cause of the lymphoedema is obstructed lymphatic vessels and making a patient dehydrated will do nothing to relieve this obstruction.

Lymphoedema of the lower legs can be treated in the same way as in the arm and support stockings are extremely helpful in these patients. When the lymphoedema extends up to the waist however, vigorous compression of the lower limbs will only tend to squeeze the fluid into the genital area resulting in grossly oedematous scrotum or penis in the male or grossly oedematous vulvae in the female. This causes more discomfort than the heavy lower limbs.

Skin care of the lymphoedematous limb is of paramount importance. Even minimal abrasions will allow bacteria to enter and a rapidly developing cellulitis will spread through lymphoedematous tissues. Chiropody and finger nail care must be meticulous to avoid a paranychia developing and any evidence of Athletes foot should be treated immediately with topical antifungal agents. The first sign of inflammation in the lymphoedematous tissues must be treated vigorously with antibiotics, remembering of course that fungi may have entered percutaneously.

Depression

Depression is a distinct clinical state. It is understandable that any patient with any illness will feel sad, angry, bitter and may seem quite 'depressed'. This must be differentiated from a clinical depression which will respond to antidepressants. Antidepressants are not 'happy making drugs'. They will do nothing for the patient who is appropriately sad. They are often slightly sedative and will therefore make the patient feel worse if given when not indicated.

So how do you differentiate the depressed patient from the sad patient? Patients with classic depression often have similar symptoms to those seen in patients with advanced cancer. Both diseases share symptoms of anorexia with consequent weight loss, weakness, lethargy and fatigue; sadness will give the flat affect also seen in the depressed patient. Early morning wakening is possibly the best indicator of a patient being depressed. Another pointer is the patient's mood on wakening in the morning; the depressed patient tends to feel dreadful at the beginning of the day whereas the patient who is sad because of all that is happening will tend to feel worse as the day goes on and the reality dawns again. Depression is often mixed with an anxiety state; this must not be confused with fear. The patient frightened of how he or she will die, when and what will happen on the way, needs to be able to talk about it, not be given diazepam.

Having decided that an antidepressant is indicated, the next choice to be made is which one. The tricyclic antidepressants such as amitriptyline do seem to have a very slight co-analgesic effect with opiates and so may be useful in a patient with pain. Prothiaden is a sedative antidepressant and this, like the tricyclics, is best given as a single nightly dose. The newer antidepressants such as flupenthixol are more anxiolytic than antidepressant and should be given in the morning. The antidepressant effect of any of these drugs takes an average of about 10 days to occur.

Fear and anxiety

The eyes are said to be the window of the mind. The patient's eyes, wide and staring describe the terror of facing the unknown. As pressures pile in on patients having to come to terms with the end of their lives, often prematurely, they need to be able to voice these fears; often some fears can be allayed. For example, many patients are very frightened of being unable to breathe in the end stages of their disease and deserve the reassurance of the knowledge that their symptoms will be kept under control and that they will maintain their dignity.

Insomnia

Insomnia can be very depressing. The tired patient copes less well the following day, making a rapidly downwards spiral of symptoms; for example if pain keeps a patient awake, the next day he or she is tired and the pain feels worse so he or she is less able to sleep and so on.

There is no hypnotic that will compensate for poor symptom control. There is no hypnotic that will make somebody feel warm, comfortable, loved, secure, at peace within themselves. The majority of patients do not need an hypnotic. Good symptom control and good attention to all psychological aspects of the patient's care deserve attention before exhaustion supervenes and compounds the situation.

Conclusion

Perhaps the first rule in treating patients is to believe the patient. The question 'What is the worst thing for you at the moment?' can get the problem list into the patient's order of priorities and often takes the professional carers by surprise. The second rule is to never abandon the patient. When health professionals feel there is nothing more that can be done, they, as carers, should review the situation as there is always comfort that can be given by caring and continuing to support.

There is no shame in needing to ask for help and advice from other colleagues and recognising honestly when other input to the clinical problem is required. The primary care team must always maintain their principal role in providing the care, calling on others when appropriate to do so. The challenge to the professional is to continue to ask the question 'Why?' to elucidate the cause of each problem so that treatment is scientific, not randomly plucked from the air like recipes from a cook-book.

References

ALLEN, S. C. (1985). Respiratory disease: managing residual symptoms. *Geriatric Medicine*, June, 15–20.

BAINES, M. (1981). The principles of symptom control. In *Hospice: The Living Idea*. C. M. Saunders, D. H. Summers and N. Teller (Eds), pp. 99–118.

DOVER, S. B. (1987). Syringe driver in terminal care. *British Medical Journal*, **294**, 553–4.

FINLAY, I. G. (1986). Oral symptoms and candida in the terminally ill. *British Medical Journal*, **292**, 592–3.

HEATH, D. E. (1989). Hypercalcaemia of malignancy. *Palliative Medicine*, **3**, 1–11.

HELLER, S. R. and HOSKING, D. J. (1986). Renal handling of calcium and sodium in metastitic and non-metastatic malignancy. *British Medical Journal*, **29**, 583–5.

IQBAL, S. J., GILES, M., LEDGER, S., NANJI, N. and HOWL, T. (1968). Need for albumin adjustments of urgent total serum calcium. *The Lancet*, December 24/31, 1477–8.

KIRKHAM, S. R. (1988). The palliation of cerebral tumours with high-dose dexamethasone: a review. *Palliative Medicine*, **2**, 27–33.

MCKILLOP, W. J., STEWART, W. E., GINSBURG, A. D. and STEWART, S. S. (1988). Cancer patients conception of their disease and its treatment. *British Journal of Cancer*, **58(3)**, 355–8.

MORRIS, J. S. (1984). Ascites. *British Medical Journal*, **289**, 209.

NEWMAN, V., ALWOOD, A. L. and OAKES, R. A. (1989). Use of metronidazole gel to control smell from fungating lesions. *Palliative Medicine*, **3**, 303–5.

OLIVER, D. J. (1985). The use of methotrimeprazine in terminal care. *British Journal of Clinical Practice*, **39(9)**, 339–40.

OLIVER, D. J. (1988). Syringe drivers in palliative care: a review. *Palliative Medicine*, **2**, 21, 26.

REGNARD, C. (1988). Constipation: an algorithm. *Palliative Medicine*, **2**, 34–5, 54–5.

SYKES, N. (1990). The management of nausea and vomiting. *The Practitioner*, **234**, 286–90.

The Lancet (1990). Editorial. Management of smell tumours. *The Lancet*, Jan. 20, 141–2.

Further reading

GALLAGHER-ALLRED, CHARLETTE, R. (1989). *Nutritional Care of the Terminally Ill.* Aspen Publishers, Maryland.

REGNARD, C. and DAVIES, A. (1986). *A Guide to Symptom Relief in Advanced Cancer.* Haigh and Hochland, Manchester.

5

Confusional states

Kathryn A. Mannix

'All the physicians and authors in the world could not give a clear account of his madness. He is mad in patches, full of lucid intervals.'
From Don Quixote, *by Miguel Cervantes (1547–1616)*

What is confusion?

'Confusion' refers to many different symptoms, such as incoherent speech, disorientation in time or place, difficulty with concentration, hallucinations or misinterpretations. Use of the word confusion can lead to confusion amongst the carers, because the word may mean something slightly different to different carers. However, all carers understand that it refers to something fundamental and constant about any patient: the thoughts this patient is expressing are different from usual. When visiting a patient who is confused we expect to find muddled thought.

Feeling muddled and being unable to make proper sense of the surroundings can be very frightening, and so to help a patient who is confused the professional carer must be able to offer two things: firstly the carer must start to calm the patient's fear, try to find the threads of reality in the jumble and help him or her to keep hold of reality as much as possible; secondly the carer must find out why the patient has become confused. Confusion is not a diagnosis, it is only a symptom of illness, and we can only hope to fully reverse the confusion by identifying and treating the underlying physical illness.

Some definitions

The language used about confused patients is very important, because we can only explain about a patient to other carers by using words we all understand.

When an illness is due to physical damage in the body it is an *organic* illness. Confusion is a psychological symptom of an organic illness. Psychiatrists call this an *organic brain syndrome*. There are two recognised organic brain syndromes, acute (sudden and usually reversible) and chronic (slow and continuing). The *chronic organic brain syndrome* is due to death of nerve cells within the brain; it is of gradual onset and gets steadily worse. It is recognised as *dementia*, and it is almost always irreversible. The *acute organic brain syndrome* is usually of fairly sudden onset, and instead of getting steadily worse it tends to fluctuate. It is always worth trying to find the physical cause of the acute organic brain syndrome because treating the cause will usually restore normal brain function. This syndrome is also called *delirium*.

Table 5.1   Differences between acute and chronic organic brain syndromes.

Acute (delirium)	Chronic (dementia)
Usually reversible	Irreversible
Clouding of consciousness	Clear consciousness
Misinterpretations Hallucinations, especially visual	Hallucinations rare
Release of emotion	Affect may be released or reduced
Fluctuating, often worse at night	Unchanging hour to hour, but slow deterioration over months/years
Sleep disturbance (not enough or too much)	Normal amount of sleep but may sleep at the wrong time
Activity change	No activity change
Global impairment	Often memory change before other changes

Table 5.1 shows the main characteristics of these two brain syndromes. Many patients with cancer are elderly and hence some may also have dementia. The important point about the acute organic brain syndrome (delirium) is that the person is *different* from a short time previously.

Observing and listening to confused patients shows that their mental processing of information ('cognitive function') is affected in all its aspects; this is called *global* impairment of cognitive function. The major aspects of psychological function are:

consciousness
attention
mood
perception
thinking
memory
behaviour

It will help to explain the changes seen in confused patients if each of these aspects is considered in turn.

● *Consciousness*   This refers to how awake and alert a person is. 'Clouding of consciousness' is the first, almost imperceptible step on a slope from normal alertness down towards coma and death. It is different from sleep, which is a normal, healthy brain function.

● *Attention*   This is the ability to select and concentrate on a particular stimulus, for example to listen to a conversation and ignore distracting noises. Confused patients often appear to be paying less attention than usual, although they may in fact be paying *more* attention, but they cannot select a particular stimulus and their attention flits between your conversation, noises in the room, thoughts in their head and the colour of the carpet.

- *Mood (affect)* Most people have a recognisable mood or *affect* which is 'normal' for them (e.g. anxious, carefree, suspicious) and this is recognised as their personality. People with dementia often display less personality than they used to, becoming rather bland. In delirious patients the opposite is seen: the personality is *'released'* and they are unable to damp down some parts of their affect. In this way, anxious individuals may become terrified, carefree people may become euphoric and suspicious people become paranoid. This may occur in dementia but it is less florid.

- *Perception* This is the process of becoming aware of the information being presented by the sensory nerves, such as a hard bed, the smell of burning toast, the sound of visitors' voices, feeling sick, or having pain. Perception can be altered by the circumstances in which the brain receives messages, and this can led to *misinterpretations*. Misinterpretations are more likely to arise in the following instances.

(i) *When the level of consciousness is reduced*, e.g. during sleep a person may dream about alarm bells ringing when they hear the alarm clock sounding.

(ii) *While attention is not focused on that sensory pathway*, e.g. while concentrating on typing (visual pathway) the sound of the radio (auditory pathway) may be misinterpreted as the telephone ringing. Darkness reduces a person's ability to attend to visual stimuli, and so visual misinterpretations are more common at night.

(iii) *If a strong emotional state is present*, e.g. after reading ghost stories a person may be frightened by a rustle of the curtains.

By 'turning up the volume' of attention and emotion people can alert themselves to particular stimuli, for example a mother may sleep through the noise of traffic but will waken instantly if her baby cries.

Emily had a long history of agitated depression, so she surprised herself and her family by how well she coped with the diagnosis of breast cancer at the age of 60 years. She did very well for eight years, but when she was admitted to the Hospice with bone pain her family asked us not to tell her that her disease was advancing.

Emily did not settle well. She was shouting and fighting with the night nurses, although she remained withdrawn during the day. The night sister noticed Emily kept referring to matches, and accusing the night staff of trying to kill her. When she asked Emily if she felt hot, Emily replied that anyone would feel hot if they had been set on fire! Her family told us that Emily had once been in hospital with depression when a schizophrenic patient set fire to the ward, and she had always been very afraid of fires at home after that.

She was found to have a high temperature. Investigations revealed a urinary tract infection, which was treated with antibiotics. One of Emily's daughters came to sleep with her at the Hospice for a few days. We explored her fear of burning to death, while her daughter was with her. Emily told us she could feel she was weaker and less well, and she thought that she might be dying. She was very afraid of losing control of herself if she got frightened during dying, because she had experienced panic attacks in the past. She was told that when the time came she was likely to lapse into a coma very gently, and found this so comforting that she told this story to all the patients who had become her friends at the Hospice, too!

She went home for a further six months, and came back to the Hospice when she was dying 'because you understand me here . . .'

• *Thinking*   A person's thought content can be recognised by their speech and behaviour. Usually thoughts are connected like links in a chain. When a person thinks, the links into 'what is happening now', 'what happened in the past', 'how I feel inside', 'how my friend seems to be feeling', can be separated out and the person can make sense of a situation.

In an organic brain syndrome the cross-linking becomes less easy to separate and to follow, and the person has difficulty separating the internal and external worlds. They may misinterpret memories for present reality, and they speak more slowly, with long pauses as they try to focus their thoughts. Later they lose ability to reason thoughts out, their ability to form abstract thoughts is impaired and they display *concrete* thinking. Usually they lose *insight* at the same time, i.e. they do not realise that their thinking has changed in the way that it has, although patients often have a vague feeling that all is not well and many express a fear of madness.

• *Memory*   The decreased ability to receive and process information accurately causes disruption of memory. New information cannot be stored and patients may require the same information to be repeated frequently, although their memory for past events remains intact. When the episode of delirium is past, patients frequently have no memory of it at all, or may only remember meaningless fragments.

• *Behaviour*   As the control of normal behaviour is lost in the muddled mind, people may display signs of their illness by becoming noisy, hyperactive and irritable. More commonly, though, people become slower. Their speech and spontaneous activity are reduced, and repetitive, purposeless movements are common. This *perseveration* of movements or speech seems to be due to an inability to turn off attention from a particular, fragmented thought. This can be very distressing for the patient and for his or her family.

Looking for a cause for confusion

Patients with advanced cancer may become confused for many reasons. If life expectancy is short it is important to see if there is a treatable cause as quickly as possible, because the last days of a patient's life will be so much more comfortable, and comforting for his or her family, if the patient is lucid and peaceful. Table 5.2 lists some of the causes of delirium which are worth looking for in cancer patients. Of course, there are other causes, but these are the most common or, for rare causes, those which can be treated easily and effectively.

Once the physical cause of delirium is treated it may take several days for the confusion to subside. During that time it is important to continue to reassure the patient and family, and to keep assessing for signs of improvement. Because delirium is a fluctuating condition there may be periods of complete normality followed by confusion again, which can reduce families to a state of emotional exhaustion as they celebrate 'recovery' only to be plunged back into despair once more. They need support and reassurance to cope with a beloved person who fails to recognise them or even blames them and accuses them of ill-treatment.

Table 5.2 Causes of acute organic brain syndrome in patients with advanced cancer.

Drugs

Any drugs acting on the CNS, particularly

— Antidepressants
— Anticonvulsants
— Sedative drugs

Corticosteroids
Opioids
β-blockers
Diuretics
Digitalis

Remember drug withdrawal, especially
Alcohol
Opioids
Benzodiazepines

Infection
(The patient may not be pyrexial, and very ill patients or those on corticosteroids may even be hypothermic)

Chest   }   most
Urinary tract }   common
Diverticulitis   (in the elderly)
Ears   }   /(in
Throat }   children)
Pressure sores
Necrotic tumours

Trauma
Head injury
Subdural haematoma

Tumour
Cerebral primary, cerebral metastases
'Paraneoplastic' (malignant disease elsewhere)
Anaemia due to bleeding or bone marrow infiltration

Cardiovascular/Respiratory disease ($\rightarrow$ cerebral hypoxia)
Stroke(s)
Myocardial infarction (classical symptoms and signs may be absent)
Heart failure/Hypotension/Arrhythmias
Deep venous thrombosis alone or with pulmonary embolism
Respiratory failure

Biochemical/Metabolic

Electrolyte disturbance (most commonly hyponatraemia, hypokalaemia, dehydration, hypercalcaemia)
Uraemia
Liver failure
Hypoglycaemia/Ketoacidosis

George visited his mother Hilda at the Hospice every day. She was dying with bladder cancer, but she 'held court' and was queen of the four-bedded bay which she shared with two other patients.

Then George stopped visiting. No-one saw him for days. One of the nurses met him in town, and he angrily told her that his mother had accused him of spending all her money on parties and disreputable women. We asked Hilda directly about this, and she assured us that it was quite true, and George was only waiting for her to die to convert her house into a brothel.

Hilda's husband had left her when George was a little boy. She was afraid that his father's traits were becoming evident in George, and that he would go off the rails when she died. In fact, George had a girlfriend but he had not told his mother, in case she worried that he would leave home while she was ill.

We attributed Hilda's muddled thoughts to the corticosteroids she was taking for painful pressure on her pelvic nerves, and explained this to George. We tried to stop the corticosteroids, but her pain came back. Gently probing her fears for George she wept to think of him living alone after her death. George was able to ask her how she would feel if he were to marry in the future, and she was overjoyed. He did not risk bringing his girlfriend to meet her, in case this was misconstrued. She continued to ask disinhibited questions about his 'love-life' from time to time, but George was able to understand that the origin of this thought was real concern for his future, and he continued to visit regularly until his mother died.

Understanding the confused patient

Definitions and some understanding of what is happening to confused patients' bodies and brains may feel reassuring to the professional carer, but it is not a great deal of help when in the room of a frightened, confused patient whose relatives are looking to the professional carers for help. It is necessary to try to understand what is happening for the patient.

Start by looking at the mind of a normal, healthy person – like yourself, perhaps. The thoughts which are reaching your consciousness are arising from three main areas: from the environment (how warm the room is, how tight your shoes are, how interesting your book is, whether there is a cup of coffee being poured for you); from your body (hunger, gritty eyes, need to sneeze, respiratory movements, posture); and

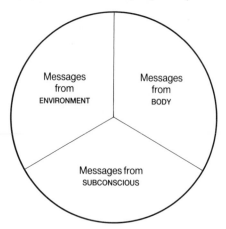

Fig. 5.1   The divisions of the conscious mind. (Based on Stedeford, 1984.)

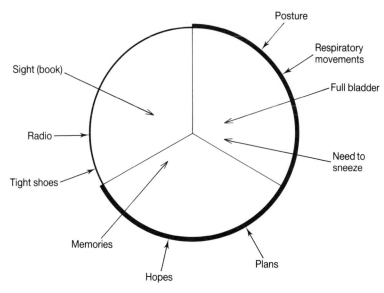

Fig. 5.2 See text for details. (Based on Stedeford, 1984.)

from your subconscious (memories of last weekend, hopes for next holiday, remember to buy some milk today, wonder if your child has got to school safely). If you pay attention to *all* those thoughts you will get no work done, remember nothing of what you are reading and be too busy getting your coffee to reach for a tissue to catch your sneeze. The mind therefore has a selective filter, which allows a person to concentrate on the job in hand and only allows other thoughts into consciousness if they are important. Fig. 5.1 shows how the conscious mind is divided.

Figure 5.2 shows an awake, well person reading a book. The filter to the body and the subconscious is thick, but it allows relevant thoughts into consciousness (remembering a patient who illustrates the problem you are studying; getting a tissue in time for the sneeze). Note that the boundaries between the different areas of the mind are clear; you can easily separate which messages came from your memory, from your book and from your nose.

Figure 5.3 shows another healthy person, but asleep this time. The boundaries of the three areas of the mind are less clearly demarcated. The environment is being filtered out; although some stimuli from the environment reach consciousness, they may be misinterpreted as part of a dream (telephone ringing becomes a dream about fire-bells). Similarly the body is also being filtered out, but some stimuli still get through (pain, full bladder) and may be misinterpreted because the boundaries are unclear. Thus a person may dream of being attacked because they have pain during sleep. The 'volume control' discussed earlier can be set to alert a person to particular stimuli, such as a full bladder, baby crying or the postman arriving.

From this model it can be seen that all the thoughts in a person's consciousness have come from somewhere. They are all rooted in reality – real physical stimuli, real memories, hopes or fears, real feelings within a person's body. It is the same for the confused person, but it seems that the boundaries have broken down and it is difficult for the person to work out where a thought came from. Their filter to the

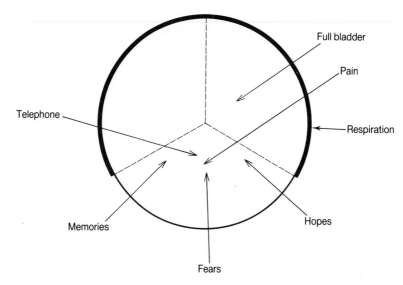

Fig. 5.3   See text for details. (Based on Stedeford, 1984.)

environment is thick so that it is difficult for another person to reach them. This is illustrated in Fig. 5.4.

With this model in mind, it becomes easier to understand why confused people have such bizarre experiences. First of all their 'volume control' is reset by their fear and anxiety, so stimuli they particularly fear or desire are perceived more readily. They may have difficulty in getting a grip on reality, or interpret reality as a dream.

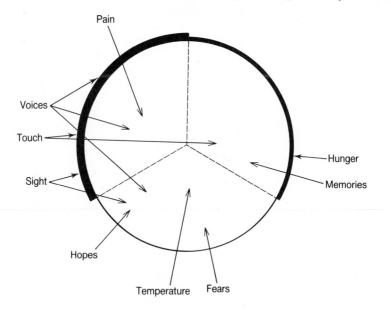

Fig. 5.4   See text for details. (Based on Stedeford, 1984.)

By trying to trace their (confused) thought back to its origin in reality, the carer may be able to help to reduce the anxiety and so to turn down the 'volume control' of their fears.

Treatment of confused patients

RECIPE

Ingredients: 1 confused patient
5 distressed family members
1 hospital room, with light switch
3 morning nurses, 2 afternoon nurses, 2 night nurses
1 ward doctor, 1 on-call doctor
2 large hospital porters
1 syringeful of chlorpromazine
1 green hypodermic needle
1 wardful of assorted sick patients

Method: Remove the confused patient from his or her familiar bedroom at home, and place in cold hard bed in unfamiliar hospital room. Ask family to leave. Ward doctor should examine patient. Change nurses regularly.

After eight hours, switch off lights. Leave patient in dark room and disturb regularly to check that he or she is asleep. When he or she protests, send for on-call doctor.

Wait until patient becomes frightened. When he or she begins to rise over the edge of the bed, apply one large hospital porter to each arm. On-call doctor should give injection of chlorpromazine into patient's bottom whilst repeating the incantation 'this won't hurt' or 'this is for your own good'.

Agitate the whole ward for four hours and await ward round. Repeat chlorpromazine if patient shows any sign of waking up. Garnish with diazepam suppositories.

It is easy to see why 'confusion' is such a common cause of admission to hospital. Sometimes the patient's behaviour is too violent for him or her to remain at home, sometimes the family is too distressed to cope. It is also easy to see where our management went wrong in retrospect. It is getting it right as we go along that is the challenge.

Refer again to Fig. 5.4. The aim of the health professional is to get the frightened, confused patient back in contact with reality. The carer is in the patient's environment, approaching the patient through his or her sight, hearing and touch. The patient's filter is blocking out the professional carer. How can the carer reach the patient? If sedative drugs are given the thickness of the filter to the environment is increased and the internal divisions of consciousness broken down even further. Sedating a patient will never improve his or her condition, only that of the carer. Sometimes this really is necessary, for example if, in their fear, the patient becomes a danger to themselves or others, or if they are becoming exhausted.

Can the patient be reached via his or her body or subconscious? A gentle touch, holding the patient's hand, smiling, all these are messages of friendship and care which may get through the filter when spoken language is not helping. There is usually comfort from the presence of a trusted friend or relative.

The priorities for management from the patient's point of view are:

1   *Stop or reduce the fear*
2   *Rationalise the underlying anxieties*
3   *Find and treat the cause of delirium*
4   *Orientation to reality*

● ***Stop or reduce the fear***   There is fear of the situation in which the patient finds him or herself. The carer must help the patient to restore reality. Explain to the patient that if they find they are muddled it is because they are not well. Keep reassuring and smiling. Keep assuming that they will understand at least some of what you say to them.

There is also fear of madness. This is very common but patients are often unable to express their fear. Patients and families need to be reassured that this muddledness is temporary and is due to the physical illness. We do not think they will go mad. We do not think they are becoming senile.

Hallucinations may occasionally occur and they are often visual. Colluding with the patient is rarely helpful because their mental state is fluctuating; if you agree that you can see the little pink frogs now, then when the patient becomes more lucid later on they may remember you 'went along with them' and stop trusting you – or even believe that you are mad for seeing those things! It is often helpful to acknowledge that the hallucination *is* real for the patient, 'Yes, I know you can see them and that they are very frightening. I can't see them, but you can. You want them to go away and I want to help you to make them go away.'

Misinterpretations are far more common, but they may be mistaken for hallucinations unless a very careful history is taken. With misinterpretations, it is useful to explore the underlying thoughts: 'Did you wish I was your mother when I came in then? Why? Tell me about her? Tell me what she would have done for you.' This should always be accompanied by re-orientating that patient and explaining why they have become muddled ('Your temperature is high, so you are delirious like small children sometimes are'. You have a chest infection, so there is less oxygen than usual getting to your brain').

Paula was 33 with two young sons and a husband who worked shifts, so when she was dying she was admitted to the Hospice to try to keep the home 'normal' for the boys. She had a single room and the whole family moved in at weekends. She slept well when they were with her, but during the week she slept badly and got increasingly tired and cross.

One afternoon she asked her Macmillan nurse, who was visiting, whether all the patients were discussed like this, because it was stopping her from taking naps. Exploring this strange comment we found that she could overhear voices in the patients' kitchen during the day. Although it was impossible to hear what was being said,. Paula misinterpreted the voices as a discussion about her illness, as the onset of renal failure made her muddled and unable to separate her own thoughts and fears about her illness from the voices she was hearing. When the family was with her, she was too busy listening to her boys to perceive the sound of voices in the kitchen.

She told us that the voices simply commented on her appearance and state of health. She had been a very attractive woman before her weight loss, and she grieved for her lost looks. Her Macmillan nurse collected her makeup and some clothes from home. The ward nurses explained that although the voices were real, the words she heard came from inside Paula's head, and she was able to understand this. Once she knew she was not going mad, she decided to make friends with the voices. When she was dressed with her makeup on the voices told her how nice she looked!

The message to the patient must be

— you are safe here
— this is not your fault
— you are not going mad.

• ***Rationalise the underlying anxieties***   Nightmares and misinterpretations are often clues to the fears in the patient's mind. If the carer can share the fear and help the patient to express it, often the fear can be reduced to more manageable proportions. During nightmares, the patient should be gently woken, re-orientated and the dream explored there and then.

Steve was a diver who worked for an oil company. He had a very rare cancer which progressed slowly and had initially responded to surgery and chemotherapy. But now he had lung deposits and damage to his pelvic nerves. Having spent long periods working way from home, he was unsure how to talk to his nine and 12 year old sons about his disease. He became angry if his doctor tried to discuss the future, saying he had fought his cancer so far and he would not allow it to beat him now.

The doctor noticed that Steve's wife was looking increasingly tired. She told the doctor that Steve was shouting in his sleep and waking everybody up, but the next morning he could not remember any of this. The doctor asked her to wake Steve up next time it happened, and ask him about his dream.

When she did this Steve woke up terrified and gasping. He was dreaming about diving. In his dream he was on a very deep dive, repairing an oil pipe. Then he became aware of difficulty breathing and realised that his air supply was about to run out. He could not attract the attention of his diving buddy. He should not surface and leave his buddy alone, but he would suffocate if he did not surface. While he was deciding what to do his air ran out.

Bravely, his wife asked him why he might have this dream. He told her that he thought it was about dying, and that time was running out. He could not stay with her to bring up their children, and he felt guilty for leaving her.

The next day they told the children about how ill Steve was. Steve said he thought he might die, but that he would never stop loving them. They all cried together. The dream never came back, and Steve died peacefully at home two months later.

• ***Find and treat the cause***   The list in Table 5.2 (p. 81) shows some of the more common causes of the acute organic brain syndrome in cancer patients. In patients who are physically very ill unnecessary investigations may cause distress and it is important to assess the patient with care, decide on the most likely causes of confusion, and look for these quickly if they are treatable. If the cause is not treatable this must be explained very carefully to the family, and to the patient if possible, and the carer must concentrate on managing the patient's distress.

• ***Orientation to reality***   Throughout the patient's confusion it should be assumed that he or she understands what is being said to them. It will be easier for the patient to be orientated in time if his or her daily schedule is regular, with meals at predictable times, few changes of faces (nursed by family and a few, familiar nurses if possible) and lots of other cues, for example wearing his or her watch, having today's newspaper near the bed. Remind patients where they are; ask them to try to remember where they are and how they came there. Keep the lights on. Remind them of the day, the date, world news, family news. It is helpful to reinforce reality by asking questions which lead the patient to the correct conclusions, for example:

'What sort of place is this?'

'I'm not sure . . . Queer sort of place if you ask me . . .'

'Do you see all those beds there? And all these people in pyjamas? So what sort of a place do you think this is?'

'It looks like a hospital to me.'

'Yes, you're right, it is a hospital. We are at the Royal Infirmary. Do you remember coming here?'

'I don't know who sent me here . . .'

'You came with your son. What is your son's name?'

'Kevin.'

'Yes, Kevin brought you here. You had been staying at Kevin's house. Do you remember?'

'So this is a hospital, eh? And Kevin knows I'm here? How long am I staying?'

'You are welcome to stay until you are stronger. You have been very ill and things got muddled in your mind. You are improving. You will be home soon.'

Above all, the confused person needs constant reassurance by calm, sympathetic and familiar people that he or she is safe, that he or she is sane and is understood.

Drug treatment for confused patients

Occasionally it becomes necessary to use drugs to manage patients with delirium. There are two particular reasons why drugs may be necessary.

- Uncontrollable terror, sometimes leading to dangerous behaviour
- Unreachable distress caused by muddled thinking

With terror or dangerous behaviour it may be necessary to *sedate* the patient. This means using a drug which is rapidly active and is unlikely to cause serious side effects. The best drugs in this category are the *benzodiazepines* which are sedative but do not cause hypotension. *Diazepam* is the drug of choice. Many people use the phenothiazine *chlorpromazine*, but it can cause hypotension and this in turn can cause myocardial infarction or stroke in at-risk patients. Also, phenothiazines lower the epileptic threshold and so many increase tendency to fitting in patients withdrawing from drugs or alcohol.

With predominantly jumbled thinking an *anti-psychotic* drug is needed. This will help to re-build the divisions within consciousness which are broken down in confusion. The problem is that these drugs all cause some sedation, which increases the barrier through which the carer is trying to reach the patient. The least sedative anti-psychotic drugs are the *butyrophenones*, and *haloperidol* is the drug of choice.

Occasionally the drug of first choice does not give the desired effect. If this happens, first check compliance: check that the prescribed drug was given at the right dose for the right number of times (see Table 5.3). If the drug of first choice is failing, there should be a drug 'in reserve'. Chlorpromazine, with all its side effects, is probably still the reserve drug of choice: it is sedative (indication 1) and anti-psychotic (indication 2). Further details of the use of drugs are given in Table 5.3.

Use of drugs should be confined to the smallest effective dose for the shortest possible time. Where possible, treatment for the cause of delirium should be carried

Table 5.3 Drug treatment in patients with acute organic brain syndrome.

Problem	Aim	Drug	
		First choice	*Second choice*
Fear due to muddled thoughts or hallucinations	Rationalise thoughts with minimal sedation, so that patient can discuss fears	Haloperidol 5–10 mg po/sc Repeat hourly until settled or until 50 mg has been given*	Chlorpromazine 25–50 mg po/im Repeat hourly until settled WATCH BLOOD PRESSURE
Paranoid behaviour		WATCH FOR CHANGES IN MUSCLE TONE	
Irreversible terror or distress Urgent behaviour control	sedation	Diazepam 10 mg po/pr Repeat hourly until settled, then observe and only repeat if necessary WATCH RESPIRATORY RATE	Chlorpromazine as above

* Maintenance dosage of haloperidol: add up the dose required in the first 24 hours, and give this as a single daily dose. Reduce this daily dose as soon as possible by 5–10 mg daily, and continue to reduce every day until the drug is discontinued or the symptoms reappear.

out at the same time. Drugs should be given with the patient's permission, and by mouth, although this is not always possible. If a patient is suspicious about medication it is important to have the drug ready, then negotiate and give the tablets/elixir as soon as the patient agrees to take it. By the time you have gone to the drug cupboard the patient may have forgotten or changed his or her mind.

The correct dose of the drug should be established by starting with small doses, assessing the response and repeating as necessary. If the oral route is not possible, diazepam works quickly by rectum (diazepam injection per rectum via a 2 ml syringe can be used if no rectal solution or suppositories are available, but remember to take the needle off!) and haloperidol can be given by relatively pain-free subcutaneous injection.

Summary

Confusion is frightening for the patient and for their family. In previously lucid cancer patients it is usually due to an acute organic brain syndrome (delirium) and so a treatable physical cause must be sought.

It is usually possible to understand where the muddled thoughts are arising from, and to comfort the patient's fears even though their thoughts may remain confused.

The priorities for treatment are to stop the patient's fear, rationalise the underlying anxieties, find and treat the physical cause for the confusion and help to re-orientate the patient to reality. This means enlisting the help of his or her family to maintain a calm, reassuring environment either at home or in hospital. The patient may need drug treatment, which should preferably be voluntary and by mouth.

Above all, it must always be assumed that a patient understands what is being said, the patient must be reassured that he or she is safe, is not insane, and that the people caring for him or her are trying to understand.

Confusion is often reversible, but even when it cannot be completely resolved it can be understood and made manageable.

Acknowledgements

Dr Claud Regnard, for enthusiasm and for checking my manuscript.
Dr Andrew Brittlebank and Sister Jeanne Gilchrist for their helpful criticisms and suggestions.
Dr Averil Stedeford, for diagrams upon which the figures are based, and Heinemann Medical Books Ltd for permission to use these.
My husband, for patience which is apparently inexhaustible.

References

STEDEFORD, A. (1984). *Facing Death. Patients, families and professionals.* William Heinemann Medical Books, Oxford.

6

Nutritional care of the terminally ill patient and family

Charlette R. Gallagher-Allred

Caring for the terminally ill patient and family is as important to any health care professional involved with palliative care as treatment of the symptoms resulting from the underlying disease. To care means that we accept the patient and family and deal with the issues and concerns that are important to them. Nutrition is often a major issue and concern of terminally ill patients and their families.

The meaning of food and nutrition during terminal illness

Food carries biological, emotional, and sociological meanings. It means different things to different people, and, within the same person it has different meanings depending on whether they are ill or well.

The act of serving food to others, regardless of setting, carries a highly symbolic value. It characterises the social and community values of 'being thy brother's keeper' (Callahan, 1983). Food also carries with it religious, cultural, and ethnic values that have meaning to patients, families, and health care professionals. In order to fully appreciate the meaning food has in the lives of patients, those involved with palliative care would do well to identify the meaning food has in their own lives.

Terminal illness can alter a patient's nutritional needs in three ways.

• The anatomical, physiological, and metabolic changes that occur because of various diseases can decrease gastrointestinal absorption and increase nutrient requirements, such as frequently occurs in patients with acquired immune deficiency syndrome (AIDS) who often develop severe diarrhoea and malabsorption.

• The dying process itself slows many body functions, including gastric emptying, which results in increased satiety, decreased hunger, and frequent food intolerances.

• Medical interventions, such as curative chemotherapy, alter metabolic processes and frequently result in increased nutrient requirements. Even palliative medications such as narcotics alter nutrient needs when side effects occur, such as nausea, vomiting, and constipation.

Overlaid on these *physical* conditions are changes in the desire for food because of the *psychological* changes that accompany the grief process. For example, the dying patient often holds different views of food depending on his or her stage of death and dying. An angry patient may express anger and guilt through statements such as, 'I ate a high fibre diet all my life and I *still* got colon cancer'. A patient during the bargaining stage of death and dying may ask, 'If I give up alcohol, will my liver cancer stop spreading?' Depressed patients are often anorectic and do not eat, but the acceptance stage may be signalled by an increase in appetite as the patient is relieved of depression, anger, and denial.

Goals of nutritional care

Overall goals of palliative care are to maximise enjoyment and minimise pain. When eating and mealtimes can accomplish either of these goals, they should be used to advantage. If eating is not an enjoyable experience, on the other hand, its practice should not be overemphasised. It is at this time that the health care professional involved with palliative care can be a strong patient advocate and family ally by reassuring both that loving care can be demonstrated in ways other than through feeding.

The goals in the provision of nutritional care to terminally ill patients and their families include the following.

- Relief of troublesome symptoms (diet can be an effective adjunct to medical and nursing interventions)
- Enhancement of pleasurable experiences of living
- Prevention or treatment of malnutrition, which could be the unavoidable cause of death, if death by starvation or dehydration is unacceptable to the patient, family, and/or health care team.

The nurse's role in achieving nutritional goals

In order to achieve the goals in the provision of nutritional care to terminally ill patients and their families, the palliative care nurse will perform several functions including the following.

- Assess the patient's physical and psychological condition for the role that curative and palliative treatments, food, and mealtimes have on causing symptoms; ascertain if dietary modifications can alleviate these symptoms and improve well-being
- Identify the patient and family's nutritional concerns and dietary questions
- Establish goals of treatment and integrate dietary intervention as appropriate into the overall plan of care
- Counsel the patient and family on specific and practical dietary modifications that can enhance well-being
- Re-evaluate nutritional goals and intervention periodically, and implement changes when appropriate

Assess the patient's condition

Assessment is the first component in the provision of nutritional care to terminally ill patients and their families. A plan of care can only be as good as the completeness and accuracy of the data collected and the assessment of the patient's condition and the family's situation.

Figure 6.1 is an assessment instrument that includes important nutrition-related questions that the palliative care nurse might ask the patient and family during an initial visit and during on-going visits. Answers to these questions will give clues about the nutritional status and eating behaviour of the patient. In addition, it might alert the palliative care nurse to the need for the services of a dietitian or nutritionist.

Identify patient and family concerns

Figure 6.1 also includes questions about specific nutrition issues and dietary concerns that patients and their families may wish to express. The palliative care nurse will want to be attentive for offhanded concerns that expose hidden fears, such as those given below.

- 'If I don't drink anything, will dehydration be painful?'
- 'I'd like to eat, but I'm afraid I'll choke and be unable to breathe if I eat too much.'
- 'If I had eaten "right" would I have avoided cancer?'
- 'I'm sure people will think I look too thin in the coffin.'

Integrate nutrition into the plan of care

After the information from the nutrition assessment tool is collected and assessed, a nutrition problem list can be delineated. Nutrition goals that are consistent with other medical and nursing goals should then be established. Following the delineation of appropriate palliative nutrition therapies to treat each nutrition problem, the problems, goals, and therapies are written into the plan of care.

When identifying goals and suggesting appropriate therapies, the palliative care nurse will want to take the patient and family's ethnic, cultural, and religious background into consideration. Despite the well-known adage that it is hazardous to apply stereotypes to individual patients, peoples of various backgrounds *do* have different views and *do* respond differently to food, symptoms, pain, health care delivery systems, and dying. The views and responses of others are often greatly different from our own. To be helpful to patients and their families, palliative care nurses must not only recognise that individual differences exist but must also be supportive of these differences (Gallagher-Allred, 1989, p. 127).

Counsel on appropriate dietary modifications

Anticipatory guidance is an important aspect of the nutrition care plan. When counselling the patient and family on how to manage the symptoms associated with dying, the palliative care nurse anticipates those problems most likely to occur and guides the patient and family in making plans to handle them, thereby alleviating their fears of future problems. Information about diet and nutrition that the patient

1. Does the patient experience any of the following problems?
   - nausea and/or vomiting   Yes ☐   No ☐
     if so, is it associated with:
     - taste of specific foods   Yes ☐   No ☐
     - sight or smell of particular foods   Yes ☐   No ☐
     - temperature of foods   Yes ☐   No ☐
   - diaorrhea   Yes ☐   No ☐
   - constipation or gastrointestinal obstruction   Yes ☐   No ☐
   - mouth sores   Yes ☐   No ☐
   - difficulty chewing   Yes ☐   No ☐
   - difficulty swallowing   Yes ☐   No ☐
   - dry mouth   Yes ☐   No ☐
   - poor appetite   Yes ☐   No ☐
     if so, is it caused by:
     - pain or other symptoms   Yes ☐   No ☐
     - depression or anxiety   Yes ☐   No ☐
     - early satiety, fatigue, or weakness   Yes ☐   No ☐
   - pressure sores   Yes ☐   No ☐

2. Does the patient take any vitamin, mineral, other food supplements?   Yes ☐   No ☐

3. Does the patient have a gastrointestinal or intravenous feeding tube in place?   Yes ☐   No ☐

4. Does the patient or family express significant remorse about weight change or food intake?   Yes ☐   No ☐
   - If the patient has lost a lot of weight, does the weight change make the patient more dependent on others?   Yes ☐   No ☐
   - Does the patient or family want to try to reverse the weight loss with enteral or parenteral nutritional support?   Yes ☐   No ☐

5. Does the family exhibit any of the following behaviours?
   - inappropriate use of food as a crutch for emotional problems   Yes ☐   No ☐
   - belief that disease is caused by what the patient did or did not eat   Yes ☐   No ☐
   - fear that if the patient doesn't eat, he or she will feel hunger pains   Yes ☐   No ☐
   - fear that if the patient becomes dehydrated, he or she will suffer   Yes ☐   No ☐
   - fear that if the patient quits eating, he or she will die soon   Yes ☐   No ☐
   - belief in unorthodox nutritional therapies such as vitamin C, laetrile, the macrobiotic diet, enzymes   Yes ☐   No ☐

Fig. 6.1 Nutrition assessment instrument.

and family will benefit from counselling by the palliative care nurse includes the following (Gallagher-Allred, 1989, p. 223).

- How the disease process and the process of dying can affect the patient's desire for food
- How changes in a patient's appetite and ability to eat can cause changes in food intake, bodily appearance, and bodily function
- Specific dietary measures for symptom control
- Relief measures that will be available as the patient's condition deteriorates
- The availability of community nutrition and food resources
- How to reach the palliative care nurse when questions arise and assistance is needed

Armed with an individualised and appropriate nutritional care plan, the palliative care nurse should experience a great deal of satisfaction in implementing the plan. An effective counsellor will use the following information and skills in carrying out the plan of care, and counselling the patient and family on their nutrition issues and dietary concerns (Gallagher-Allred, 1989, p. 261).

- Knowledge about what losses mean to patients and their families
- Knowledge of the stage of dying of the patient and the individual members of the patient's family
- Ability to listen actively
- Well-honed communication techniques

Counselling and communication techniques are discussed further in Chapters 13 and 14.

Re-evaluate goals and intervention

Self-evaluation, evaluation of the established plan of care, and evaluation of the ability of the patient and the patient's family to achieve desired goals should be a part of the palliative care nurse's standard procedure during and after each visit. It is only with such evaluation that progress can be noted and the care plan be modified as necessary.

Two dietary situations that palliative care nurses frequently are (*i*) the patient who cannot and will not eat (the family often wants to push this patient to eat more than the patient can or is willing); and (*ii*) the patient who can and wants to eat but needs assistance in knowing what to eat and how to maximise the quality of mealtimes.

Helping the patient who cannot and will not eat

Anorexia and cachexia are hallmark conditions of many end-stage chronic diseases. This is particularly true for patients with incurable cancer, renal disease, pulmonary disease, AIDS, and heart failure. Suggested causes include abnormal host metabolism of protein, carbohydrate, fat, hormones, fluids, and electrolytes; diseases elaboration of cachexia-inducing substances; and debilitating effects of various therapies.

Cancer-related anorexia and cachexia are particularly common phenomena that health care professionals concerned with palliative care must address. Tumours cause early satiety (especially with lung, stomach, and pancreatic tumours), specific food aversions (particularly to protein-containing foods such as beef and pork with almost all tumours), nausea and vomiting (especially with liver cancer or metastases to the liver and as a result of narcotics and other therapies), and decreased interest in foods (particularly with any external tumour compression or partial obstruction of any part of the gastrointestinal tract). Although weight loss in the cancer patient is a worrisome sign, treatment unfortunately does not necessarily improve the patient's well-being or survival (DeWys *et al.*, 1981; Nixon *et al.*, 1981).

Although anorexia and cachexia commonly occur with incurable disease, they are not always problems to the patient and family. Indeed, one task of the palliative care health professional is to ascertain whether either or both are of significant concern and, if so, whether the problem is the patient's, the family's, or both. Often anorexia and cachexia are more problematic for the family than the patient.

Cachexia may be a problem for patients and families because they do not understand what causes it or how it occurs. Patients and their families should be told that, contrary to the popular misconception, cancer does not cause loss of body weight by eating away body parts like a worm eats a leaf. Hearing this can help alleviate the fear that something ugly is happening inside the body.

In working with an anxious family with a patient who cannot or will not eat, the health care professional should attempt to diminish the effects of the no-win situation. Treatment is best directed at ameliorating social consequences such as embarrassment of the patient at his or her gaunt appearance and physical complications. Teaching the family about the effects that the disease and dying process have is also important. The family's anxieties can be diminished and the patient can be freed from the pressure to eat when attention is shifted from maintaining the patient's nutritional status to enhancing patient comfort through providing small appetising meals. Sometimes it is most appropriate to offer the patient no food unless the patient requests it. Although this shift may be difficult at first for the family, it brings considerable relief to both patient and family in the long run (Gallagher-Allred, 1989, p. 220).

Helpful phrases in discouraging the 'he must eat or he will die' snydrome include the following.

- 'The disease controls his appetite; pushing him to eat will cause the tumour to grow and won't do him any good now.'
- 'He's sick and will be sick even if he eats.'
- 'Pushing him to eat will only make him uncomfortable.'
- 'It's important to show him you love him in ways other than through food.'
- 'Let him sit with you and eat what he wants.'
- 'Try not to worry that he eats poorly; it doesn't seem to bother him.'

Dehydration has been called a natural anaesthesia for terminally ill patients because it appears to decrease the patient's perception of suffering by reducing the level of consciousness. The concomitant dry mouth effect associated with dehydration can be relieved through ice chips, lubricants, and other simple suggestions (Zerwelch, 1983).

If the patient's life expectancy is measured in weeks or days, dehydration, as a natural course of events, may be preferred to aggressive nutritional support through tube feedings and/or total parenteral nutrition (TPN) if such feedings cause discomfort. By foregoing aggressive therapy, the following conditions may result which will benefit the patient (Cataldi-Betcher *et al.*, 1983; Dresser and Boisaubin, 1985; Hacklor Fetsch and Shandor Miles, 1986; Zerwelch, 1984; 1987).

- Decreased gastrointestinal and venous distension
- Decreased nausea, vomiting, and potential for aspiration
- Decreased diarrhoea
- Decreased oedema and tumour pressure
- Decreased pulmonary secretions resulting in less coughing, less fear of choking and drowning, and less rattling secretions
- Decreased urine flow and need to void

For some patients the procedures required in order to avert malnutrition and dehydration are so onerous that the benefits are inconsequential or meaningless. Is not to intervene acceptable, or is it tantamount to murder? The choice lies in doing what is in the patient's best interests after the goals to be accomplished have been considered and the expected benefits and burdens have been analysed by the patient, the patient's family, and competent health care professionals (President's Commission for the Study of Ethical Problems in Medicine and Biomedical and Behavioral Research, 1983, pp. 1–12). Ethical issues have been discussed further in Chapter 2.

It has been the experience of this author and others (Lynn and Osterweiss, 1985) that most terminally ill patients rarely find any advantage to aggressive nutritional support via tube or parenteral feedings. Instead, terminally ill anorectic patients who are allowed to eat and drink as desired, and who are not pushed to do so if they do not desire or are unable, is a viable alternative. A previously placed tube for enteral feedings or an intravenous line for TPN may not need to be discontinued, however, unless the patient desires. Even though the feeding tube may be in place, there is no moral reason for using the tube for feeding (President's Commission for the Study of Ethical Problems in Medicine and Biomedical and Behavioral Research, 1983, pp. 1–12; Boisaubin, 1984; Lo and Jonsen, 1980).

Helping the patient who can and wants to eat

For patients who want to eat and who can be helped to eat better, the importance of improving appetite and enabling them to eat as normally as possible cannot be overestimated. The palliative care nurse's role is of paramount importance in this patient situation. Medications, such as corticosteroids, alcohol as an aperitif, and tricyclic antidepressants, can be administered to improve appetite and mood. Improving a poor self-image through suggestions such as clothes that are worn, a hairdresser appointment, or a dental appointment, can also improve a patient's appetite.

Table 6.1   Suggestions for improving oral intake. (Adapted from Gallagher-Allred, 1989, pp. 221 and 269, with permission of Aspen Publishers, Inc.)

- Feed the patient when hungry, changing mealtimes if needed. Note the patient's best meals and make there the largest meals.
- Serve a small serving of the patient's favourite foods on a small plate.
- Gently encourage, but do not nag, the patient to eat; remove uneaten food without undue comment.
- Cold foods are generally preferred to hot foods. Reassure parents of a dying child that they do not have to serve a hot, nutritious meal daily for the child; encourage them not to feel guilty if the child wants nothing or only wants a fast-food hamburger or fries.
- Set an attractive table and plate, using a plate garnish or table flower if enjoyed by the patient. In an institutional setting, serve the patient's food on trays set with embroidered tray cloths and pretty china or stoneware, rather than on traditional paper underliners and dishes. Allow the patient's personal china and utensils from home to be used if feasible.
- Make mealtimes sociable and enjoyable, vary the place of eating and remove bedpans from the room.
- Children can be encouraged to drink by playing games; it is fun for a child to drink fluids in out-of-the-ordinary ways, such as through a syringe, in small medicine cups, and by eating juice bars or ice lollies. Remove toys from the bed, turn off the television, bring in friends for a meal. Children will enjoy a packed lunch on occasion, and they enjoy eating foods that have been cut into interesting shapes or look like favourite characters.
- Suggest the patient rest before eating; most children and adults feel more like eating when they are relaxed.
- Encourage high-calorie foods day or night, including eggnog, milkshake, custard, pudding, peanut butter, cream soups, cheese, fizzy drinks, pie, sherbet, and cheesecake. In an institutional setting, consider serving foods from a hot trolley instead of or in addition to allowing patients to choose their meals in advance. Consider soup and soft sandwiches for midday meals. Try to supply as much variety in food selection as possible, including regional favourites.
- Provide lipped dishes for those patients who have arm and hand weakness; use rubber grips on ordinary cutlery for those with a weak grip.
- In an institutional setting, have a dining room available, with a home-like atmosphere, where patients can eat and patients and families can eat together. Allow the family to eat with the patient in the patient's room if desired. Have staff available to feed patients who are unable to feed themselves. Do not hurry patients to eat.
- Liberalise diets as much as possible; rarely are diabetic or low-sodium diets essential, but if they are, consider low simple sugar foods and no regular salt packets instead of more restricted diets.

If anorexia is due to correctable causes and the patient has a predicted life expectancy of several months, the correctable causes should be treated aggressively if desired by the patient. Likewise, treatment should be aggressive if the patient's anorexia appears to be an isolated symptom and the suspected consequence is malnutrition that could compromise both the quality and quantity of the patient's remaining days. Suggestions for improving oral intake of adults and children have been summarised in Table 6.1.

Over-the-counter medical nutritional supplements also may be warranted for terminally ill adults and children who want a high calorie intake in a small volume. Medical nutritional supplements are often appreciated by weak patients and their families because the patient can drink the highly-fortified liquid products with minimal effort and the family members feel that they are providing 'something special'.

Enteral tube feedings, in addition to oral intake or as the sole source of nutrition, may also be appropriate in feeding the patient who can and wants to eat. Liquid commercial nutritional products are usually administered from a small-bore, flexible catheter that in most terminally ill patients is passed through the nose into the stomach or upper small intestine. The tube may also be passed directly into the stomach through the abdominal wall.

If tube feedings are desired, the palliative care nurse will need to make decisions concerning the osmolality of the solution, whether the solution will be administered by continuous drip or by intermittent feeding, and the rate the solution is to be delivered. In general, the formulas to be administered should be isotonic solutions. Depending on the patient's ability to tolerate the solution, feedings should be started with a continuous drip at half or full strength if isotonic solutions are used, or at quarter or half strength if hypertonic solutions are used. An appropriate beginning rate is usually 50 ml/hr (up to a final rate of 100–125 ml/hr), or the concentration can be increased (quarter to half to three-quarter to full strength), depending on patient tolerance and nutritional goals. Many patients and families prefer intermittent tube feedings to continuous drip because that method seems more like a meal than drip delivery via pump.

In theory, a continuous drip administration of 100–125 ml/hr of full-strength (1 kcal/ml) solution is the maximum amount needed if weight maintenance is the goal (2400–3000 kcal) for terminally ill patients. In practice, however, only 1000–1800 kcal/day (continuous drip for 10–15 hours) is generally needed to achieve satiety and comfort. Greater amounts frequently cause complications in terminally ill patients, including fluid overload, cramps, diaorrhea, reflux, and aspiration. Raising the head of the patient's bed 30 degrees helps prevent reflux and aspiration. Unless commercially prefilled bags are used, the solution should hang no longer than 4–6 hours and the tubing should be changed daily; commercially prefilled bags and tubing can be hung for 24 hours.

Total parenteral nutrition is generally not well-tolerated by terminally ill patients, and rarely does parenteral feeding reduce the distress of anorexia and cachexia. Instead, it often subjects the patient to new problems that are more distressing and to prolong suffering that would not have been faced had parenteral feeding been foregone (Billings, 1985). If TPN is desired, it is best begun in the hospital setting before the patient is returned to the home or long-term care facility. Home and long-term care facility administration should be under close monitoring of a specially-trained care team.

When aggressive nutritional therapy in the form of enteral or parenteral feedings is implemented in an attempt to overcome a particular problem, such as weakness so that a patient can attend a family member's graduation or wedding, the feedings should generally be stopped in about ten days if the weakness does not lessen.

Dietary therapy for common nutrition problems

Although dying often brings many less-than-desirable side effects, it would be wrong to view dying as a 'disease' hungry for medical 'remedies'. However, the palliative care health professional can give the patient and family many helpful dietary suggestions for symptom control, so that they can maximise comfort during the dying patient's remaining days.

Table 6.2 provides suggestions for appropriate dietary therapy for common symptoms in terminal illness. Because the majority of terminally ill patients that we currently care for are diagnosed with incurable cancer, the suggestions are primarily based on responses from treating cancer patients. As the world's population ages and chronic degenerative diseases, including renal disease, cardiovascular failure, pulmonary failure, and organic brain syndrome, have more time to exert their ravishing effects, we may be caring more for these patients in the future. In Table 6.2, reference is made to specific diseases but the diaorrhea associated with postsurgical dumping and AIDS, and the nausea and vomiting associated with gastrointestinal obstruction and narcotic use, are included under the symptoms of diaorrhea and nausea and vomiting, respectively. The reader is cautioned that not all of the identified treatments may be appropriate for all diseases or conditions.

Ethical and legal considerations in nutritional support of terminally ill patients

The ethical and legal considerations in nutritional support of terminally ill patients are increasingly being debated, and those involved with palliative care will want to become familiar with legal decisions that affect feeding issues. 'To feed or not to feed', as with other methods of treatment, requires that those involved with the palliative care ask the underlying question, 'What good will it accomplish for the patient?' Three conditions when nutritional support might result in disproportionate burden to the patient include (*i*) when nutritional support would be a futile treatment, (*ii*) when no possibility of benefit could occur with nutritional support, and (*iii*) when the burden outweighs the benefit (Lynn and Childress, 1983). Chapter 2 provides further discussion of ethical issues.

In working with patients and families who may consider the use of aggressive nutritional support, the palliative care nurse's role is to undertake the following (Gallagher-Allred, 1989, p. 240).

- Listen carefully to the patient and family
- Clarify options
- Provide pros and cons of aggressive nutritional support
- Support the patient-family choice
- Encourage deliberative palliative care team decisions that are consistent with patient and family wishes

Health care professionals concerned with palliative care are often asked questions about unorthodox nutritional therapies or claims that have not been scientifically validated. For several reasons – including ignorance, hope, and fear of abandonment – many people cling to nutritional claims that have no proven basis or may have been disproved. The first goals of those concerned with palliative care are to understand the patient's point of view and then to acknowledge the patient's concern as real. After identifying the patient's concerns, it will be necessary to deal

Table 6.2 Dietary therapy for common symptoms in terminal illness. Note that not all of the identified treatments may be appropriate for all diseases or conditions. (Adapted from Gallagher-Allred, 1989, pp. 221 and 269, with permission of Aspen Publishers, Inc.)

Belching

- Allow the patient to make the final choice of foods to eat and avoid, but consider testing the patient's tolerance to gas-producing foods, such as the following: beer, carbonated beverages, alcohol, dairy products if lactose intolerant, nuts, beans, onions, peas, corn, cucumbers, radishes, cabbage, broccoli, Brussels sprouts, spinach, cauliflower, high-fat foods, yeast, and mushrooms.

- Encourage the patient to eat solids at mealtimes and drink liquids between meals instead of with solid foods.

- Advise the patient to avoid eating quickly and reclining immediately after eating; encourage the patient to relax before, during, and after meals.

- Advise the patient to avoid overeating, avoid sucking through straws, avoid chewing gum, and to keep the mouth closed when chewing and swallowing.

Constipation

- Encourage the patient to eat foods high in fibre (bran; whole grains; fruits, especially pineapple, prunes, and raisins; vegetables; nuts; and legumes) if adequate fluid intake can be maintained. Avoid high-fibre foods if dehydration, severe constipation, or obstruction are anticipated.

- Increase fluid intake as tolerated; encourage fruit juices, prune juice, and cider. If liked by the patient, a recipe (1–2 ounces with the evening meal of a mixture of 2 cups apple-sauce, 2 cups unprocessed bran, and 1 cup 100% prune juice) is effective and may reduce laxative use.

- Discontinue calcium and iron supplementation if used; limit cheese, rich desserts, and other foods if constipating.

Diarrhoea

- Let the patient make the final choice of foods to eat and avoid, but suggest omission of the following foods if they cause diarrhoea: milk, ice cream, whole-grain breads and cereals, nuts, beans, peas, greens, fruits with seeds and skins, fresh pineapple, raisins, cider, prune juice, raw vegetables, gas-forming vegetables, alcohol, and caffeine-containing beverages.

- Encourage the patient to eat bananas, apple-sauce, peeled apple, tapioca, rice, peanut butter, refined grains, crackers, pasta, cream of wheat, oatmeal, and cooked vegetables.

- Encourage the patient to avoid liquids with a meal and instead to drink liquids an hour after a meal.

- Encourage the patient to relax before, during, and after a meal.

- Enteral and/or parenteral nutritional support in the AIDS patient may be appropriate if the patient has a lengthy life expectancy and the cause of the diarrhoea is known and treatable; if tube feedings or oral diet is appropriate, they should be high in calories and protein and low in fibre, lactose, and fat.

- If dehydration is a problem, encourage high-potassium foods.

Hypercalcaemia

- Allow the hypercalcaemic patient to eat foods high in calcium such as dairy products if desired, but encourage the patient to avoid calcium and vitamin D supplementation; restriction of high-calcium foods is rarely helpful.

- Encourage the patient to drink lots of fluids, particularly carbonated beverages containing phosphoric acid if the patient enjoys them.

Mental disorders

- Encourage the patient to avoid alcohol and caffeine-containing foods, such as coffee, tea, and chocolate, if they contribute to anxiety, sleep deprivation, or depression.

- If the patient is *drowsy* or *apathetic*, suggest that the family may need to feed the patient. Encourage them to prepare the patient's favourite foods, usually in soft form to be served with a spoon or bite-size so the patient might self-feed. Help the family protect the patient and others from the patient by shutting off or removing knobs from stoves, removing matches, and locking doors to cabinets or closets that contain poisons, alcohol, or medications. Put away electrical appliances, such as mixers, food processors, can openers, and waffle irons; unplug microwave ovens.

- If the patient is *agitated* or *confused*, caution the family about the dangers of hand-feeding the patient. Suggest feeding with a spoon and not allowing the patient to handle feeding utensils, plates, glass, etc. Encourage the family to tell the patient what time of day it is, what meal is served, and what foods are served. Remind the patient that the foods served are favourites. Make mealtimes enjoyable by reminiscing about pleasant events in the patient's life. Consider the pros and cons of waking the patient if asleep at mealtimes.

- If the patient is *stuporous* or *comatose*, counsel the family that semi-starvation and dehydration are not painful to the patient; explore with them the pros and cons of enteral and parenteral nutritional support if they request information.

Mouth problems

- If the patient says that foods taste *bitter*, encourage poultry, fish, dairy products, eggs, milk, and cheese; bitter-tasting foods usually include red meat, sour juices, coffee, tea, tomatoes, and chocolate. Suggest cooking foods in glass or porcelain instead of in metal containers, and avoid serving foods on metal or with metallic utensils. Encourage sweet fruit drinks, carbonated beverages, ice lollies and seasonings, herbs, and spices to enhance flavours.

- If the patient says that foods taste '*old*', try adding sugar; sour and salty tastes often taste 'old'.

- If the patient says that foods taste *too sweet*, suggest drinking sour juices, and cooking with lemon juice, vinegar, spices, herbs, and mint; add pickles to appropriate foods.

- If the patient says that foods have *no taste*, suggest marinating appropriate foods, serving highly seasoned foods, adding sugar, and eating foods at room temperature.

- If the patient has *difficulty swallowing*, suggest small frequent meals of soft foods (pureed if needed); advise against foods that might irritate the mouth and oesophagus, such as acidic juices or fruits, spicy foods, very hot or cold foods, alcohol, and carbonated beverages.

- If the patient has *mouth sores*, suggest blenderised and cold foods; gravies, cream soups, eggnog, milkshakes, cream pies, cheesecake, macaroni and cheese, and casseroles are well-liked. Suggest the patient avoid alcohol and acidic, spicy, rough, hot, and highly salted foods.

- If the patient has a *dry mouth*, suggest frequent sips of water, juice, ice chips, ice lollies, ice cream, fruitades, or slushy-frozen baby foods mixed with fruit juice. Sucking on hard sweets may stimulate saliva. Solid foods should be moist, pureed as needed, and not too tart or too hot or cold if mouth sores are present.

Nausea and vomiting

- Encourage the patient to avoid eating if nauseated or if nausea is anticipated.

- Suggest small meals of cool non-odourous foods. Many patients find it helpful to avoid fatty, greasy, or fried foods; avoid mixing hot and cold foods at the same meal; avoid high-bulk meals; and avoid nausea-precipitating foods, such as overly sweet foods, alcohol, spicy foods, and tobacco with meals.

- Encourage the patient to eat slowly and avoid overeating. Relaxing before and after meals and avoiding physical activity and lying flat for two hours after eating may also help.
- Suggest that the patient not prepare own food.

Obstruction (gastrointestinal)

- If oral intake is not contraindicated, encourage the patient to eat small meals that are low in fibre, low in residue, and blenderised or strained. Many patients will prefer to eat their favourite foods, enjoy large meals, and then vomit frequently. A gastric tube, open to straight or intermittent drain, may alleviate the need for regular vomiting.
- With 'squashed stomach syndrome', encourage the patient to eat small frequent meals, avoid nausea-producing foods, odourous foods, gas-producing foods, and high-fat or fried foods. Limit fluid with meals, taking fluids an hour before and after meals.

---

with the patient's ignorance or feelings in a caring manner. Discuss the treatment fully and outline the pros and cons dispassionately and in a nonjudgmental way (Gallagher-Allred, 1989, pp. 226–7).

Although it may be appropriate to do so, there is no obligation on the part of the professional carer to dispel the hopes that an unorthodox nutritional therapy or claim may bring a patient, unless what is being practiced is harmful or unless the costs outweigh the benefits. Try to identify whether the unorthodox practice is producing a positive psychological effect. If so, then the cost-to-benefit ratio can be determined and a decision whether to discuss the practice with the patient can be made somewhat objectively (Gallagher-Allred, 1989, p. 227).

In closing, the palliative care nurse should discuss with dying patients and their families any guilt feelings they may have that they caused the patient's incurable illness by foods that were or were not eaten. Not to dispel these feelings is to leave in place an inhumane weight of guilt. The goal of palliative care nurses is to comfort patients and their families. Relieving them of this possible guilt is consistent with this goal (Cassileth *et al.*, 1985).

Acknowledgement

Acknowledgement is due to Aspen Publishers, Inc., Maryland, for permission to include material based on, and Fig. 6.1, Table 6.1 and 6.2, from Gallagher-Allred (1989).

References

BILLINGS, J. A. (1985). *Outpatient Management of Advanced Cancer: Symptom Control, Support and Hospice-in-the-Home.* J. B. Lippincott Co., Philadelphia.
BOISAUBIN, E. V. (1984). Ethical issues in the nutritional support of the terminal patient. *Journal of the American Dietetic Association*, 84, 529–31.
CALLAHAN, D. (1983). On feeding the dying. *Hastings Center Report*, 13, 20–2.
CASSILETH, B., LUSK, E. J., MILLER, D. S., BROWN, LORRAINE L. and MILLER, C.

104 *Nutritional care of the terminally ill patient and family*

(1985). Psychosocial correlates for survival in advanced malignant disease. *New England Journal of Medicine*, **312(24)**, 1551–5.

CATALDI-BETCHER, EMMA L., SELTZER, M. H., SLOCUM, BERNADETTE, A. *et al.* (1983). Complications occurring during enteral nutrition support: a prospective study. *Journal of Parenteral and Enteral Nutrition*, **7**, 546–52.

DEWYS, W. D. and KUBOTA, T. T. (1981). Enteral and parenteral nutrition in the care of the cancer patient. *Journal of the American Medical Association*, **246(15)**, 1725–7.

DRESSER, REBECCA S. and BOISAUBIN, E. V. (1985). Ethics, law and nutritional support. *Archives of Internal Medicine*, **145**, 122–4.

GALLAGHER-ALLRED, CHARLETTE R. (1989). *Nutritional Care of the Terminally Ill.* Aspen Publishers, Inc., Rockville, Maryland.

HACKLER FETSCH, SUSAN and SHANDOR MILES, MARGARET (1986). Children and death. In *Nursing Care of the Terminally Ill*, Madalon O'Rawe Amenta and Nancy L. Bohnet (Eds), pp. 215–16. Little, Brown & Co., Boston, Massachusetts.

LO, B. and JONSEN, A. R. (1980). Ethical decisions in the care of the patient terminally ill with metastatic cancer. *Annals of Internal Medicine*, **92**, 107–11.

LYNN, JOANNE and CHILDRESS, J. F. (1983). Must patients always be given food and water? *Hastings Center Report*, **13**, 17–21.

LYNN, JOANNE and OSTERWEISS, MARIAN (1985). Ethical issues arising in hospice care. In *Hospice Programs and Public Policy*, Paul Torrens (Ed.), p. 205. American Hospital Association, Chicago.

NIXON, D. W., LAWSON, D. H., KUTNER, M. *et al.* (1981). Hyperalimentation of the cancer patient with protein-calorie undernutrition. *Cancer Research*, **41**, 2038–45.

President's Commission for the Study of Ethical Problems in Medicine and Biomedical and Behavioral Research (1983). *Deciding to Forego Life-sustaining Treatment.* United States Government Printing Office.

ZERWEKH, JOYCE V. (1983). The dehydration question. *Nursing '83*, **13**, 47–51.

ZERWEKH, JOYCE V. (1984). The last few days. In *Hospice and Palliative Nursing Care*, Ann G. Blues and Joyce V. Zerwekh (Eds), p. 180. Grune & Stratton, Orlando, Florida.

ZERWEKH, JOYCE V. (1987). Should fluid and nutritional support be withheld from terminally ill patients? Another opinion. *American Journal of Hospice Care*, **4(4)**, 37–8.

7

Complementary therapies

Jenny Penson

'There are more things in Heaven and Earth, Horatio, than are dreamt of in your philosophy'

Shakespeare, 'Hamlet'

Patient care today, even in its most modern and technological forms, still contains an element of mystery. There is always a degree of unpredictability about the outcome of even the most scientific treatment and nurses are aware that faith, willpower and the wish to be well all affect recovery for any individual. The function of the human spirit in healing may be not only mysterious but, quite possibly, mystical.

All professional health carers have tried to act as healers at certain times, with particular patients and in their own different ways. From earliest times human beings have striven to heal each other physically, emotionally and spiritually. A desire for wholeness and harmony both as an individual and as part of a community appears to be a fundamental human need.

In one sense carers are all healers, simply because they have the desire to alleviate suffering and to reach out a little to their fellow human beings. But how people should learn to heal or how they should practice healing may be difficult issues. Many paths may seem to lead to the same place. Sometimes orthodox ways seem best, at other times other less orthodox approaches may seem appropriate. How should a person choose?

The therapies discussed in this chapter are all 'complementary' therapies in the sense that they can all complement orthodox approaches to treatment and care, although each may also stand alone. Other phrases used to describe them seem, to the author, to confuse and mislead. 'Alternative Therapies' for instance suggests that the unorthodox can and must replace the orthodox. In the same way 'Fringe Medicine' suggests that the therapies discussed here must, by definition, remain peripheral, to orthodox medicine. Since the world 'medicine' itself can be defined either as 'the art and science of prevention of disease' or, alternatively, as 'a charm or anything of magical power' it may be concluded that medicine can refer to any remedy which heals or cures, or makes the patient feel better. Anyone who can do any of these things is therefore practising medicine. Complementary therapies may properly be a part of that practice.

Knowledge and approval of complementary therapies is implicit in the concept of holistic care as it applies to nursing. Holistic care acknowledges the constant interactions between body, mind, emotions and spirit and maintains that any individual is a totality greater than the sum of these parts. Therefore in holistic nursing neither symptom nor condition is treated, rather the whole individual is the focus of attention. Holistic nursing provides an obvious link with complementary therapies and this may be one reason why nurses are often sympathetic to them. In both systems, as Whitehorn (1983) has pointed out, 'mobilising the patient's own powers becomes the central issue in cure and care'.

The recently increasing prominence of complementary therapies may be seen first of all as a response to the changing needs of the consumer. Patients may indeed be mobilising their own powers. Nowadays the average patient seems to be better informed, more aware that he or she has choices, and therefore more willing and capable of making them. In society generally, attitudes to authority figures are changing with less reliance on institutionalised knowledge, and there is less passive acceptance of advice given. Also, the current political ideology stresses individual responsibility which extends, of course, to all aspects of health care. At the same time as these phenomena are becoming apparent, a certain mistrust or scepticism appears to have grown up around orthodox medical systems. Scepticism has been fuelled by the media with much publicity being given to the potential harm of eating certain foods and to the negative effects of prescribed drugs. This probably began with the Thalidomide tragedies of the 1960s, but has since encompassed a wide range of medications from Opren to Valium, and from the use of Cortisone to the over-frequent prescribing of antibiotics. The contraceptive pill provides a particularly good example of such changed attitudes. Once heralded as the panacea for all birth control problems, its use has steadily declined as more women return to less convenient methods because they fear the long term effects of taking synthetic hormones.

A further case for complementary therapies is made by considering the plight of people suffering chronic illness. In spite of great advances in the treatment of acute conditions, far less has changed in the care of those with the classic chronic illnesses. Patients who are told that 'nothing more can be done' or 'you must learn to live with it', are understandably motivated to seek out alternatives. Indeed complementary therapies are often resorted to only when all else has failed to provide relief. But there may be some real therapeutic value in patients taking control of their conditions and one way of doing this is to actively seek out a system of treatment which is both hopeful and personalised. There may, however, be difficulties in doing this since it involves making choices and this may be especially demanding for people who are feeling ill and vulnerable.

The need for payment can be another problem; it can prohibit choice for some people while giving a sense of control and positive feelings to those who can afford to pay. In the United Kingdom, some complementary therapies may be available under the National Health Service, notably homeopathy and sometimes acupuncture.

Common to all complementary therapies is the belief in the body's own power to heal itself, although this may be defined in different ways. Each recognises the part the mind plays in health and disease. There is also a further belief among therapists and users of complementary therapies that they are safer and kinder than some orthodox treatments. When considering complementary therapies for the first time both patients and nurses can easily become bewildered by the choice that is available. Everyone may find that the boundaries of what can be considered as alternatives or adjuncts to orthodox medicine are very ill defined. For example, do colour therapy, crystal healing, radionics or dowsing appear to be viable alternatives? Is there a difference between these and, for example, homeopathy, osteopathy or acupuncture? Are relaxation techniques and biofeedback alternatives, or part of orthodox medicine? Which complementary therapies can fit into the repertoire of skills of nurses and other health care professionals? Can the skills of massage, aromatherapy, therapeutic touch or relaxation techniques become part or orthodox nursing care? And if so, are there margins to what is or is not acceptable for nurses to include within nursing care? Answers to these questions depend on a variety of factors; personal preferences, aptitude, length of training required, the kind of settings in which nurses practice and the views of both professional colleagues and patients.

The first group of complementary therapies considered are below those that appear, from both the literature and from experience, to be the most frequently used by patients with advanced cancer. They are also therapies which usually require extensive training as preparation for practice: they may properly be called Major Complementary Therapies.

Major complementary therapies used in treating patients with cancer

Homeopathy

Homeopathy is a system of treatment developed by Dr Hahnemann in the late 1780s. Hahnemann was a conventionally trained doctor who became interested, in the course of his normal work, by the idea that the symptoms produced by the drug quinine in a well person were the same as those caused by the disease malaria. Quinine did indeed cure but was curiously able to produce the same symptoms as those that it removed. Hahnemann resurrected the ancient idea that 'like likes to be treated by like' as a principle of treatment. Drugs that simulate the symptoms of a disease when taken by someone who is well may be remedies for the same disease. Homeopaths believe that their drugs somehow enhance the body's own defences against disease and so accelerate healing, although this has not been proven by controlled trials.

A second principle of homeopathy is that the *lower* the concentration of any remedy used, the more effective it will be: this is probably because the body is more able to absorb low concentrations and because an ill body will reject strong substances. Homeopathic remedies are therefore available in different levels of potency but all contain extremely small amounts of the active ingredient. At a homeopathic first aid course attended by the author, the question 'When would you prescribe arsenic?' was asked – this illustrates this point.

Homeopathy is regarded as a very safe form of intervention, because the remedies used produce no side-effects. Homeopathic treatment is a truly holistic approach which takes account of external factors such as the patients living habits and the home environment. It does not, however, require faith in the remedies on the part of the patient. Homeopathy is available under the National Health Service in the United Kingdom. There are four homeopathic hospitals in Scotland and two in England.

Acupuncture

Acupuncture is a form of Chinese medicine which originated over 2000 years ago, and is sometimes used in combination with herbal medicine, special diets and attention to psychological needs. In the West it tends to be used on its own as an alternative method of pain relief. It has been suggested that the way in which acupuncture works is by the release of endorphins, the body's natural pain relievers. Acupuncture is based on the idea that there are meridians in the body which carry an energy or life-force known as Chi. At certain points along these meridians there are junctures where it is necessary for energies to be in balance to maintain health. There are 365 such points where the balance may be harmonised by the insertion of acupuncture needles into the skin. It is the act of interference and not the form it takes which is important: finger pressure may be used at the critical points instead of needles in the techniques known as Shiatsu. Additionally heat may be applied to the balance points through the technique called moxibustion. Electrical stimulation of the points may also be used.

Acupuncture points are often very close together. There are 50 points in the ear alone for example: its shape is considered to correspond to that of the human foetus. The needles used in acupuncture are made from stainless steel and need to be flexible. They are manipulated or rotated at times during treatment and may be left in situ for 15–30 minuts. It has been suggested that the new-found respectability of acupuncture in medical circles is due to the fact that sticking needles into people makes doctors feel at home!

Herbalism

Herbalism is one of the oldest systems of healing and was in use in primitive civilisations long before Christ. It aims to treat the whole person and therefore considers the whole life-style of the patient. The most famous herbal published in Britain is that by Culpepper which, though written over 300 years ago, is still consulted today.

Although many drugs used by orthodox medicine today derive from herbs and plants (vincristine from the periwinkle, digoxin from the foxglove) there is an important difference between manufactured drugs and the herbal original. Herbalists stress that, in their natural form, the active ingredients of medicines are buffered with other substances from the plant: chemically extracted and isolated elements may be too strong for the body to absorb usefully.

When herbal remedies are prescribed by qualified herbalists they can be seen as being safe and free from side-effects. However, at present in the United Kingdom there is no regulating legislation which limits the sale of herbal remedies and concern is sometimes expressed, not least by the medical profession, about the dangers of easy access to these substances. The general public may think that anything labelled as 'herbal' may be intrinsically safe and may not appreciate that some remedies may be toxic if used indiscriminately.

The popularity of herbalism may be seen as being in tune with the current Green Movement where there is a growing 'feel' for natural materials and a life-style that is in harmony with nature. The consumer interest in country living has also caused many people to plant their own herb gardens. Growing and using herbs for healing as well as cooking is an attractive idea; one example is the cultivation of feverfew plants, the leaves of which may be eaten in a sandwich to prevent the recurrence of migraine headaches.

Dr Bach's Flower Remedies

These are a variety of herbal treatment since they are all based on flower extracts. Bach was a conventionally trained doctor at the turn of the century, whose system of healing is based on the notion that mental states such as fear, anxiety, uncertainty etc. open up pathways that allow the body to be invaded by illnesses. By treating these emotions, rather than the physical manifestations of illness, the individual is freed from them and so recovers.

No extensive body of knowledge is necessary to use Dr Bach's remedies. Individuals can often treat themselves by consulting Bach's guide which describes various outlooks on life and suggests one of his 38 remedies to treat them. Remedies can be used separately or in combination. The best known is called Rescue Remedy which can be used for all kinds of sudden shock. The remedies can be diluted in pure water and sipped, dropped on the tongue in an emergency or rubbed on the skin. They tend to be used by cancer patients as part of a strategy for healing, rather than as a treatment complete in itself.

Naturopathy

Naturopathy (or Nature Cure) is a system of healing, developed by Dr Lindlah, which brings various, and sometimes disparate, methods together as a whole. Naturopathy is thought of not only as a means of eradicating illness, but also as a positive way of living that promotes health generally. The underlying philosophy of the system is the law of cause and effect,' what a man sows, so he must reap'. Illness is seen as being only to be expected when the laws of nature are violated by unhealthy living or behaviour.

Naturopathy emphasises the idea that ultimately the individual is the only one who can heal himself. Healing can be aided by treatment to purify the blood, by encouraging the body to eliminate poisons and by a gradual build up of vitality resulting from changes in life-style and outlook. The system recognises that a positive mental attitude to life affects health and healing which can be enhanced by a balanced diet, exercise, pure water, sunshine and fresh air.

The Bristol Programme

This is probably the most widely known system of complementary therapies of cancer. Started by Penny Brohn, who had been a cancer patient, and Dr Alec Forbes in 1979 the programme shows some similarity to naturopathy in philosophy. The Bristol Programme is a registered charity and its patients pay only what they can reasonably afford: inability to pay does not prohibit treatment.

The approach is essentially holistic, acknowledging the fact that cancer of the body is often cancer of the mind and soul as well. It aims to encourage patients to take as much responsibility as possible for their own health and promotes the idea that a healthy body is able to reject all illness, even cancer. The Programme also sees itself as having a preventive role.

The Bristol Programme is sometimes referred to as the Gentle Method of cancer treatment. It is, in reality, not one system but a 'cocktail' of therapies individually chosen by patients themselves and tailored to their needs. For example good nutrition, food supplements, relaxation techniques, counselling, meditation, creative visualisation, art therapy, 'faith' healing and herbal treatments may be used in different combinations.

In the Bristol Programme it is not suggested that there is any single preferred way of treating a person with cancer which will work for anyone else. The Centre is presently taking part in research in an attempt to evaluate the effectiveness of its approach compared with conventional methods. The Bristol team is currently making regular visits to Professor Sikora's Unit at Hammersmith Hospital, working out how therapies such as healing and meditation can be combined with conventional medicine (Kent, 1989). Results so far have put a question mark over the effectiveness of the Programme in terms of life expectancy and further research is required to assess its' value.

Anthroposophical medicine

Anthroposophy, a system devised by the Swiss philosopher Rudolf Steiner, is an approach to living which emphasises the need of every individual to express creativity, something which is not always acknowledged in the rush of modern life. A particular kind of dance therapy known as eurhythmy and a type of artistic expression called veil painting are two examples of Steiner's approach to creative release. Steiner saw modern man as being beset by many fears. The fear of cancer is very commonplace and may be exacerbated by conventional approaches to prevention. For instance, campaigns for changes to life-style which appeal to fear, and even screening programmes aimed at making healthy people more aware of pre-cancerous conditions would be counter-productive according to Steiner. He perceived cancer as being a 'cold' disease linked to his idea that fear makes us feel cold The opposites of fear are excitement, enthusiasm and zest for living which Steiner thought of as warming. A specific anthroposophical remedy for cancer is Iscador, prepared from varieties of mistletoe and having 'warming' or stimulating properties. It is of interest too that mistletoe, like cancer, is a parasite which grows on its host.

Complementary Therapies compatible with nursing

A second group of therapies are those which are either being practised by nurses or which could be easily compatible with nursing care. Nurses know that much can be communicated and shared in the simplest of bodily ministrations. The intimacy which can develop between two people when one of them is incapacitated by illness and the other is attempting to meet their needs is rarely achieved in other kinds of relationships. Within the high levels of security that patients experience when being blanket bathed or when having a painful dressing changed, searching questions can be asked and the deepest fears can be shared. Campbell (1987) describes this kind of nurse/patient relationship as 'graceful care' which is not about 'anxious people trying to earn love, but about sensitive people who release us from bonds of our own making in spontaneous and often surprising ways'. I suggest that the use of touch may be described like this.

Touch

Touch is described by Le May (1986) as being 'the earliest and most primitive form of communication'. The process of attachment in early life emphasises the signifi-cance of touch for healthy development. It is suggested by some that the need for this kind of human contact continues throughout life. Morris (1973) goes so far as to suggest that all individuals require a regular quota of body contact, the 'body quotient', to stay healthy. Barnett (1972) and others hold the view that becoming a patient may result in a greater need for touch.

Therapeutic Touch

This is a term first used by Krieger in 1975, and is described as an act of healing or helping which can be likened to the laying on of hands used in faith healing. The process of therapeutic touch has also been described as a 'healing meditation' and refers to the healer as being in a state of consciousness which is quiet and focused on the patient. The healer's hands 'listen' to the patient as they scan the body, tuning in to areas of accumulated tension and redirecting energies experienced there. Krieger believes that the energy is closely linked to the concept of 'prana' in Sanskrit literature, which is often translated as vigour or vitality. Eastern literature says that prana derives from the sun. Krieger points out that this idea is not at variance with modern thinking about the crucial chemical basis of life: photons coming from the sun are the driving force for the primary synthesis of organic matter. Krieger was also influenced by the work of Martha Rogers (1980) whose model of Unitary Man contains the assumption that man is an open system in continual interaction with his environment.

Research by Krieger (1986) on the use of therapeutic touch as a means of altering haemoglobin levels, showed statistical support for the hypothesis that following treatment by therapeutic touch, mean haemoglobin values in patients in an experi-mental group would change significantly from pre-test levels. There would be no such significant changes of level in a control group. Her further research on therapeutic touch performed by husbands during their wives labour showed that labour was shorter and deliveries were less complicated. Other research cited by Krieger suggests that therapeutic touch was also effective in relieving chronic pain.

Krieger has been practising and teaching nurses therapeutic touch for over 15 years. Writing about this learning experience, Quinn (1984) describes the changes that took place within her as a manifestation of the 'principle of sychrony'. This states that 'Change in the human field depends only upon the state of the human field and the simultaneous state of the environmental field, at any given point in space-time'. This means that if healers are completely centered and open to the universal energy then they are left feeling quiet, peaceful and energised themselves. If, however, they are not open to the environment, much of the energy given to the patient is their own and they can be left feeling tired, sad and ineffectual I think most of us have been left like this on occasions where we have reached out to someone in a crisis and have ended up feeling drained, just as if we had given away our energy. It is therefore of great importance that the healer acts as a transmitter of energy rather than a generator. This point has been reiterated by the healer Matthew Manning who emphasises that he does not feel exhausted and depleted when he tries to heal someone. Therapeutic touch is therefore a useful kind of healing that can be practiced by nurses: it does not apparently require a belief in spiritual healing and may properly be explained eventually in some orthodox scientific way.

(See also chapter 6, p. 256.)

Massage

Massage has taken place ever since earliest times when cave dwellers rubbed their bruises! The systematic use of massage appears to have originated in China, and French translations of Chinese texts on the subject appeared about 100 years ago. Because of this much of the terminology used in massage is French.

Massage is a very effective means of communicating. It provides physical contact in a very acceptable way which can be particularly valuable for those who receive little human touch. Massage can be a way of conveying acceptance to patients whose body image has been altered by cancer. To be touched in a gentle and unembarassed way can be very comforting and is also a good way of getting to know someone well by developing a relationship based on honesty and trust. While doing this there needs to be awareness, however, of personal differences in both the need for touch and acceptance of touch. Those with defences against the intimacy of touch may more easily accept it in the form of massage because its purpose is unambiguous and premeditated. Victor Brewer, a patient with advanced cancer, is quoted by Pembrey (1989) as describing the effect of massage as, 'You unwind with the gentleness of the human touch. It would be marvellous if nurses could do it in hospital . . . With massage, as soon as the hands go on, you know she's there, she's calm, she has time for you . . . It helps you think positive.' Sims (1988) carried out a small study on the effects of slow stroke back massage on the perceived well-being of patients with breast cancer. Overall these patients reported less symptom distress and higher degrees of tranquillity and vitality than the control group.

Nevertheless, massage is not a panacea and must be used with caution on patients with cancer. It has been suggested that massage may promote tumour extension and metastases (Knapp, 1971). Therefore the nurse must be careful to ensure that no disease is present at the site which is to be massaged and gentle touch must always be used. The feet are a safe place to massage. Inherent in this notion of sharing and safety is the need for nurses to be willing to break down psychological barriers between themselves and the patient. This may not always be easy to achieve. The use of massage emphasises the need for people within the caring professional role to develop their own self-awareness and personalised relationships with the people for whom they are caring.

Aromatherapy

The art and science of using essential plant oils in massage treatments or as inhalations can be used alone or to complement other therapies or orthodox medical treatments. Aromatherapy claims to be a truly holistic therapy taking into account the life-styles of individuals as well as mind, body, spirit, eating patterns and relationships.

The history of the use of aromatic oil on the body goes back at least to 2000 years before Christ, and is, of course, frequently mentioned in the Bible both as treatment for illness and for religious uses. The earliest use recorded in England was apparently in the 13th century. Culpepper's herbal published in 1652 mentions the aromatic properties of many plants. Although aromatherapy is usually applied through massaging oils into the skin, the oils can also be absorbed by inhalation. Patients can use oils themselves by rubbing them into the skin or by putting them in bath water. The oil extracts are usually referred to as 'essential' oils and are pure concentrated essences of plants, flowers, trees, fruits and herbs. They are considered to act not only on the body by stimulating organs and physiological processes, but also by affecting the mind by stimulation or calming and sedating. They are also said to restore the balance of vital energies. Passant (1990), describing a holistic approach to the care of the elderly, mentions how the need for conventional sedatives could be reduced when essential oils were used on a ward. A bath containing essential oils followed by massage and a few drops of oil on the patient's pillow often induced deep and peaceful sleep. Using the oils intuitively, Passant found that lavender and rose geranium were helpful to patients with dementia, cedarwood helped mood swings and chest problems, cardamom helped failing memory and lavender was useful for headaches and muscular pain. Passant also used a garlic ointment for patients with persistent skin problems; results were so good that they eventually convinced the Consultant of its effectiveness.

Knowledge and care are needed in using aromatherapy, in the same way required of all herbal preparations given by mouth, because it is not always realised that these substances can be potent. Mixtures of different oils also need to be carefully made up for the individual, under supervision, in order for prospective practitioners to prescribe remedies safely. Many nurses appear to be taking advantage of the growing number of courses in massage and/or aromatherapy which are available and are incorporating these skills into their nursing care.

Visualisation

Visualisation techniques to help fight cancer are associated with the work of Carl and Stephanie Simonton and are based on work by Silva (1978). The underlying idea is that the patient should conjure up a picture in his or her mind of his or her body being able to heal and take care of itself. Patients who are interested in this approach are helped to visualise their cancer in whatever terms seem meaningful to them; they may be encouraged to draw pictures to help them focus on it. They then need to explore ways in which they can visualise their immune system fighting the cancer, and winning. Brohn (1987) makes the important point that the cancer must be represented by something that is weaker than the immune system. The aim is to imagine a strong powerful force which is battling against a very feeble and weak opponent. It is also very helpful and positive for patients to imagine themselves being well in the future, which may mean beginning by remembering themselves well in the past.

Visualisations give a feeling of control back to the patient with cancer: they are a positive therapy which can counteract the negativity which surrounds the disease itself. It seems feasible that nurses could be involved in assisting patients who are interested in using visualisations, since the technique is easy and quick to learn.

Biofeedback

This is a way of learning how to control body states which are not normally considered to be under the control of the mind. In biofeedback training, the individual is attached to a device which feeds back to him or her information on his or her physiological processes. By watching some kind of visual display, or hearing a signal the patient is able to use the alterations which the body makes in response to his or her thought processes. This gives a very positive experience of being in control and has been shown to be an effective way of relaxing and affecting the body's immune system. Stress monitors are an example of this technique by anyone at any time, without professional help. Biofeedback can also be combined with meditation techniques to induce deep relaxation or control of the immune response.

Relaxation

Body and mind need regular deep relaxation. Watching television or dozing may not be sufficient to reduce habituated tension which may continue unconsciously.

Patients, carers and nurses themselves will benefit from regular relaxation for perhaps 30 minutes each day. Techniques to achieve deep relaxation can be learned quickly in classes or from tapes. Simple biofeedback machines can help enormously in learning relaxation. Deep relaxation is a *skill* that nurses can easily pass on to their patients.

(See also chapter 16, p. 260–1.)

Meditation

Everyone has the ability to meditate but Western culture, with its concern for busyness and *doing*, seems to militate against this practice. Meditation techniques help the individual towards an inner state of peace by changing their customary thought patterns. Thoughts are allowed to drift into mind and then are released or 'thrown away'. Eventually calm and peacefulness replaces our customary busy 'mind chatter'. 'Scripts' for meditation can be found in Bond (1986). Meditation has been shown to have beneficial effects, including lowered blood pressure and slower pulse rates.

Music therapy

Music has been used as a way of expressing emotion and for therapeutic purposes throughout history. Over 500 years BC Pythagoras put forward the theory that music could be used in daily life to make a significant contribution to health. Many dentists now use music as a way of promoting relaxation and controlling pain.

Music can be used as a means of social exchange through singing or playing instruments. Music appreciation can include listening to live or recorded music on one's own or with others; listening may be followed by discussion about the kinds of feeling that particular music evokes in the individual or about how music can express spirituality.

When using music in patient care the likes and dislikes of individuals need to be discussed and time should be set aside for discussion when listening sessions are completed. Music should probably be considered together with other means of meeting patients needs for creative expression like art, literature and poetry, all of which are essentials in palliative care.

Other complementary therapies

Osteopathy and chiropractic

These are two different kinds of manipulative technique without which no review of complementary therapies could be complete, even though their function in the treatment of cancer is smaller than the others discussed so far. Many people involved in orthodox medicine such as physiotherapists, doctors and sometimes nurses, also practice manipulation.

Osteopathy was founded by Dr Still in the 1890s and, allegedly, a patient of his called Daniel Palmer went off to found the rival system of Chiropractic. A great attraction of osteopathy is that it is possible for patients to feel almost instantaneous relief from it. Osteopathy works by isolating the precise point in the spine or joint which is causing trouble and treating it with manipulation or massage, always using the minimum of force necessary. Many osteopaths use X-rays to aid diagnosis. Their view is that any musculo-skeletal abnormality can cause symptoms even when there appears to be no evidence of disease as such. Osteopaths may give general advice with particular reference to posture and methods of relaxation.

Chiropractic was established by Daniel Palmer in America. Unlike osteopathy which deals with all joints, chiropractic deals only with the spine. It is said that Palmer made his discoveries about the importance of misaligned vertebrae following his dealing with a miner who had suddenly gone deaf. Palmer thought that working in cramped condition for long periods might somehow have contributed to the man's condition and discovered that one of the patient's vertebrae was badly displaced. On manipulating it to the correct position, the man's hearing was restored. The whole system of chiropractic is based on the possibility that any misalignments of the vertebrae can produce an almost limitless array of symptoms in any part of the body. For instance, digestive disturbances might be cured by manipulating the appropriate vertebra.

Radionics

This very ancient approach to healing utilises a tool such as a pendulum or dowsing rod to detect illness. The assumption is made that all forms of life share an electro-magnetic field, and so the rod or pendulum can be used to diagnose diseases and to answer questions made by the conscious mind. I well remember a lady who would never take any prescribed medicine until she had swung her pendulum over it. If the response was positive she would take the drug and if negative she would not. Radionics is said to be useful in the early detection of illness. Pendulum responses may reveal disorder well before any overt symptoms appear.

Reflexology

Reflexology is another form of Chinese medicine concerned with massage of the feet. Each part of the foot is said to correspond to a part of the body, so that tenderness or discomfort of the foot will reflect problems in other parts of the patient. It can be used to aid diagnosis and also to treat conditions by massage and acupressure (Shiatsu) to the feet.

Faith healing

Practitioners of faith healing tell us that this term is a misnomer. It implies that the individual needs faith in order to be healed. This is not so and no-one advocates any kind of penitence in order to earn the necessary amount of grace required for healing. However healers may well encourage self-awareness in those they treat. By the laying on of hands or by simply being near the patient, healers believe they become channels through which healing may take place. The source of the healing is outside of the healers themselves, coming from God or Universal Consciousness or by some other external power which is meaningful to the healer. The power or energy which is transmitted is often described by the recipient as 'heat' and has been explained by some in terms of energy fields, radiation or magnetism: others talk of extra-sensory perception. Whatever the explanation, all healers and recipients agree on its existence.

Healing may also take place from a distance. An optimum time for this phenomenon is when the patient is actually asleep. Healing has been described by Matthew Manning, the modern British healer, as 'reprogramming'. He gives, as an example, a patient who said 'If I live I have to confront my problems. If I die, I don't.' Manning feels that some of the people with cancer who turn to him have already decided to die. They may want release or to let go of life, but find that their families try to keep them surviving: then they may feel stressed and guilty. Healing, like medicine, is surrounded by much mystique. It does appear however to have much to offer people with cancer either as a cure or halting to the progress of the disease or else as a way of helping patients to feel peaceful and whole.

Nursing care and complementary therapies

Complementary therapies can be, perceived by nurses as fostering a more active therapeutic relationship between nurse and patient and so aiding the healing process. Healing may be defined either in terms of cure or of making real improvements to the quality of patients lives. Nurses' use of complementary therapies may help both patient and nurse to fill in some of the gaps left by orthodox medicine. It is important to notice however that, although I believe that the current enthusiasm for these ideas should be encouraged, issues such as appropriate insurance, adequate preparation and training to perform the therapy and how it can be incorporated into nursing care need careful consideration. Research is important too: results must be evaluated by nurses and other members of the health care team in order to justify the use of these methods. Perhaps the last point to make however is that when nurses are responding to the wishes of their patients in using complementary therapies, they may be doing a great deal to assist orthodox medicine. The use of complementary therapies may well mean that patients are being offered the best of both worlds by receiving care that is truly holistic.

References

BARNETT, K. (1972). A survey of the current utilisation of touch by health team personnel with hospitalised patients. *International Journal of Nursing Studies*, **3**, 195–209.

BOND, MEG (1986). *Stress and Self-Awareness: a Guide for Nurses.* Heinemann, London.
BROHN, P. (1987). *The Bristol Programme.* Century Hutchinson, London.
CAMPBELL, A. (1987). *Moderated Love: a Theology of Professional Care.* SPCK, London.
KENT, A, (1989). Mind and body care. *The Times*, 11.5.89.
KNAPP, M. (1971). In *Handbook of Physical Medicine and Rehabilitation*, F. Knusen (Ed.) W. B. Saunders, London.
KRIEGER, D. (1986). *The Therapeutic Touch: How to use your hands to help or to heal.* Prentice Hall Press, New York.
LE MAY, A. (1986). The human connection. *Nursing times*, **82**, 49, 56–7.
MANNING, M. (1989). *Guide to Self-Healing.* Thorsons, Wellingborough, Northants.
MORRIS, D. (1973). *Intimate Behaviour.* Bantam Books, London.
PASSANT, H. (1990). The holistic approach in the ward. *Nursing Times*, **86(4)**, 24–6.
PEMBREY, S. (1989). The development of nursing practice: a new contribution. *Senior Nurse*, **9**, 8.
QUINN, J. (1984). Therapeutic touch as energy exchange. *Advances in Nursing Science*, 46–8.
ROGERS, M. (1980). Nursing – a science of unitary man. In *Conceptual Models for Nursing Practice*, V. P. Riehl and C. Roy (Eds). Appleton Century Crofts, New York.
SAGAR, E. (1990). Therapeutic touch – a healing meditation. *Nursing Practice*, **3**, 2.
SILVA, J. & MIELE. P. (1978). *The Silva Mind Control Method.* Souvenir Press Ltd, London.
SIMS, S. (1988). The significance of touch in palliative care. *Palliative Medicine*, **2**, 58–61.
WHITEHORN, K. (1983). Your life in their hands. *Observer Review*, Nov. 13.

Further reading

AUTTON, N. (1989). *Touch: An Exploration.* Darton, Longman and Todd, London.
BAUM, M. (1983). Quack cancer cures or scientific remedies. *Clinical Oncology*, **3**, 275–80.
CHAITLOW, L. (1983). *Relaxation and Meditation Techniques.* Thorsons, Wellingborough.
COWARD, R. (1989). *The Whole Truth: The Myth of Alternative Health.* Faber and Faber, London.
FULDER, S. (1988). *Handbook of Complementary Medicine.* Oxford University Press, London.
FULDER, S. AND MUNRO, R. (1981). *The State of Complementary Medicine.* The Threshold Foundation, London.
KRIEGER, S. (1981). *The Renaissance Nurse: Foundations of Holistic Health Practices.* J. B. Lippincott, Philadelphia.

PENSON, J. AND HOLLOWAY, I. (1989). Fringe benefits: alternative medicine in patient care. *Senior Nurse*, **9**, 8.
PRICE, S. (1987). *Practical Aromatherapy*. Thorsons, Wellingborough.
SIMONTON, O. C. (1984). *The Healing Family*. Bantam Books, London.
TAPPAN, F. (1988). *Healing Massage Techniques: Holistic, Classic and Emerging Methods*. Appleton and Lange, Connecticut.

Journals

Attitudes
Holistic Medicine
Journal of Alternative and Complementary Medicine
Kindred Spirit

8

The care of the patient near the end of life

Ann Newbury

'I shall live a year, barely longer. During that year let as much as possible be done'.
Joan of Arc

Very many people with a progressive malignant illness have a year or much less to live. During this period realistic advice, attention and support can make a vast difference to the remaining life. Today there is increasing professional interest and concern for these people. However, on discovering that the disease is progressive and curative procedures are no longer appropriate, it is all too easy for the patients and their families to embark on an awesome, lonely venture full of apprehension, threats and fears. Facing death is probably the most profound experience any one of us will ever have to cope with and, it is said, emotions aroused by it are legion (Hinton, 1967).

When considering the holistic care of the patient with a limited life span, he or she must be viewed as a member of a wider circle of family and friends within the cultural and environmental setting. Therefore when planning and delivering care the needs of the whole family must be considered (see Fig. 8.1).

Every patient with cancer has the right to appropriate care by experienced nurses whether at home, in palliative care units or hospital. In the case of the patient who will ultimately die, it is especially important that the professional carer supports the

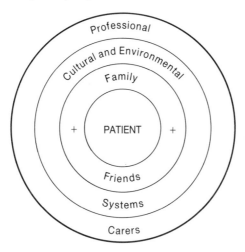

Fig. 8.1 Total care of the patient which includes care of the family and friends within their own cultural and environmental circle.

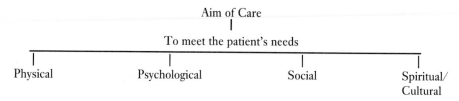

Fig. 8.2   The aim of care.

family and friends also, for it is often the latter who are left caring for the patient 24 hours a day.

The goal of care is to help the person to 'continue life as usual, work, being with the family, doing what is especially significant before life comes to a close, and feeling a part of ongoing life' (Craven and Wald, 1975). Hopefully this will give a sense of achievement and fulfilment.

When the cure role is changed to a comfort and care role, it is important that the quality of the person's life is improved and that that improvement is maintained for as long as possible by monitoring and controlling symptoms, and by building a stable relationship so offering support to both the patient and their family. Ultimately the patient must be able to experience a dignified, peaceful death which is free from distressing symptoms and, hopefully, in the company of those he or she loves and certainly not in isolation.

Every nurse has many responsibilities in respect to providing for, or facilitating the general well being of the patient. Besides ensuring adequate general care the patient near to, or at the end of life may have specific needs, which must be met, whether the duration of the illness is days, weeks or months. Wherever these patients are cared for they will have similar needs throughout the illness, and if nurses are to be efficient in their caring role there must be a full understanding of these needs. Not only should the nurse understand the total care required and the needs of the patient, but also the role of relatives and friends and the care which they may require, and the role of the nurse and the nurse's needs.

The total care and needs of the patient

Many patients with incurable cancer are not confined to bed until the last stages of the illness and, then, more indepth nursing care may be required. Initially they may be comparatively well and able to enjoy a fairly normal life. The aim of care must always be to provide for the patient's total needs (Fig. 8.2).

Physical care and needs of the patient

Relief of pain
Pain due to malignancy is usually chronic in nature with a tendency to get worse if uncontrolled. It serves no useful purpose as it does not warn of, or protect from danger. Twycross (1975) observes that chronic pain 'frequently expands to occupy the patient's whole attention, isolating him from the world around'. Fear, anxiety

and unrelieved physical symptoms may intensify the patient's perception of pain. Pain is a dual phenomenon, involving perception of the sensation, and the patient's emotional reaction to it (Saunders, 1978). Therefore it is necessary to treat the 'whole pain' and understand the need to alleviate other problems. Poor pain relief is often caused by inadequate or irregular medication. Administration of analgesia for chronic pain must be regular and the doctor will adjust the dose according to the patient's level of pain, slowly increasing the dose until the patient is painfree; the principle being to give the next dose of analgesia before the previous one wears off. (See Chapter 3 for further discussion of the analgesic staircase.) It is often difficult to help the patient and the family to appreciate this principle when the pain has been relieved, and sometimes the patient has to prove the point for themselves by delaying the next dose.

More than one drug may be used and some non-drug therapies such as transcutaneous nerve stimulation may be employed (see Chapter 3). Psychological dependance to opiates does not appear to be a problem in these patients (Regnard *et al.*, 1983). The patient who is given irregular, insufficient medication may crave more for relief, but it has proved possible to reduce, and even discontinue opiates when pain is no longer present. Fear of dependancy is more of a concern to the professional carer than the patient. All too often opiates are seen as only to be given at the very end of life and the full potential of use is never realised.

Controlled pain will usually eliminate the fear of pain allowing the patient to get on once more with living. The aim of pain control 'is to relieve the pain without compromising the consciousness' (Alderman, 1988). A patient's pain threshold will vary according to mood and morale (Corr and Corr, 1983). Therefore every effort must be made to raise the pain threshold.

Raising the pain threshold
The professional carer can assist in raising the pain threshold to improve relief by ensuring the following.

- The medication regime is understood and adhered to
- Other symptoms are reported and controlled
- The patient has a good night's sleep and adequate rest
- Understanding to relieve fear and anxiety
- Prevention of isolation and loneliness
- That opportunity is given for expression using listening and counselling skills
- Relief of boredom
- Comfort by application of heat and use of special equipment as required

Other common symptoms
There are other physical symptoms which may need to be controlled and the nurse can assist in this control. The symptoms mentioned below are some of the more common ones which may be experienced by patients with a progressive malignant illness, however many other symptoms are discussed in detail in Chapter 4 and other works (Twycross and Lack, 1990).

Nausea and vomiting
Regnard *et al.* (1983) point out that 'the vomiting centre in the medulla can be stimulated in several ways'. Treatment depends on the cause. Predisposing factors

should be eliminated in addition to the use of antiemetic drugs are prescribed by the doctor. The nurses role should be to control nauseous odours, prevent unpleasant sights, eliminate constipation, ensure pain control and to see that an appropriate diet is provided. If diet is not tolerated soda water or iced water may be helpful to minimise dehydration. The patient will need reassurance as these symptoms are very distressing and exhausting especially in the latter stages of illness, when he or she may already be very weak and anxious.

Constipation

This distressing symptom, unless monitored and carefully controlled, may cause other problems such as nausea, anorexia, and abdominal discomfort.

As the patient's condition deteriorates and he or she becomes weaker and less mobile, the risk of constipation can increase. It is aggravated by poor dietary and fluid intake which frequently occurs with the progression of the illness. Increased analgesic therapy, which must not be denied to ensure the patient's comfort, may slow down the motility of the gut. The nurses role is to ensure the appropriate use of aperients, provide a suitable diet and to encourage an increased fluid intake if the patient is able to tolerate it.

If simple measures do not control constipation then it may be necessary to resort to suppositories or enemas. If these are required great care must be taken to minimise exhaustion and discomfort to an already weakened patient. Dignity must be preserved at all times.

Anorexia

This is a frequent symptom and patients unable to eat adequately as their disease progresses may become fearful, because the inability to eat may be viewed as a threat to life. Antiemetic therapy should be given as prescribed. This is very significant when the fear of vomiting still lingers, having been the original cause of anorexia. Fear may precipitate vomiting. Carers should do all in their power to encourage the maximum enjoyment of food, but as the person becomes more ill food often becomes less important to them. This is natural.

A calm positive attitude is helpful but the patient should never be forced, and should be allowed to take as much time as required over meals. Unwanted food should be removed quickly without critical comment.

Meals should be served attractively. Small frequent meals or snacks will be greatly appreciated especially when the patient experiences gastric fullness.

Other symptoms such as pain and nausea must be controlled. Unpleasant odours should be eliminated and it is helpful if offensive wounds are attended to at least half an hour before meals to allow the patient to settle down, promote comfort and prevent embarrassment. The use of charcoal type dressings help. An alcoholic aperitif may stimulate the appetite. In the earlier stages of illness the doctor may prescribe a trial of appetite stimulant, but as the person becomes more ill this is less appropriate.

The person whose general health is deteriorating is susceptible to mouth infections and ulcers making it painful to eat. If present they should be treated appropriately. It is also significant that with loss of weight dentures may become ill fitting and cause eating to be difficult. (See also Mouth problems, below.)

If the patient's desire for food lessens it may be beneficial to substitute one or more meals with a high calorie drink. Several are available. Reasonable fluid intake will prevent the distress of dehydration and, even when the patient is very ill, frequent sips of fluid will prevent thirst. The nurse has to be vigilant as the patient may be too ill to help themself.

The family may need help to undersand and accept the patient not eating, as it may be seen as a failure on their part, or a giving up on the patient's side. Sometimes relatives feel that a patient should be fed at all costs – 'the eat to survive syndrome'. They may even inappropriately request intravenous feeding.

Insomnia

Sedation is not necessarily the answer to insomnia. Pain, nausea and other physical symptoms need to be controlled or else wakeful, restless periods will occur. When the person is near to the end of life they may be afraid to go to sleep in case they do not waken up, they may also become anxious and fearful in the night. The greatest need then is probably for a cup of tea and the opportunity to voice his or her fears to an understanding listener who will not brush aside the anxieties, making light of the process of dying and just offer more sedation. Night nurses have an important role to play.

Sleep disturbance may also indicate depression but this has to be recognised and differentiated from the normal understandable sadness of the dying person.

Mouth problems

In the last few weeks of life, as the patient becomes weaker, they are prone to develop sore mouths and regular oral toilet should be routine. Condition of the teeth may have deteriorated or dentures become ill fitting so a visit to, or from, the dentist may be beneficial, even though the person may not have long to live – quality is important. Mouth infections commonly occur in debilitated people because they have little reserve to fight the infection. Therefore infections must be treated. Mediction in orobase, soothing gels or medicated pellets can give relief if ulcers are present.

Dry mouths can also be troublesome and may aggravate anorexia. Dryness can be indicative of dehydration, infection, mouth breathing or may be related to medication. Frequent mouth washes, mouth care and attention to diet will help to minimise problems. Sucking boiled sweets, citrus fruit slices or pineapple chunks can be refreshing. Artificial saliva, special lozenges, frequent drinks, crushed ice or frozen tonic water cubes to suck may help. Medication may need to be reviewed with the doctor.

Pressure area care

Care of the skin is essential, because patients with a cancerous condition, nearing the end of life often become very debilitated, and their skin may be friable from corticosteroid therapy. There may be marked loss of weight, cachexia and immobility. It is crucial that the skin is kept clean and most patients appreciate a daily bath or shower, even when they become very frail. Regular massaging of pressure areas is comforting and aids circulation. The use of special mattresses, sheepskins, alternating air beds, and water beds all play a part in protecting pressure areas and should be used as a preventative measure for 'at risk' patients. Patients should be encouraged to change position at regular intervals. As they become more immobile and perhaps confined to bed, it is the nurse's responsibility to turn the patient regularly and treat pressure areas to minimise damage.

Weakness

In the last weeks and days of life weakness may become one of the most frustrating symptoms. The mind is often willing and active but the body is too exhausted to respond to the demands made upon it. Uncontrolled symptoms will slowly weaken and distress the person, so effective symptom control is of paramount importance, and the nurse must act as the patient's advocate as necessary.

There is a place for the realistic, caring physiotherapist who may be able to assist in making the patient feel stronger, become more mobile, and teach ways of doing things to preserve energy. Some patients, even in the last weeks of life, may benefit from hydrotherapy because water gives buoyancy, is relaxing and enables easier movement. Rehabilitation is ongoing and involes the person understanding their disability, regaining confidence and incentive to do what they are able for as long as they can. They are encouraged not to be left out or forgotten. The person needs to be taught to reserve energy for the things they wish to do, and not waste it on unimportant things. Alternating periods of rest with activity helps the person to live within their limitations. As they become more weak and ill the periods of rest usually need to lengthen and activity lessens, which is yet another sad reminder that they are not getting better.

When uncontrolled symptoms are severe the patient may wish to die but as they become controlled, even though the patient may be very ill, the desire to go on living is often revived. It is important to control symptoms so that the patient can invest the energy they may have in living until they die.

Psychological care and needs

Caring for people who are near to the end of life extends beyond physical care to supporting them emotionally as they adjust to an increasing physical weakness, and cope with grief. There must be a bond of honest trust between the patient and all carers by respecting privacy, showing concern and empathy. Cancer is an emotive word and can conjure up many fears and anxieties in the mind, especially when the patient becomes aware that curative procedures are exhausted. Having perhaps completed surgery, radiotherapy or chemotherapy, they may well feel 'no more can be done', which of course may be applied to 'cure' but never to 'care'. This can leave the patient feeling anxious, frightened and disillusioned, convinced they will suffer pain or perhaps die at any moment. Realistic hope must be restored and although cure is no longer an option, the patient must be assured that help is available and every effort will be made to control the situation, making the remainder of life worthwhile and meaningful. They also need to understand and be reassured that all forms of palliative care will be employed where appropriate, for example radio-therapy for some types of bone pain.

It may be at this point that the person considers complementary therapies (see Chapter 7). Alternative methods of treatment may 'enrich our interventions and bring comfort and better health to patients with cancer' (Dobbs, 1985).

A kaleidescope of negative and potentially destructive emotions might be experienced (Fig. 8.3). Patients may well need to express any of the feelings indicated in Fig. 8.3 should they experience them, and should be given the opportunity to work through them. It is important to take the cue from the patient as to when, and how much, they wish to discuss at a time. For the carer to impose upon the patient their

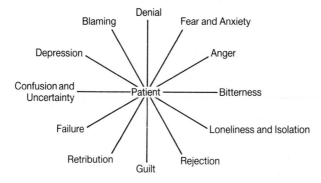

Fig. 8.3   Explosion of emotions which may occur in the cancer patient with a limited life span.

own interpretation of the patient's need to talk is presumptive, and may be quite the wrong timing. Some people ask, want to know and be totally involved in all decision making, whereas others know but are not prepared to discuss the matter further and may not even be willing to make decisions. However, 'not everyone wants to know' (Hinton, 1967). Some people live in a make-believe world where all is well, never acknowledging to themselves, let alone others, that they may be very ill. Professional carers have no right to forcibly break down a person's denial defence mechanism. This could be detrimental as denial may be the patient's way of dealing with the situation for the moment, until more positive coping strategies can be mustered. The decision must be the patient's as to when he or she is ready to abandon denial. There are gentle ways of imparting the truth – it is not necessary to be blunt. Frequently, given opportunity, the patient will answer his or her own questions.

Unexpressed fear may cause great anxiety culminating in depression. There may be fear of pain, loneliness and meaninglessness (Chaney, 1976). Uncertainty, inability to cope with the process of the illness and fear of lack of help from medical and nursing staff may all give rise to added anxiety. Patients need to be able to voice their fears, and work through their emotions with an understanding, empathetic person who is able to answer their questions, hopefully giving support, reassurance and encouragement. Everyone needs to be able to give and receive love (Summers and Young).

Each person needs to 'live' until they die, and wherever they are cared for this should be the nurse's prime consideration. The person must be helped to forget the things they cannot do and learn to set goals for themselves, so there may be a sense of achievement. The goals must be the patient's and not the nurse's. Encouragement to do the normal things of life, even dressing in day clothes when most of the day is spent resting, will improve the morale.

Gill was a young woman who struggled valiantly to make up her face each day for her husband and young children. When she was becoming too weak to manage this she taught her husband what to do. He continued to do this for her until she died so retaining normality, and for Gill, dignity.

Ben was an independent, middle aged gentleman who, for a long time, declined to attend the day centre. Eventually he came and began to develop latent talents. He continued to attend even after admission to the unit. He became very weak and ill but, late the afternoon before he died, he busily beavered away at making a plate for his wife. He worked into the early evening and saw it put into the kiln saying 'please give it to my wife'. He died that night but left this 'love gift' for his partner, which she cherishes. It can be said of Ben 'he lived until he died' and was in control of the situation throughout, even though it took great effort and courage.

In providing psychological care nurses' aims should be to use their listening, communication and counselling skills to support, encourage and give incentive to the patient hopefully helping them to feel fulfilled. Communication and counselling skills are discussed further in Chapter 14 and 15 respectively.

Social care and needs

Social needs must be met so that the patient can remain as independent as possible, for as long as possible, preferably within their normal social setting. Fulfilment of social needs enhances safety and security and is an intrinsic part of total care.

In the early part of the illness it is hoped that the person will continue normal employment, but as the illness progresses and this is no longer possible replacement by some form of occupational therapy may be helpful if, and for as long as, the person wishes it. This will often bridge the gap between employment and illness. Occupation within the patient's capability, even when frail or in hospital, helps to prevent boredom and withdrawal. It minimises feelings of uselessness and helplessness.

Each person needs to feel socially acceptable, of use to others, and that opinions and company are important. Life style and identity need to be maintained, and recognition of social status within the home and every other area of life, such as being a father, mother, chairman, business woman, sportsman, seamstress. Independence should be encouraged for as long as possible. It is often very hard to admit to needing help. As the patient becomes weaker practical help may be necessary to aid daily living, especially within the home.

The ill person may experience financial embarrassment if they can no longer be the breadwinner, or perhaps it is the working wife whose financial contribution to the home has been essential. The professional health carer can direct them to the appropriate Social Services department who can advise and help, possibly assisting in the application of allowances and grants.

Praising anything the person attempts or achieves will make them feel good and boost self esteem. Investing in a new wardrobe of clothes when they have lost weight markedly will improve body image and self worth – it is worthwhile even when time is limited.

When a patient is admitted to a palliative care unit or hospital the nurse may need to adopt a preventative role to protect the patient from personal problems. One such problem is 'role stripping' (Smith, 1981) when the 'person' becomes a 'patient'. The patient must always remain a person with their own identity and specific place in society. Wherever they are cared for the title to be used by staff should be agreed.

Not all patients are comfortable being called by their Christian name, equally so it could be alien to some to be addressed more formally. The patient should decide. The nurse can prevent role stripping by recognition of the individual, respecting views, likes and dislikes, allowing the patient to use their own clothing and to be up and dressed by day if they are able. Clothes are a symbol of personal identification. People are quickly dehumanised by diagnostic labelling such as the patient in bed 2 with carcinoma of the pancreas instead of Andrew Green who is still a person. It is the responsibility of the nurse to respond to the human being, who happens to be a patient, in such a way as to maintain their unique personality.

Social interaction is enhanced by early introduction to other patients, staff and volunteers, allowing freedom of choice as to with whom the patient wishes to communicate.

It is helpful if bed, ward and faces become familiar as quickly as possible and that the patient is encouraged to make his or her own space personal, perhaps by displaying a photograph or cards which have meaning for them as an individual.

Taking on the 'patient' role can be a form of escapism (Smith, 1981). This sometimes happens when the personal or social situation becomes hard to tolerate. Maintainance of social role can be aided by the nurse showing a genuine interest in family, friends, job and hobbies, so keeping the patient in touch with the outside world.

A 'dependancy syndrome' may develop (Smith, 1981). Sometimes this is imposed unintentionally by the carer out of genuine fear for the patient's safety, or the need to feel needed. Every effort should be made to allow as much independance as is safe, reasonable and desirable to the patient. Views need to be recognised, acknowledged and permission asked of the person rather than 'taking over' by the carer imposing his or her own will. This is very important as the patient becomes weaker. When a person is admitted to any form of residential care it involves the transfer of the patient's 'home' for that period of time and the staff become an extended family.

Day centres
Attendance at a centre can be helpful for the person with cancer even in the latter stages of the illness. Many palliative care units have a day centre attached to them. It can be a place for 'time out' from home or ward where people can be themselves, gain relief from boredom, loneliness, pursue hobbies and boost self esteem. It may give the patient an opportunity to talk away from family and friends at home, about the things that really concern them. They may not talk at home for fear of upsetting those they love. Attendance can be a means of developing latent talents, promoting social acceptance, interaction, and mealtimes can be regarded as eating out. Socialisation can be enhanced by provision of pre-lunch drinks as an appetiser, and then meals being eaten around a dining room table. Outings are a great asset as they help to ensure that patients remain a part of a wider society. Much satisfaction is derived from being able to help one another.

Day centres play an important role in providing social care for cancer patients whose illness is progressive, and respite care for relatives, but it must be remembered that they may not be beneficial for everyone.

Spiritual/Cultural care and needs

Spiritual care is the care, given to the patient, which is not tangible or material. It is the care of the innermost being which, generally, people feel is concerned with or affects the soul. Every person has a need to feel fulfilled and an opportunity to work out their own beliefs and confirm them for themselves. 'With the contemplation of death come thoughts of what life means; family, friends, work, talents, potentials, accomplishments, failures and beliefs about life after death' (Caughill, 1976). It may be a time when life is reviewed, re-evaluated and the things that matter often become very important. According to Corr and Corr (1983) everything gets doubly precious.

In multi-racial countries there are many religions and philosophies present. When caring for patients with a short while to live it is important to be aware of and acknowledge the needs of people of other cultures and customs, and to provide opportunity for them to fulfil these needs. (See also Chapter 12.)

Hope is a part of spiritual care, being revealed as a feeling that one's existence is in some way worthwhile and desirable, and which spurs on the will to live. (See also Chapter 11.)

Spiritual care involves the nurse in helping the patient to cope with disappointment, losses, uncertainty and allowing them to talk of the meaning of life after death, if they so wish. For some people religion can be of great support, particularly if they have a deep meaningful faith, but even people with an apparently unshakeable faith may question. Faith is not a guarantee against all the ills of life but, hopefully, will give support and meaning to the situation. Those with little or no faith may seek something deeper. It may be that the nurse caring for the very ill patient can offer help in the spiritual realm, but, if the nurse feels inadequate in this role there is a responsibility to employ the services of someone who is able to help.

Spiritual care and wellbeing is an important part of total care.

Throughout the illness the patients need to feel that they are coping and in full control of the situation, with symptoms controlled and needs met. It is important that they participate in decision making. During the weeks or months of illness many services may be involved, both hospital and community, hopefully enhancing life, encouraging the patient to live it fully and not to be just waiting for death. Each day is a bonus to be enjoyed. Relatives and friends can join with and be supported in the caring role by General Practitioners, doctors, community and hospital nurses, cancer care nurse specialists, Social Service workers and others. Equipment needs must be met urgently as the patient's requirement is now, not next week or next month. That may be too late to bring the extra comfort and opportunity to maintain as normal a life as possible. Sometimes during the course of their illness the person may need to be admitted for a period of assessment and stabilisation of symptoms, respite care, rehabilitation or more permanently for Tender Loving Care (TLC).

It is desirable and advantageous that every patient has an individualised care plan which identifies needs, problems, action taken and outcomes. Recording goals and achievements are also important. This plan should be regularly evaluated and updated.

Where should the patient be cared for in the last days of life

The patient may have been deteriorating almost imperceptibly over weeks or months but quite suddenly a change may occur and the actual process of dying is recognised. When this change occurs, and the forseeable end is in view, relatives caring for the patient at home, and the patient him or herself, may become very aware that plans need to be made accordingly. Hopefully there will have been some discussion between the patient, family and the caring professional team, and desires for future care will have been expressed and wishes be known. It may be that admission to a palliative care unit or hospital is requested or, alternatively, the patient and carers may wish to continue at home. Sometimes the patient who is actually in hospital may request to go home to die. It is all too easy to tell the patient that he, or she is too ill, and yet with the coordination of all services available, and laying on of adequate caring facilities at home, it may be possible to grant that last wish.

Caring at home

Certainly admission is not necessarily best unless physical and emotional needs cannot be met at home. Where possible it should be the patient's choice. At home 'the patient is in familiar surroundings and the family are left with a sense of having done their best' (Saunders, 1978). It may be a more peaceful, relaxed, informal atmosphere in which to be cared for with those the patient cares about around him or her, and it encourages family participation.

Patients being cared for at home require adequate provision of the following.

- **Time** Time for both patients and their families to express their fears, anxieties and difficulties. The nurses communication skills are a valuable asset here.

- **Personnel** Community nursing staff are of prime importance in offering time, professional skills and support. In many areas the community nurses may be supported in their role by a specialist nurse who is experienced in symptom control and the support of patients at home who have cancer. It is essential that all members of the caring team liaise closely with the patient's General Practitioner. Night nursing services and Marie Curie Foundation Services have an important contribution to make where they are available. Relief at night eases the pressure on relatives and ensures continuity of care.

- **Equipment** Availability of loans are essential to aid the provision of quality care. The patient may require material items such as mattress covers, commodes, wheelchairs, urinals, bedcradles, anti-pressure devices and feeding cups.

- **Comfort** Room temperature must be maintained so extra heating may be required. Grants may be available to help finance this need. Sometimes the provision of extra bedding will be necessary and some areas have a laundry service.

- **Resources** Caring for patients at home can make greater demands on available resources as more frequent visits may be required to ensure effective symptom control and care. Four hourly injections may be necessary however, in many areas, the need for regular intramuscular therapy has been largely eliminated with the advent of the 24-hour syringe driver (see Chapter 3, p. 33 for further information on syringe drivers).

Within the home it is especially important to ensure that drug therapy is readily available, with clear instructions and controlled drug records. As the patient's condition deteriorates and he or she is unable to take oral medication, a supply of subcutaneous or intramuscular analgesic drugs, such as Diamorphine, should be available in the home. It is also helpful to have a supply of antiemetics, and some form of sedation for use as necessary in suppository or injection form. Hyoscine may be helpful to minimise the 'death rattle'.

● **Professional carers**   The basis of good care at home is reliant on having an efficient, knowledgeable, empathetic team, who are communicating well and able to anticipate and so prevent problems. They must be able to work with and support the family.

Apart from the specific needs associated with home, of which community nurses are well aware, the care of the person at home, in a palliative care unit, or ward is very similar. 'If a dying person can have adequate care in his own home there is much to be said in favour of ending his days there' (Hinton, 1967).

Admission to palliative care unit or ward
Remaining at home may not be practical or possible for some patients. Reasons for admission include the following.

- Patient's request not to die at home
- Exhaustion of carers
- Lack of suitable accommodation
- Beyond the family and friends ability to carry on
- Lack of support
- Difficulty in controlling symptoms
- Fear of the unknown
- The need for 24 hour medical or nursing care

Timing for admission, if carefully planned, will allow the person an adequate period to settle in and become familiar with surroundings and staff. Leaving it too late may cause confusion and restlessness. The move must be seen as both acceptable and desirable to the patient and the family so as to minimise feelings of failure and guilt.

This may prove a difficult period for the patient who has inevitably had to face many losses associated with the illness. A rising proportion of people now die in some type of residential care and consequently have had to face the loss of their home, and now the prospect of losing life itself.

Admission – ward versus single room
Most nurses acknowledge that patients nursed in side wards may have increased psychological and physical needs, especially if they are afraid of being alone. Equally it may be a comfort and less distressing if relatives are able to remain with them – isolation should be avoided. It may be desirable to move a patient to a side room for medical reasons, or if the situation is particularly distressing. The patient or relatives sometimes request it for privacy. Moves should only be made after careful con-

sideration of the reason and implications. It is not necessarily in the best interests of the patient or those around them to remove them from familiar surroundings and companionship. For other patients it may conjure up an air of unease, suspicion and mystery if the person is suddenly removed, without explanation never to be heard of again. Most nurses have observed the fear of the person moved suddenly to a corner bed in a general ward, near the door or to a cubicle. The patient may recognise this is a final move and feel as though he or she is being shown the door before they are ready to leave. Sensitive explanation will avoid this and care must be taken to keep ward morale up, as other patients may fear this move for themselves. Fears of a distressing death may be eliminated by the observation of a quiet, peaceful death of the patient well supported by caring staff. It has been known for a patient to say 'If that is what death is like I am no longer afraid', and so a service to other patients may be done. However the repeated deaths of those with whom a relationship has been established may be demoralising and depressing, so a willingness on behalf of the nurse to spend time with remaining patients, encouraging them to express their feelings and fears in a positive way is appreciated.

It may be possible to provide a quieter, more peaceful atmosphere at home or in a palliative care unit rather than in a busy general ward.

The dying patient's needs

Loneliness can be a frightening experience, and may well be increased if people avoid the patient because they don't know what or how to say things. There is a need for companionship. Death is probably the loneliest experience for any of us (Twycross, 1975). Loneliness can be worse in a busy ward where the patient is surrounded by hustle and bustle, and they see others getting well but their own life is slipping away.

Dying patients often accept the approach of death but may need help to express themselves. The sensitive nurse can encourage them to talk and questions will often be of the type needing reassurance, such as when and how they will die. The nurse has a responsibility to face up to questions with quiet honest reassurance, but she may need help from a more experienced person if she feels inadequate. Denying death will only bring more distress (see Chapter 2).

Most experienced nurses can recognise when the patient is entering the final stage of the illness and is likely to die in the near future. Maintaining the comfort of the patient remains very important throughout.

Position

When patients become weaker and are unable to move their position, assistance will be greatly appreciated. Frequent gentle massage and change of position will relieve stiffness and discomfort and may ease restlessness. Many patients prefer to be propped up a little with the head well supported and dislike the supine position intensely.

Skin

Some people perspire profusely and feel cold to the touch as peripheral circulation fails. The skin often becomes discoloured and mottled. Gentle sponging is helpful, also regular care to pressure areas. The use of special mattress, sheepskins and alternating air beds will ease pressure.

Thirst
This may be a last craving and can be eased with frequent small sips of water or by allowing the patient to suck fluid from a sponge. Keeping the lips moist is essential and protection with lip salve or a little vaseline helps.

Mouths
Mouth care is essential to the end. The mouth should be kept moist; dry mouths soon become dirty mouths and, unless attended to, dirty mouths will become sore and infected. Dry mouths can often be eased by giving drinks which increase the flow of saliva, such as citrus fruits, or sucking pieces of ice or frozen tonic water.

Treatment to the mouth should be carried out as often as required. Dirty mouths can be cleaned with sodium bicarbonate or hydrogen peroxide solution. Teeth sholud be kept clean, whether false or not. Infections should be treated and, at this stage, Nystatin suspension is often the easiest to administer.

Restlessness
There may be many causes of restlessness in the dying patient and before resorting to sedation the elementary care of the patient should be checked. Most patients hate being imprisoned by the bedclothes being tucked in too tightly and they may become restless in order to rid themselves of their burden. A change of position may help. A full bladder will aggravate restlessness. Pain must be controlled. Patients are more restful if they have put their house in order and it may be that, even at this late stage, if they are capable, they need to make a will, or repair a broken relationship.

Eyes
Frequent bathing with normal saline will help, especially when a patient is sleeping deeply or is unconscious with eyes part opened. If the eyes become sore installation of 'artificial tears' may help.

Spiritual
The chaplain or clergyman's visit may be appreciated and bring comfort to both the patients and their families. The nurses' respect for the person does not permit them to impose their own faith or views upon the patient, but they may be able to bring comfort verbally or by unspoken presence and reassurance so helping the person to find peace of mind.

Support
When the patient deteriorates and becomes more ill, it may be that less time gets spent with him or her. On a busy general ward with other needs pressing, the entourage of doctore may pass by leaving the patient disillusioned. The visits of the doctor, however short, can be a great comfort to the person, as they realise they are still important and not forgotten.

At the end of life the dying person will often appreciate a family member or friend sitting with them. If this is not possible a nurse should fill this role. No patient should be left to die alone.

Medication
As the patient draws near to the end of life most medications can be discontinued with the exception of analgesia, antiemetics and some drugs made available for

specific individual problems. The latter are usually given on an as required basis.

Analgesia should never be abruptly discontinued, even when the patient appears deeply unconscious. Restlessness and marked distress can occur if pain is allowed to break through. At this stage the patient may not be able to communicate, so unknown suffering can be caused if analgesia is thoughtlessly withheld. It must be remembered that the patient may have been taking opiates for pain relief for many months.

During the last period of life it may be valuable to use a 24-hour syringe driver (Regnard and Newbury, 1983) to administer regular medications, so abolishing the need of four hourly injections to a person who is probably very thin and frail. Diamorphine hydrochloride is often used for injections as 'its high water solubility allows small volume injection' (Regnard *et al.*, 1983), which is an advantage. The use of the syringe driver entails multiplying the single injection dose by the number of times it is to be given in 24 hours, and administering that dose by the syringe driver over a 24 hour period.

'Death rattle'
This is when secretions collect in the throat and oscillate with respiration. The patient no longer has the strength to expectorate so a bubbling sound occurs. Hyoscine given by injection at the earliest detection may prevent this situation from developing. It may need to be repeated at regular intervals. If the 'death rattle' is marked, Hyoscine is unlikely to be effective because its action is to prevent secretions from forming. The patient generally appears oblivious of the situation but it is the relative who becomes distressed and needs explanation and reassurance. 'Cheyne Stoke' breathing may occur and again may be worrying to the family so should be explained.

Senses
It is a well known phenomena to put curtains around a bed and nurse the patient in a semi-darkened room. However most patients, when they are dying, have a fear of the dark and desire gentle light and fresh air. They have a need to experience quiet feelings of life around them. Throughout the final period of life there is a need for contact by touch and through hearing. If the patient lingers he or she may be aware who is with them although unable to communicate. Care must be taken in regard to what is said in the presence of the apparently unconscious person as hearing is one of the last senses to be lost.

At the point of death most people are unconscious and have been for some time. There are a small number who drift in and out of consciousness and, although weary, are usually peaceful, relaxed and seem accepting of the situation. Most people wish to die in their sleep.

Sedation may be necessary for the restless person when other causes have been excluded.

When death has occurred the relatives may appreciate a few quiet moments alone with the patient to pay their last respects. Simple prayers, said at the bedside after death, with the family if they so wish, may bring great comfort.

The role and care of relatives and friends

The very ill person cannot be helped really effectively if the family and friends are forgotten. Many events may cause stress in a family – every member interacts with each other so any problems will affect them all. Equally, the patient's response will be affected by the relatives and friends reaction to the illness. The average person encounters and copes with many stresses in a 'normal life' and it is worth remembering that most people do cope. In caring for the person who is near to the end of life, the family often draw on strengths they did not know they possessed. A very stressful time for the family is being told of a diagnosis or prognosis. This may be done at visiting time when they must remain composed to visit the patient. This may inhibit further questions which, in turn, may lead to confusion over already revealed facts. There are of course some relatives who prefer not to know and never ask, or only want to know if the news is favourable. It is helpful if the telling can be done in a quiet, calm atmosphere by someone who has set time aside and has the authority to answer questions and can help the person to express their feelings. This is difficult in a ward office where they may be many interruptions. One problem area for the relatives to cope with is when the patient has been given information very optimistically, and they pessimistically. It often helps and minimises problems if the patient and family are seen together. After being told bad news a relative may become over-protective. As they cannot protect the patient from his or her illness this may lead to feelings of guilt and resentment and, in its turn, to criticism of care – almost that by the telling of a diagnosis the staff are the cause of the illness, they allowed it to happen. Twycross (1975) observes that the patient's relatives experience a variety of emotions which vary according to the depth of the relationship, the duration of the illness and mode of death.

In caring for the person at home there is considerable physical and emotional strain on the carers as the continuous caring role and patient demands may be very exhausting. Therefore it is important that all appropriate support services are involved. Hospital visiting can be tiring, especially if it is necessery for the visitor to travel long distances. Conversation may not be easy and relatives often need to be encouraged to sit quietly with the patient. They also need to realise that it is not essential to be there all the time, however they must be assured that the patient will be cared for and kept comfortable in their absence. The present situation may be a sad reminder of other losses, especially if the person has never worked through the grieving process effectively.

Many families have difficulty in talking about dying and may deny the facts and be unrealistically optimistic with the patient, being unable to be sensitive and perceptive to the patient's feelings. Even in the early stages of the illness, care must be directed to those looking after the patient, because this can be a particularly distressing period for them as they travel along the road with the ill person, unable to alter the direction, and they frequently feel helpless and very vulnerable. Sometimes relatives may try to make amends for the past, accomplish uncompleted tasks, unfulfilled promises. No relationship is perfect and relatives often find something to feel guilty about just as everyone can. Some people try to justify their own existence whereas there may be secret relief for others at the expected demise of the patient. They will naturally feel guilty about that. They may feel responsible if they have at sometime wished the person dead. Throughout the illness the fears of the patient, family and friends are intertwined, and they may each experience the same emotions. The nurse can encourage them to express and work through these feelings.

Relatives often need help to understand the patient's needs with regard to information and that, at times, he or she may deny their situation, or at others be very angry instead of accepting as they had hoped. They may need to be helped to see that if the patient is asking and genuinely wants to know then it is important not to lie but, in telling, hope must not be destroyed.

> A lady who was told her husband's diagnosis, was also told she should not tell him. She kept this secret for two years even though he asked, but eventually when he became more ill it was impossible to keep up the pretence and he was told. This gentleman was not angry or bitter, only hurt. Hurt that he had not been told. Hurt that his wife had kept this secret from him all that time, when their marriage had previously been loving, open and shared. For the last seven months of his life they were able to share again, both the good and the bad spells. His wife was a very capable lady who set goals with her husband and together they achieved many things. However the experience of hurt has never left this lady.

Throughout the patient's illness relatives need to have careful explanation regarding treatments, care and drugs in order that they can fully understand what is happening, what to look for, and how best to cope. They also need encouragement in their caring role. It certainly helps if their role is recognised, acknowledged and praised.

Relatives sometimes try to shield the patient from participating in everyday matters, which in turn makes the patient feel useless and does not give them the incentive to lead as normal a life as possible. This may lead to a more rapid loss of physical health, and mental stagnation. Relatives need to be helped to accept that human contact is necessary, otherwise boredom, insomnia and premature withdrawal may occur.

As the patient's condition deteriorates withdrawal from that person by the relative may occur, which is understandable as they now lead different lives and, the relative has to think about a future that does not exist for the patient. According to Hinton (1967) growing emotional separation is revealed to the dying person by uncertain behaviour of others, such as excluded whispers and hollow cheerfulness. Withdrawal from the patient can be very distressing but, equally so, the withdrawal by the patient from the relative who wants to prolong life and perhaps has not come to terms with the situation. The nurse needs to help both patient and relative to accept that withdrawal is natural. Silent support is important. Some families find it hard to let go; they may not be ready to do so.

The family are not guests but an essential part of any caring team and as key members should be welcomed and encouraged to take an active role in decision making. They need to feel useful and helpful. Confidence in their caring role and encouragement shown by the staff will help them to cope more effectively. When nurses are talking to relatives silences must be tolerated as these give them opportunity to collect their thoughts, and a chance to think through what has been said. Relatives frequently feel guilty about taking up a professional carer's time and comments such as 'I mustn't go on so' or 'You're too busy to listen to me' must not be used as escape routes for the nurse. It is the nurse's role to help them to find their own meaning in the situation, but not to impose the nurse's own views.

The relative may find it hard to cope with the illness, especially when the one they love appears difficult, irrationally angry or hostile towards them. These emotions and their own fears may cause physical manifestations such as weight loss, sleep disturbances, anorexia and lack of concentration, being unable to settle to anything. The nurse must allow time for them in order to help them through this difficult period.

The latter period of time leading up to the death may be particularly distressing to the relatives and friends. It is frequently a time when they need added support and reassurance. Over the telephone a little personal information and reference to the patient by name can be very comforting rather than 'comfortable' or 'as well as can be expected'. This may be a time when they appear dazed and may not really comprehend what is actually happening. A friendly welcome makes the relative feel needed and wanted. They may need encouragement to show natural affection and maintain contact by touch. Even in the last stages of life relatives and friends have a very important role to play, a job to do, perhaps sitting holding a hand, moistening a mouth or helping with practical care. They need to witness a peaceful death and hopefully the professional carers will have built up a relationship of trust with the family which will give comfort and support in the last hours. Some relatives need to remain with the dying person throughout. Some may have other responsibilities and are deprived of staying. Others may be weary from caring and giving and may not be able to stand any more. Respect must be given to each person and there should be no disapproval, but reassurance that they have done all they could, if that is so, and endeavour to help them not to feel a failure. If the relative wishes to stay, the nurse should not misguidedly discourage them from this last caring act by urging them to go home and get a good nights rest. This may be their last opportunity to give of themselves to the patient and, if possible, a room should be provided for them to stay.

The patient's physical distress will cause emotional suffering of the family and friends and therefore, for their sakes as well as the patient, it must be controlled. The final willingness of the patient to die should not be seen by the grieving person as a rejection of them by the patient. If the relative was not present it is often helpful to reassure them of the comfort and peacefulness of the patient. It also helps to remind them that they were there when the patient could enjoy their company. After death relatives have to be helped back along the road to a normal life.

A quiet understanding chat over a cup of tea can be helpful at this time. The grieving one should be allowed to cry even though it might be very uncomfortable for the professional carer to observe. There will be pain and distress before healing can begin. Time to listen to relatives is essential. Time to share the grief, the memories, the good times and the bad. Available support from staff they already know is tremendously helpful, a sharing between relatives and staff, both professional and lay is appreciated. The nurses must allow the bereaved to express their concern and even sharing in silence with the grieving one can bring comfort and be important. All too often people feel they must talk and sometimes this can be inappropriate and causes more distress. Support is very important at this time and the need to be busy and leave the person can be hurtful. Real caring is unmistakeable to the bereaved. A caring person can give more help than is realised.

There are some practical matters associated with the death which the nurse needs to understand in order to advise the family. There is a need to explain to the family what is likely to happen and what they should do if there are any problems. This is especially important if they are caring for a person at home. If the death is to occur at home the family need to be told to call the General Practitioner as soon as possible after the person has died. The doctor will visit to confirm death and may write the medical certificate of death at the house but, if not, the family may be asked to collect it from the surgery later. If the death occurred in a palliative care unit or ward the attending doctor will sign the medical certificate of death. It is important that the family or next of kin understands what to do when they leave the ward after the death, with regard to collecting the certificate and the personal belongings of the patient. It can be helpful if there are written instructions because people often forget when stressed. Once the doctor has confirmed death and has issued the appropriate certificate, the death can be registered. This is done at the registrar's office of the district in which the patient actually died. It is usually done by a near relative. It is helpful for the nurse to be aware of the office opening times for informing relatives if this is not dealt with by the administration department. After certification of death a funeral director can be contacted and he or she will make arrangements for the deceased to be removed to a Chapel of Rest, but until registration takes place the funeral director can proceed no further. Funeral directors act on behalf of the family, making all necessary arrangements and are very helpful and caring, paying attention to detail. The family can be sure they will guide them through this difficult period. (See also Chapter 13 on bereavement.)

The role and care of the nurse

It is important to summarise the role of the nurse in caring for patients with a limited life span. The nurse's role is to assist the person to live life as fully as possible, within the limitations imposed by the illness, until they die, maintaining hope, achieving goals and coping with the everyday situation. Today nursing has progressed to concentrate on the whole person and the family. The nurse should be a provider of quality care, using his or her nursing expertise and skills at the appropriate times throughout the person's life. The nurse must be able to assess symptoms and other needs effectively, and is the most likely person to observe changing needs or symptoms breaking through, because of spending longer periods of time with the patient than other team members. It is essential to act upon observation and here the nurse can be the eyes and ears of the medical staff and the rest of the team, as well as the patient's advocate.

It helps if the nurse understands the hierarchy of needs and Maslow (Quinn, 1980) formulated a theory.

Hierarchy of needs   (with special emphasis on those with a limited life span)

- Physiological   Basic survival and comfort needs
- Safety and security   Helped if patient and nurse form a partnership of care giving explanations and information
- Love and belonging   Being understood, accepted and comfortable in place of care; sharing with family and staff help

- Self esteem   Recognition of need for independence and dignity by planning individualised care and helping patient to achieve goals

- Self actualisation   Finding a meaning in death and working towards acceptance and disengagement from environment

Fulfilment of physical, psychological, social and spiritual needs are all equally important, therefore all services to the patient must be coordinated to achieve quality care. Communication between patient, family, nurse and the whole caring team must be effective or misunderstanding, anxiety and unnecessary suffering may be caused. The nurse is often required to give advice on a variety of issues such as rest, diet, exercise etc., but she or he must know when and how to refer to others. The nurse is not an expert on everything. Frequently the nurse teaches both patients and relatives simple nursing procedures and techniques and also has a responsibility to share his or her expertise with colleagues and others.

Counselling and facilitating are important roles. The nurse needs to be a positive listener, giving the person encouragement to identify problems, and find their own acceptable solutions, by knowing available resources. Counselling also involves dealing with feelings and the nurse must control the natural response to console and calm, but rather encourage the person to get the feelings out. Negative feelings may have to be dealt with. It is crucial that nurses do not take over and impose their own views. (See also Chapter 15 on counselling.) Relatives must be kept fully informed and the nurse must have the ability to involve them, and friends, in care as appropriate. This will be appreciated and may well help to minimise the patient's social loss. The support role involves many other roles and will bring much comfort. It is said that just being there, willing to listen, share and show concern is all that matters, but support must not be a prop which, when taken away, causes everything to collapse.

Frequently, in caring for very ill people over a period of time, a very close relationship can be formed with them and their relatives and friends. It is a time when the nurse is permitted to share a very personal part of that person's life, when barriers are stripped and the real person is apparent. This is a great privilege for any nurse but also a responsibility. The effect on the nurse when the patient dies can be one of grief as though a friend has been lost. Professional people are often expected to be detached and uninvolved (Summers), but nurses are ordinary caring people, with feelings like everyone else. They too may feel helpless, upset, moved or even relieved when a person dies and should be encouraged to share their feelings at this time. Shame should never be felt at a damp eye. This often reveals to the grieving relative just how much the nurse really cared. Caring for these patients is intensive, personal care rather than curative care (Summers and Young). So it is important that nurses look at themselves, their philosophy of life and death, their feelings, and how and why they react as they do. In so doing, hopefully, they will understand those they care for better, and be able to help patients to look at themselves, and share with them.

'No one is an island' (Chaney, 1976). We all need each other. Just as the nurse needs support he or she must be willing to give it, and the whole team should support each other. Frank discussion about feelings is often helpful. It is important that the nurse develops his or her own coping mechanisms and has a balanced life outside caring for these people.

'Let as much as possible be done'. Caring for the patient near the end of life is a great challenge and, if nurses provide total care and support, the patient will achieve much in their limited life span.

References

ALDERMAN, C. (1988). Controlling pain. *Nursing Standard*, 8 August, 31–2.

CAUGHILL, R. E. (Ed.) (1976). *The Dying Patient: a Supportive Approach*. Little, Brown & Co., Boston.

CHANEY, P. S. (Ed.) (1976). *Dealing with Death and Dying*. Ravenswood Publications.

CORR, D. A. and Corr, D. M. (1983). *Hospice Care: Principles and Practice*. Faber and Faber.

CRAVEN, J. and WALD, F. (1975). Hospice care for dying patients. *American Journal of Nursing*, **75(10)**, 1816–22.

DOBBS, B. Z. (1985). Alternative health approaches. *Nursing Mirror*, **160(9)**, 41–2.

HINTON, J. (1967). *Dying*. Penguin, Harmondsworth.

QUINN, F. M. (1980). *The Principles and Practice of Nurse Education*. Croom Helm Ltd.

REGNARD, C. F. B., DAVIES, A. and RANDALL, F. (1983). *A Guide to Symptom Relief in Advanced Cancer*. Drogher Press.

REGNARD, C. F. B. and NEWBURY, A. (1983). Pain and the portable syringe pump. *Nursing Times*, **79(26)**, 25–8.

SAUNDERS, C. M. (Ed.) (1978). *The Management of Terminal Disease*. Edward Arnold, London.

SMITH, J. P. (1981). *Sociology and Nursing*. Churchill Livingstone, Edinburgh.

SUMMERS, D. H. *Staff Support*. Leaflet produced by St Christopher's Hospice, Sydenham, London.

SUMMERS, D. H. and YOUNG, J. M. *To Comfort Always*. Booklet produced by St Christopher's Hospice, Sydenham, London.

TWYCROSS, R. G. (1975). *The Dying Patient*. CMF Publications.

TWYCROSS, R. G. and LACK, S. A. (1990). *Therapeutics in Terminal Cancer*, second edition. Chruchill Livingstone, Edinburgh.

Further reading

AUTTON, N. (1986). *Pain: an Exploration*. Darton, Longman and Todd Ltd.

BUCKMAN, R. (1988). *I Don't Know What to Say*. Papermac.

CASSIDY, S. (1988). *Sharing the Darkness*. Darton, Longman and Todd Ltd.

CORR, C. A. and CORR, D. M. (1983). *Hospice Care: Principles and Practice*. Faber and Faber.

EGAN, G. (1986). *The Skilled Helper*. Brooks/Cole.
HINTON, J. (1967). *Dying*. Penguin, Harmondsworth.
TWYCROSS, R. G. and LACK, S. A. (1990). *Therapeutics in Terminal Cancer*, second edition. Churchill Livingstone, Edinburgh.

Coping strategies: the nurse as a facilitator

9

The special needs of children and adolescents

Denise Hodson

'To cure sometimes, to relieve often, to comfort always.'

Strauss

Background

The last twenty years have seen great advances in the diagnosis, treatment and survival of children with cancer. Each year, in the United Kingdom approximately 1200 children are diagnosed as having a malignant disease. Childhood malignancies differ from adult cancers. Childhood tumours are commonly sarcomas or blastomas, unlike those of adults which are principally carcinomas. The most commonly treated childhood cancer is lymphoblastic leukaemia. However, childhood cancer is rare. Only one child in 10 000 per year under 15 years of age develops a malignant disease. The rarity of these diseases led to the development in the United Kingdom of regionally based paediatric oncology units in the 1970s, to facilitate research, diagnosis, treatment and the evaluation necessary in order to provide the optimal chance of cure for this small group of children. Of children with malignant disease, 75% receive all or part of their therapy in these units. Over 60% are now expected to survive (Fig. 9.1). The reduction in mortality has seen cancer as a cause of death in childhood fall from second to third, after accidents and congenital abnormalities (Office of Population and Census Survey, 1987).

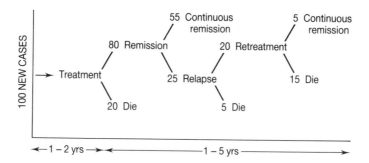

Fig. 9.1 One hundred typical oncology patients. Of the 60 who remain in continuous complete remission, 50 will be normal and 10 may have varying degrees of handicap. (Reproduced with permission of the UKCCSG, based on The Report on Cancer Services for Children, March 1987.)

The intensive treatment regimes necessitate repeated hospitalisation for many children, with their parents, sometimes for lengthy periods. For most children frequent outpatient visits are necessary, travelling to the Oncology Unit which may be many miles away. Oncology units may 'share-care' with district general hospitals to alleviate some of the problems caused by distance, to promote communication and establish confidence in the care-givers in the patients own community.

Paediatric Oncology units employ a multidisciplinary team approach, involving health visitors/liaison nurses, social workers, psychologists, dieticians and others, in caring for the child and his family. Spinetta and Deasey-Spinetta (1981) have shown that the whole family is affected when a diagnosis of cancer is made in a child. The unit aim is to help families in whatever way they feel appropriate, to be able to understand and cope with their child's illness, enabling them to continue their natural role as primary care-givers and support them through the treatment and the uncertainty of the eventual outcome (Koocher and O'Malley, 1981). It is the aim of the units to adopt an honest and realistic approach from the time of diagnosis, an approach that facilitates discussion and understanding between parents, children and staff.

Although the outlook for most children is encouraging, there remains approximately one third for whom a cure will not be achieved. A small number of these will die in the earlier stages of treatment from their disease, from infection or complications of the drug therapy, usually in hospital. For others, relapse or failure to achieve a remission may have meant further treatment programmes. Advancement of the disease necessitates a reassessment of aims and values and a change in expectations, that a cure will not be achieved and a period of palliative care is beginning.

Decision to end curative treatment

The decision to end attempts at curative therapy is not one made lightly. Where there is a progression of disease or the adverse effects of further treatment outweigh the benefits which can realistically be achieved, the need for on-going open communication between the parents, the child if he or she is old enough and the oncology unit is essential. It is important that all aspects of the treatment and the progression of disease are discussed so that the subsequent decision that active therapy has no further value is understood and made jointly with the professional carers. Open communication allows older children or teenagers to participate in these discussions, so that they too can be helped to decide if they want to try new drug treatments or, if they wish, to set their own agenda in making new goals for their future. No family should be left to make the decision alone.

Children and parents develop close ties and relationships with carers in the oncology units over many months, often years. Once the decision to end therapy has been made, there is a real need for the assurance of continuing support and expression of the carers concern for the childs continuing quality of life. Fears of being 'abandoned' or no longer part of the unit's immediate priorities are real anxieties many parents experience, with fears of what the future will hold and worries about their abilities to cope. The goals set for future care will involve re-establishing and making new contacts at home, symptom control and to help the family resume a normality of family life. There is a need to help them make plans and to 'invest' in the time left and make this final time of caring a positive one for living.

Regional oncology units encompass many districts and health authorities. Families may live in densely populated industrial areas or in rural districts. It is the practise of oncology centres to establish communication with community carers at an early stage of treatment. Contact with the general practitioner is made at the time of initial diagnosis, by phone and letter. Links will also have been made by the units health visitor or liaison nurse to those already involved with the family at home – their health visitor or school nurse and the teachers. The first contact is important not only to establish a link but to allow the exchange of relevant information. The rarity of childhood malignancies means that most general practitioners will only see one or two cases of cancer in a child throughout their career. Opportunities to meet and discuss cases are usually welcomed by both hospital and community staff.

It is at the time of relapse of the disease and the decision to end attempts at curative therapy that the framework of contact made at diagnosis establishes its importance. By building on the lines of communication, the feasibility of care that is needed can realistically be offered. Martinson *et al.* (1986) and Chambers *et al.* (1989) have demonstrated that, by working together, the hospital and community carers can establish a plan of joint care to support the child and family in any way the family deems appropriate to enable them to care for the child.

The availability of carers and facilities differs widely from district to district. Health visitors, district nurses, paediatric community nurses, Macmillan or Marie Curie nurses are but a few of the appropriate professionals whose skills may be sought but of course not all are available as a resource in any given area. The resources of oncology units also differs. Most can offer visits from liaison nurses/ health visitors and social workers. Hospital doctors may also visit. For some units, distance may mean the majority of contact with families and home carers is made by telephone. The most important factor is that appropriate care and support is given by those most acceptable to the family

Establishing the pattern of care

Where the needs of the dying child and his or her family are best met has been the subject of much discussion and research (Wilson, 1985; Armstrong and Martinson, 1980). At the turn of the century home was the natural and obvious place to be born and to die, with family and friends around. Medical advances over the years changed expectations as treatments were developed for many previously life-threatening illnesses. The specialist care centres for children with cancer were presumed to be the most appropriate place for these children to be. Now, however, options other than the acute busy hospital setting are considered. Dying children especially want to be cared for at home (Armstrong and Martinson, 1980), care which can be given by parents in familiar surroundings, if they are helped by nursing and medical staff, even though they are living with the knowledge that their child will die soon (Martinson *et al.*, 1984).

Many factors can influence the decision: duration of terminal illness, distance from the hospital, availability of local support and the immediate medical/nursing needs of the child are but a few. There may be anxieties expressed by parents about their own ability to deliver adequate care, about the response of other children and fears of uncontrolled symptoms, especially pain. They may be reticent to discuss these fears unless specifically given the opportunity to do so. Parents and children who choose to remain or return to hospital should not be left with feelings of failure – it may be right for them and it is important they feel they have done the best for their child.

Whatever the outcome, parents should know that no decision is irreversible and that an open-door policy is maintained, so that children can be cared for in the most appropriate way and place at any given time. For most families home is preferable, where family, friends and the familiar surroundings provide the comfort and support throughout this difficult time.

For some children hospice care may provide the alternative to home/hospital care. The concept of hospice care for adults is well-established, with emphasis on the quality of life and symptom control to enable the person to live their life with dignity, control and fulfilment. There are few childrens hospices in Britain. The first to be established to care for children who were dying was Helen House in Oxford. A retrospective study of 25 families who attended the hospice examined their perceptions of the care offered and of the impact of a life threatening disease on the family (Stein *et al.*, 1989). Most families felt they were greatly helped by the individualised family-orientated care and atmosphere. However, the fact that the care was delivered in a setting solely for terminally-ill children was considered a drawback. The home-from-home atmosphere where all the family could be together was deemed particularly appropriate for those whose child or children suffered a degenerative condition, and for whom periods of respite care could be offered. The impact experienced by families, caused by illness, was substantial and felt by all members. This included psychological difficulties, worries about symptom control, emotional and behavioural difficulties of siblings, financial and employment problems.

Figures show that the largest group of children to benefit from the care of Helen House in its first year were those with central nervous disorders, followed by those with mucopolysaccharidosis (Burne *et al.*, 1984). Children with a malignant disease formed a much smaller group. Most children were admitted for respite care either as a planned admission or as a crisis-situation intervention.

The duration of terminal illness in children with malignant disease differs widely from those with degenerative disorders. For most, the timespan can be measured in weeks to short months, establishing care at home as a feasible option. The role of the childrens hospice is as yet uncertain but it should remain an option to be considered when care for a child is being planned.

Caring for a dying child is one of the most difficult and emotional times in which professional carers are all involved. For nurses and practitioners in the community their previous experience will probably be limited. Many have expressed their feelings of anxiety in caring for a child and in their ability to deliver appropriate care and symptom control. The initial reaction is often that children are 'different' and that they lack the necessary expertise. The actual principles of caring for the terminally ill are similar no matter what the age of the patient. The practises may differ when the patient is a child, but community carers have a wealth of experience and skills to offer.

Over long months or years the parents have become 'specialists' in their childs disease and treatment and have usually participated actively in general procedures, treatments and care. Their dependence on the oncology unit has already been described. Feelings of inadequacy experienced by some carers are understandable as families may bypass their General Practitioner or nurse and contact the hospital unit directly. This can lead to feelings of 'exclusiveness' and make involvement seem difficult. If pathways of communication are kept open and contact is freely made by both hospital and home carers some of these difficulties can be minimised through active discussion and sharing of problems.

Principles of care

The principles of palliative care remain constant.

● To continue meaningful *communication* with the child and family. Research has shown that the majority of time spent in the childs home is spent listening to worries, fears and feelings expressed by families and in providing a 'listening' support (Norman and Bennet, 1986; Martinson, 1980). To be able to sit and listen is probably the most valuable contribution any carer can make. It asks carers to question their own attitudes to the process of dying and death, and to acknowledge the grief felt within this family.

● *Symptom control* when necessary. As symptoms arise through the pro-gression of disease it is important that they are not considered in isolation but that the physical and emotional needs of the child as a whole are considered. There may be more than one specific cause and younger children may have difficulties explaining how they feel. Various tools are available to assist in assessing symptoms especially pain (Eland, 1985; Jerret and Evans, 1986). Parents will describe changes in physical or emotional needs or abilities which often provide a valuable guide.

● To respond appropriately to their *on-going needs*. The needs of the child and family can change quickly as palliative care evolves. The duration of care is variable and input in practical terms dependant on the advancement of disease and the symptoms experienced. Subjects discussed may relate to other family members or friends or to practical issues such as finance, heating, bills or other needs. It may be appropriate to draw on the particular skills of other carers in the hospital or community to address specific problems.

● Effective *liaison and sharing of information* between hospital and com-munity carers. Throughout this time and after death the oncology unit will maintain contact by telephone calls and visits to the child and family. Joint visits with community carers can reassure parents that everyone is working in close coopera-tion for their childs comfort and support. Maintaining contact between the hospital and community can lessen the feelings of isolation for staff and families alike.

Communication

Communicating with parents

The families of dying children are generally more extended than those of adults in similar circumstances, including grandparents, relatives, close friends and the childs peers in their family unit. Younger members may not have experienced death before and the experience is made more intensive and felt more strongly when the death is that of a child (Wilson, 1988). The needs of the family and their child have been identified as similar to, but not identical, to those of dying adults and their families (Wilson, 1985).

Parents may again feel all the emotions that surrounded the time of initial diagnosis; those of shock, anger and of disbelief, 'Perhaps the doctors have made a mistake, perhaps the scan is wrong, or not my childs'. For many, these feelings are entwined in a deeper knowledge gained by living with his or her disease and its treatment over many months or years, and an acknowledgement that the grief began at diagnosis and has only been suppressed. A general observation is that mothers may be more pessimistic throughout treatment and fathers more optimistic. This may be a result of more mothers being resident with their child in hospital and forming close relationships with other parents. They seek information, not only about their child, and share good and bad times with other parents. Fathers may prefer to remain optimistic for their childs recovery, as they continue to work and organise normal activities at home for other children, and prefer to concentrate only on their childs progress.

Parents are individuals in their own right and their needs will differ throughout this time. They may find it difficult to relate to one another, as the impact of their differing emotions falls on the person they are closest to. They need to be given time to talk freely together, and individually, with carers. A common reaction is to blame either themselves for not preventing the disease or the impending death, or to blame others for not diagnosing the disease earlier.

Their hopes and expectations are forced to change direction, from the hopes of a cure to being able to give their child a peaceful, happy and painfree time to come. In a study to try to identify the needs of families with a terminally ill relative, O'Brian (1983) noted (*i*) their need for information, and (*ii*) the need to be assured of their relatives comfort and that appropriate care was being given. The same opportunities to talk to medical and nursing staff should be open to the childs siblings and relatives, as they may have questions which they feel are inappropriate to be asked of the parents at this time.

In conversation with parents, some have said that their relatives make the situation more difficult to cope with. They seem entwined in their own grief and their need to 'put things right' and in expressing false hopes. Repeated explanations about changes in the childs condition and treatment become tiresome in the battle of maintaining a normality of family life. Parents express a need to talk to people who understand what is happening and for whom explanations are not necessary.

All parents will ask when their child will die, 'How long do we have with him?' A question that is impossible to answer in absolute terms. We can only answer in the very broadest sense in the light of our past experiences. No one can answer in definitive terms of weeks or months, only maybe in the final hours.

Other questions will explore the way in which death will occur, 'Will it be sudden?' and, most importantly, 'Will he be in pain?' The professional carer is more able to discuss the answers to these questions at length, with knowledge about the most likely developments of a childs particular disease. It is difficult to describe these developments as options which may or may not happen to families, but parents feel better prepared to deal with symptoms or situations as they arise. They know that individual possibilities have been anticipated and that measures have been planned that will ensure their childs comfort.

Communicating with the patient

Childhood encompasses a wide age-range, from babies up to adolescence. The individuals age, development, both physically and psychologically, and experiences are all important factors to be considered. During illness and hospitalisation childrens need for their parents increases as they fear separation from the people and places they know best. Children are happiest in their own home, with the normality of family-life providing a secure environment (Armstrong and Martinson, 1980). Concepts of death are directly related to age and to personal experiences, and one needs to know about the child's understanding of death to be able to hold a meaningful discussion with them.

Children
In the healthy child up to three years of age the word 'death' has little meaning. The most frightening thought is that of separation from his or her parents and of being left alone. Between three and five years of age a curiosity about death and 'being dead' develops. Seeing birds or animals who have died promotes the idea of not moving, or eating, maybe sleeping? Whatever – it is not permanent. They feel invincible. Children will associate death with heaven. Heaven seems a real place where dead people go to be with others. The concept of not being able to visit, or of those who have died not returning at some time, seems strange.

From six years of age there is a gradual understanding that being dead is permanent although, for many, games played or television programmes watched reiterate the fact that their heroes recover to fight another battle next week or they can 'begin again' in a different game. Death can be thought of as a 'ghost' or associated with acts of violence or being 'bad'.

The development of children from ten years upwards and the wider experiences they have gained leads them towards a more adult reasoning of dying and death and an awareness that one day they too will die and that it will be permanent.

The ages and above outline are very broad and generalised. Children will vary widely in their understanding of death, as in their physical development and their intellectual ability at any age. Children who are very ill and have experienced repeated hospitalisation, traumatic procedures and possibly the loss of a friend through death will experience a much greater awareness of the meaning, possibly at a younger age than most of their peers.

It was thought that ill young children had little or no concept of their own death, but research has shown much higher anxiety levels and feelings of isolation, possibly as parents seek to protect their child by avoiding addressing the issue or by changes in their normal attitude toward the child (Spinetta *et al.*, 1974). Parents may have prepared themselves, however subconsciously, for the time when curative treatment ends. This preparation has been defined as anticipatory mourning, a set of processes that are directly related to the awareness of impending loss, to the emotional impact and to the adaptive mechanisms whereby emotional attachment to the child is relinquished over time (Futterman and Hoffman, 1973). The depth and degree of this mourning period will vary in intensity between families and between the individuals involved. Difficulties arise when a child dies suddenly in the early stages of his or her disease or during treatment, where parents have not had this time to prepare themselves and their families. Research has shown more long term psychological, behavioural and physical problems are experienced by parents and siblings following the sudden death of their child. Children can also demonstrate this distancing from those around from a young age. They want to protect their parents from answers or situations they perceive will cause distress.

It is not unusual for a child to choose a person with whom they will discuss what is happening to them, their fears and thoughts, and then deny the reality with others by their silence. Not all children feel the need to have their impending death confirmed. What is important is that children are listened to, that statements they make may be questions to be answered and that they are answered as honestly, sensitively and openly as possible. A lie or concealment will prevent further open communication and increase feelings of loneliness and isolation.

Parents and carers express their anxieties about what to tell a child and when. They are understandably frightened about saying the wrong thing or not being able to answer because of their own emotions. Children do not commonly ask outright if they are going to die. They may make a statement, draw pictures which can be discussed or ask a series of questions over a period of time which will provide a telling picture of their knowledge of their disease and of dying. When answering children one need only answer what is being asked. If unsure of the question then a simple return of the question to the child may clarify the thoughts behind it. It is better to say an honest 'I don't know' to a question than avoid the issue or make up what appears to be a suitable answer.

It should be remembered that children are most concerned with living. When they feel well, however weak, they want to resume their normal activities. For some this may mean a return to school for all or part of the week. They need to have their siblings and friends to play with or just to be with them. They also need the discipline that is the norm within their family unit. Where acceptable boundaries of behaviour are lifted the child becomes more uncertain of his role and limits within the family and feels insecure.

Adolescents

It is difficult to define an age-range which totally encompasses the adolescent years. For most, it includes the ages of 12 – 19 years. It is a time of great change in the physiological, psychological and social development of the individual. 'No two individuals are alike and at no age are these differences more apparent than during the adolescent years' (Crow and Crow, 1965). They are not yet adults but neither can they be treated as dependant children.

Life for a teenager becomes a challenge. It is a time of questioning the limits enforced by parents, schools and society in an effort to establish their place and identity. Their appearance assumes a great importance as they become heavily dependant on the approval and acceptance of their peer group, and as new personal relationships are formed. In the process of establishing their identity and independence, moods swing to extremes. They can be sad, uncertain, rebellious and argumentative (McCallum and Carr-Gregg, 1987).

Cancer and its treatment has an enormous impact on the teenagers self-image, identity and on their relationships within the family and with their peers. The necessity for repeated hospitalisation increases their dependence on parents when normally they would be moving away from it. Schooling is interrupted frequently, often when the most important study programmes for examinations are to be undertaken. Long or frequent spells in hospital result in a loss in ones place in the peer group. This is enhanced with changes in appearance: alopecia, weight gain or loss, all reinforce feelings of worthlessness

Teenagers may regress emotionally and display more childish behaviour. Others may exhibit a maturity and more adult understanding. Many want to take on new experiences and opportunities 'to put themselves on an accelerated track for experiencing life. Denial can be part of this race with time' (Johansen, 1988).

Carers come face-to-face with their own attitudes towards death and dying, especially when faced with a teenager who is dying. 'For health professionals to successfully work with dying adolescents they must first confront their own mortality' (Blum, 1984). Knowing that adolescent dreams and ambitions for the future will not be fulfilled, life seems unfair and unjust. Carers may be close to the patient in age or have teenage relatives, and the situation can become more personal.

'Dying adolescents grieve not only for the life they have lived but also for the life they have not lived. Grieving over their lack of future involves a process of discarding their unfulfilled dreams, expectations and goals' (Papadatou, 1989). Questions such as 'Why me', 'What did I do', 'Why can't I be . . .' can be bitter and painful and have no answers. Anger and resentment for lost opportunities may follow. Very ill adolescents know they are dying but will fluctuate between acknowledging this, either to themselves or others, and denial. The knowledge doesn't mean that they accept it. However, by being able to express their worries to a chosen person, they may gain a freedom to live their lives and reassert their independence (Papadatou, 1989). Figure 9.2 demonstrates how two teenagers chose to describe their feelings in writing, in a letter and a poem.

Adolescents especially need to be involved in open discussions about their disease, symptoms and care, to be given control and share in decision-making. Free communication between family members may be difficult to facilitate where parents try to protect their son or daughter (and themselves), and a conspiracy of silence and isolation can develop. Opportunities for communication that is honest and caring allows the adolescent to express his or her anxieties and concerns. Research shows that much of their concerns are with the actuality of dying – 'Will I be in pain?', 'How long?' and 'When will it be?'. These questions are most likely to be asked of medical or nursing carers, with their professional knowledge, than of their family. Again, these questions will only be asked where there is the trust and confidence that an honest answer will be given. Opportunities for the teenager to talk alone with medical staff should be made. This can sometimes be difficult to achieve as parental wishes must also be acknowledged, but sensitive exchanges can help them to understand their child's need for independent discussions. The individual may have certain tasks he or she wishes to complete: to say goodbye to friends, give presents, make a will or decisions about his or her funeral. Adolescents need reassurance that they will not be forgotten by their friends and that their life has made an impact on others.

Communicating with other family members

Siblings

Many parents describe real difficulties in approaching the subject of death with their child and his or her siblings. They may be anxious not to say too much too soon, or,

'I am writing about this because I daren't talk about it. My tumour had gone – the Chemo had killed it off, but what if my new tumour doesn't respond to treatment and grows. I keep thinking about Tracy and then about this tumour. I might die as well.
I know I shouldn't think about this but I just can't help it.'

Lynne

Reaching the limit

Got to go fast,
Head for the hill,
Don't seem to move,
Feeling ill.

Want to drop,
Feet do ache,
Have to stop,
Just can't wait.

Getting close,
Nearly there,
Reached the limit,
People stare.

John

Fig. 9.2   A letter and a poem by two teenagers with cancer.

of leaving explanations and the chance to talk too late. One can only offer the advice to answer questions honestly, as and when they arise. Teenage brothers and sisters will be more aware and involved than younger children, and need to talk about their feelings. Where siblings are encouraged to participate in their brother or sisters care, questions may arise more naturally over time.

Questions may be asked more than once by siblings. This may relate directly to their age, understanding and concepts of death. There may also be changes in their emotional and behavioural responses, relating to the perceived anxieties of their parents. Where the sick child becomes the focus of the parents attentions and where his or her needs and wishes seem paramount, siblings may feel left out, unimportant and isolated. Their behaviour may change to being clinging, attention-seeking or withdrawn. In promoting a more normal family life, one can encourage parents to include siblings in care-giving in planning treats or visits for the whole family to participate in and enjoy.

Grandparents

The needs of grandparents should not be forgotten in caring for the family. Their grief encompasses many losses. They grieve for the impending loss of their grandchild's life, and for their own childs sadness. One does not expect ones child to die first, certainly not ones grandchild, who should have many years before him or her. There is a loss of hopes and investment in their future.

Many will have played an active role during the hospitalisation and treatment of their grandchild, either in relieving parents by the bedside or in caring for other children at home. The relationship of grandparents and grandchildren can be a very special, close one.

It should not be assumed that returning home and re-establishing day-to-day living when a child is dying is always fraught with difficulties and communication problems. The belief that open communication about dying was an essential task for the family – held by health professionals – has been challenged (Northouse, 1984). 'Not all families need to communicate about death, especially those who have comfortable, agreed upon patterns of not discussing feelings within the family system' (Lewandowski and Jones, 1988).

The families who are identified as needing help are those who want to talk but are uncertain of how to approach the subject, or those where the needs of one member are at variance with the rest of the family. This should not, however, provide an excuse for carers not to explore the need to talk as the palliative care stage progresses. Over time and as symptoms change, carers may become aware of changes in the needs of individuals in the family.

For many parents they now have the opportunity to give the ultimate care that any parent can give. The long periods in hospital or throughout treatment may have felt safe with support from other parents and professionals around, but when the therapy has ended, home with its comforts and familiar belongings can offer its own respite.

Symptom control

Pain

Identification and assessment

In the past there have been many myths and misconceptions relating to a child's ability to feel pain. Many assumed it was not experienced with the same intensity as that perceived by adults. Subsequent research shows this assumption to be unfounded, no evidence being available to substantiate it (Reape, 1990). The child's age, development, behaviour and ability to express his or her feelings are some of the factors which must be taken into consideration when assessing and managing pain control.

Various age-related tools are available to assist in this management. One of the most reliable is the Eland colour tool (Eland, 1985), where children use different coloured pens to draw on a body outline (Fig. 9.3). They choose their own colours to describe different intensities of pain felt in different parts of the body. Other scales used utilise colours, a range of 'smiling to sad' faces, numbers and visual linear analogues, where points are drawn on a straight line indicating 'least' pain at one end and 'worst' pain at the other. Results have shown varying degrees of reliability associated with the age and development of the child when using some of these methods (Eland, 1985).

The language which children employ to describe pain varies considerably with age. The actual word 'pain' may not be understood by over half the children aged between five ane eight years (Eland, 1985). It is important that specific words used by the child and family are known in order to help communicate at the child's level of understanding. For example, some of the words more commonly used many include 'owie', 'sore', 'little hurts', and 'big hurts', also specific noises made by some children. Mothers naturally identify cries made by their babies or toddlers as being 'hungry', 'tired' or 'in pain'. Studies show us that children can and do express pain in their own way (Jerret and Evans, 1986). They do not imagine or pretend to have pain but difficulties can sometimes arise in identifying its intensity.

The behavioural changes of young children, often described by parents, such as sleeplessness, irritability, anorexia and general unhappiness at being moved or touched may all indicate that the child is in pain. These symptoms, of course, may also be described in older children and teenagers. One must always listen carefully to what is being said by parents, the issues which cause them concern may be

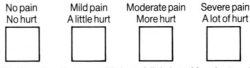

| No pain | Mild pain | Moderate pain | Severe pain |
| No hurt | A little hurt | More hurt | A lot of hurt |

Pick the colors that mean *No hurt, A little hurt, More hurt,* and *A lot of hurt* to you and color in the boxes. Now, using those colors, color in the body to show how you feel. Where you have no hurt, use the *No hurt* color to color your body. If you have hurt or pain, use the color that tells how much hurt you have.

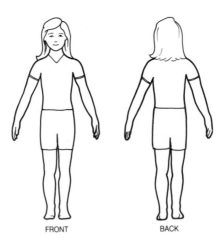

FRONT   BACK

Fig. 9.3   Body outline. A tool to describe pain intensity and sites for children.

indicative of pain in their child. Professional carers should also be aware that older children and teenagers can be reluctant to say they are in pain, if they are anticipating a return to hospital or injections as a consequence.

When the decision of where palliative care is to be given is being made, the major cause of anxiety for parents is the fear of uncontrollable symptoms, especially pain (Kohler and Radford, 1985). Children who are terminally ill do not all experience severe pain and do not all require strong opiates. Personal experience has seen, for example, that many children who have brain tumours require little or no opiate treatment although other symptom control is often necessary. This contrasts sharply with some children who have bone or soft tissue tumours for whom opiate drugs are usually needed in large doses for long periods of time.

If the care of these children is to be effective in ensuring their comfort, the professional carer must learn to listen, to recognise their symptoms then threat them appropriately and quickly.

The principles of assessing pain are well known. Pain may be related directly or indirectly to the disease or to previous anti-cancer therapy, and can be experienced in more than one site. The difference between these pains can be difficult to describe especially for a child.

It is possible to anticipate some of the types of pain which can be attributed directly to the nature and progression of disease (Miser and Miser, 1989). Severe headaches, with nausea and vomiting especially on rising, is most often seen in children with brain tumours and in leukaemia patients who have infiltration of the cerebral-spinal fluid by blasts cells, both giving rise to raised intracranial pressure.

Bone pains are commonly experienced by children with leukaemia or metastatic neuroblastoma. The pain results from invasion of bone and bone marrow and may be described as dull, aching and constant, progressively increasing in its severity. Invasion of bone and bone marrow also occcur in Ewings sarcoma and osteo-sarcoma. Occasionally this may lead to a pathological fracture. Very sharp severe pain may be indicative of rapidly growing tumour or of an intra-tumour bleed. The spread of tumour from soft tissue into adjacent nervous tissue results in a localised pain, described as sharp or burning, or in a more diffuse pain along the affected nerves pathway.

Treatment
Each pain requires separate consideration and assessment of its history, severity and nature before a diagnosis can be made. Any treatment previously prescribed and its efficacy must also be noted. When treating the pain, it is vital that an adequate dose is prescribed for the individual child.

Most drugs for children are prescribed on a 'milligram per kilogram' basis, but it must be stressed that when opiates are prescribed, this guide only provides a baseline. Drugs may need to be increased quickly to maintain pain control. The dosage increase should also be appropriate, increased of 50% or more may be necessary to regain control of symptoms.

Where pain is constant then analgesia must be prescribed regularly. There is no place for 'as required' doses for any patient in pain. Co-analgesics will often be necessary and will be described briefly later.

The most careful assessment, diagnosis and treatment is of little value if it is not monitored and reviewed often, with empathy and understanding. This may initially necessitate return visits to the home within short hours or of regular telephone calls to establish the effectiveness of the treatment. A contact, no matter how brief, is always reassuring and welcomed by the family. Where an immediate control of symptoms is necessary, contact that is once or twice weekly is insufficient and may result in panic calls or return visits to hospital which could be avoided. It can be a very demanding time for community nurses and practitioners.

The decision of which analgesic agent is most appropriate should not be difficult if pain control is commenced early and in effective doses. There is a wide choice of drugs available but a useful recommendations is to restrict ones choice to a limited number, with which one becomes familiar (Oakhill, 1988).

The widely-used 'analgesic staircase' (see p. 28) provides a useful reminder that when one form of analgesia fails, changing from one non-opiate drug to another will not regain pain control, and that to progress to a weak opiate is the next logical step.

The practise of our unit is to obtain pain control, initially, in younger children by prescribing paracetamol elixir, usually in one of the well-known proprietary forms such as 'Calpol' or 'Calpol 6 plus' (Wellcome Foundation Ltd). These are more acceptably flavoured and usually well known to the child. Where stronger analgesics are needed, progression is made to dihydrocodeine then to morphine elixir four hourly. Care should be taken when flavouring any medications that favourite acceptable foods or drinks are not used in an attempt to disguise the taste. This may only make the foods unpalatable with the result they are rejected totally.

Tablets should not be discounted by physicians because of the age of the child. Many children from a young age may prefer to take tablets, whole or crushed, and have become accustomed to doing so throughout their chemotherapy regimes.

The use of Buprenorphine (Temgesic) as a moderate strength opiate tablet which is absorbed sublingually would appear to be suitable for children. However, the use of this must be carefully considered as the drug binds to opiate receptors, making them inaccessible to morphine and diamorphine, sometimes for up to three weeks. Where the child is experiencing increasing levels of pain, the previous use of this drug may make it impossible to regain pain control during this time. Pethidine is not appropriate for patients who have cancer as it is short-acting and therefore not suitable for chronic pain. In addition, patients may experience loss of control and hallucinations.

Many children aged five years and upwards requiring strong opiate therapy have found MST Continus (controlled release morphine) tablets more acceptable. Where this is prescribed, morphine elixir should also be available to control any breakthrough pain until the appropriate MST Continus dose is achieved, as there is a delay of up to four hours before peak plasma concentrations occur. It is our experience that MST Continus tablets need to be prescribed eight hourly for children under ten years of age and twelve hourly for older children and teenagers. The drug appears to be metabolised faster in the younger age group. For children on relatively long term opioid therapy this can significantly simplify their drug taking and allows for longer periods of rest, especially through the night, for both child and parents between medication.

For the majority of children, utilising oral morphine preparations provides good pain control throughout their palliative care. However there are a small number of children for whom the oral route becomes inappropriate or insufficient. An alternative method may be necessary where the level of consciousness of the child deteriorates, where difficulty in swallowing for other reasons exists, for uncontrolled pain or where large repeated doses of oral drugs become difficult to tolerate. Failure to comply with any form of oral medication by the child is also a possibility!

Pain relief may be obtained by administering morphine as a suppository. With the exception of a few drugs such as anticonvulsants, the rectal route is not one commonly used in the United Kingdom. It is effective, but requires careful explanation to the child and parents for it to be accepted. Parents will often learn to administer the suppositories when shown by a nurse. Consideration of the childs diagnosis and condition must be taken into account where this method is to be used. Thrombocytopenia in a child with leukaemia, especially where episodes of bleeding have already occurred, may demand an alternative method of drug delivery. Morphine suppositories are available in 15 mg and 30 mg strengths, but pharmacies may be able to prepare other strengths should they be necessary.

In the past, lack of adequate pain control necessitated a return to hospital for intravenous analgesia for many children, with their families, usually hours or short days before the childs death. Anxiety at the childs condition, the urgency of the situation and failure to comply with the child and parents wishes to remain at home have all led to feelings of helplessness, lack of control, anger and extreme sadness by parents and carers at this already stressful time.

Over more recent years, parental administration of opiates at home by sub-cutaneous or venous routes have become more widely used. This method of drug delivery has been utilised for many years for adult patients and the principles for care remain the same for children. Some of the children for whom this method is appropriate will already have a venous access device in situ. Skin-tunnelled catheters, for example 'Hickman' or 'Broviac lines', or implanted devices, for example 'Portacath' or 'Implant-a-port' are widely used in oncology centres for the administration of chemotherapy, blood products, parental feeding and for blood sampling, so negating the need for repeated venepunctures and re-siting of infusions (Hollingsworth, 1987; Speechly, 1986).

A strictly-aseptic procedure is essential when these devices are to be accessed. Parents are taught how to clean, dress and flush, with saline and heparinised saline the skin-tunnelled catheter at home in order to maintain its patency between use (Clarke and Cox, 1988). When chemotherapy is discontinued the lines are usually left in situ to provide immediate access should some supportive intravenous therapy be needed.

The administration of diamorphine utilising the central venous line and a battery-operated syringe driver is a very effective method of controlling pain. Despite the very slow delivery of the drug, it is rare for these lines to occlude. Should this occur, advice should be sought from the oncology unit.

When changing from oral morphine to intravenous diamorphine, the dosage should initially be titrated to one third of the oral daily dose, although personal experience had noted that a subsequent increase in dosage has often been required quickly.

When introducing new and more technical methods of drug administration the health professional must always be aware of the increased stresses experienced by families. In our experience, with the support of hospital and, most especially, community carers, parents increasingly take over much of the care associated with drug preparation and charging of syringes. It is of course essential that parents and community nurses have full knowledge and confidence in the equipment and techniques used. Sharing information and resources between oncology units and community carers can only increase this knowledge and so benefit the child.

Where a central venous line is not available, subcutaneous diamorphine by infusion is a viable alternative, using a fine-gauge 'butterfly' needle. To help allay anxieties relating to the use of needles in hospital, many children are accustomed to, (and demand), the application of a local anaesthetic cream (EMLA) (Maunuksela and Kolpela, 1986) under an occlusive dressing, applied an hour before the needle is inserted. This practise is recommended prior to needle insertion into subcutaneous sites. The sites most commonly used are abdominal or chest wall. A transparent dressing over the needle can then be applied to secure the needle and provide easy observation of the site. Sites should be changed immediately there is any sign of inflammation or if the child complains of any discomfort.

S.H. was diagnosed as having stage III neuroblastoma at the age of eight years. After receiving chemotherapy and surgery, he remained well for two years. He then relapsed twice and was treated with chemotherapy and radiotherapy. His tumour failed to respond to the second relapse treatment and a joint decision was made to end attempts at curative therapy. At this time, he had extensive lymph node disease and two areas of bony metastases. Paracetamol controlled his pain well for some weeks, but towards the end of April he developed pain associated with one of his bony metastases. He was given a short course of radiotherapy and commenced Morphine Sulphate controlled release tablets (MST Continus). Throughout this time he had been mobile and able to attend school on a part-time basis, as his symptoms of tiredness and lethargy increased he was less able to go out. He required an increased dose of analgesia which caused some nausea. This was well controlled by Chlorpromazine and he remained pain-free until his death a few weeks later.

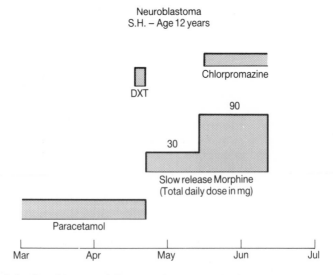

Fig. 9.4   Case history and diagram of pain control of a child with neuroblastoma.

C.K. presented as a 10 year old girl with Ewings Sarcoma of her femur. Originally treated with systemic chemotherapy and radiotherapy to the primary tumour, two years after completing treatment she suffered an extensive local relapse. The question of further therapy was discussed, but after consideration, the decision was made to adopt a palliative approach. She was started on oral paracetamol but this failed to control her pain for more than a few weeks so Morphine elixir was commenced. Her localised pain was well controlled by a relatively small dose of morphine, and she remained mobile, attending school with a relatively good quality of life.

During late October and early November, her tumour grew and began to encase her pelvis. This period of time required very close monitoring of the situation with periods of relative stability followed by fairly sharp increases in her analgesic dose.

She became anorexic, cachectic and immobilised by her tumour. She refused to take oral medication, preferring ot change to a subcutaneous diamorphine infusion. With close monitoring and appropriate dose increases, her pain appeared well-controlled for a further five months, until her death.

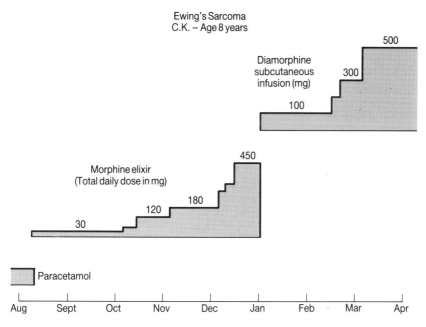

Fig. 9.5 Case history and diagram of pain control of a child with Ewing's Sarcoma of the femur.

Most children and teenagers will tolerate the use of syringe drivers well, where the need for this method of administration has been fully explained. It is not unusual to see a child or teenager who has previously appeared withdrawn, uncomfortable or in obvious acute pain, become alert and interested in his or her surroundings. Syringe drivers which have a 'boost' control of a preset bolus dose allows the child or parent to administer an isolated increased dose should there be an acute episode of pain. For those less able to participate in family life, it is comforting for them and for their family, to be able to hold and cuddle them without causing signs of distress. There is no need or reason for repeated, painful intramuscular injections of opiates, when other methods of drug administration are available. Figures 9.4 and 9.5 are brief case histories of two children, describing their different needs and the ways in which pain control was achieved.

Pain control using opiate therapy is ineffective when symptoms are not recognised or there is a failure to prescribe adequate doses. The question of addiction to these drugs does not arise where pain exists. Children, like adults, will become tolerant of the drugs over a period of time and, for this reason, dosage must be increased to achieve the same level of good pain control as before. Reluctance to prescribe large doses may be expressed by some practitioners who are concerned about depression of the respiratory centre. This is not a problem as tolerance develops in the same way as the analgesic effect. Parents may also be concerned about increasing the treatment, sometimes by substantial amounts. Children can tolerate high doses of

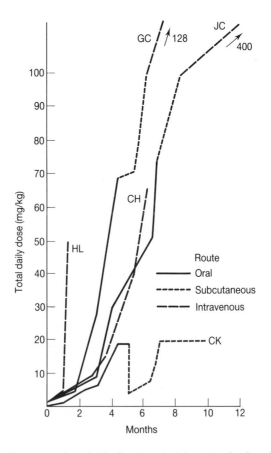

Fig. 9.6   Dosage and method of opiate administration for five children.

opiates and it is a difficult and very different concept for parents that there is no real upper-limit to the dose, only that which controls their child's pain (Fig. 9.6).

Time should be spent by nurses and physicians to explain how the drug works and in what amounts it should be increased at the time. The social and media implications of opiate drug-taking have great impact on the general public. Parents may have to be reassured that the drugs are most effective and appropriate for their child.

Adverse effects of opiate therapy

A side effect of opiate therapy which is to be anticipated in all patients is that of constipation. Appropriate laxatives should be prescribed in conjunction with opiate drugs, for example Lactulose and Senokot. Advice should be given to parents about active measures they can take with diet. Most children and teenagers will become drowsy when opiate drugs are begun. This is usually temporary, decreasing after a few days as they become more tolerant of the drug. It is essential that children who are old enough and parents are advised of this. It can be frightening for parents who are not informed, as death may seem to be more imminent when they are faced with a sleepy, less-responsive child. It can also be frightening for the child who may relate it to his or her own death or to previous experiences of chemotherapy, where antiemetics and sedatives give rise to the same feelings and memories of impending nausea. For both reasons they may be reluctant to start opiate treatment.

Nausea and vomiting caused by morphine preparations are not commonly experienced by children, but where it is directly related to opiates, drugs such as Metoclopramide or Chlorpromazine can be effective in relieving symptoms.

A more common side-effect is that of pruritus. Children may complain of severe itching which can be very distressing. This again will last only a few days and the prescribing of an antihistamine will offer relief over these first days. Unfortunately, a side-effect of most antihistamines is drowsiness.

Adjuvant therapy

Analgesic agents form the basis of pain control but other drugs may also be used for specific symptom control.

Corticosteroids, for example Dexamethasone, are frequently used to reduce cerebral oedema and thus relieve raised intracranial pressure caused by tumour. The reduction in pressure may relieve headaches, nausea and vomiting and may also cause a raising of the conscious level of the child. Corticosteroids are also effective where nerve pressure or soft tissue involvement gives rise to 'burning' symptoms. These drugs should be prescribed with care, as the features of Cushings Syndrome and overt weight gain are distressing, disfiguring and increase nursing problems. Dosage should be maintained at the lowest possible level at which the drug is effective for the child. Non-steroidal anti-inflammatory drugs (NSAID), for example Aspirin and Ibuprofen, may be indicated where bone pain or soft tissue infiltration exists.

Nerve pain may be experienced as burning and tingling or as sharp, shooting pains. The use of tricyclic antidepressants, for example amitriptyline, or anticonvulsants, for example Carbamazepine, have proved effective in reducing these symptoms. The use of antidepressants for children or teenagers for psychological reasons may be questioned, but for an individual child they can be beneficial, in small doses. The need to look at reasons why the child remains depressed once his or her general condition is improved should not be forgotten, and time should be spent in helping the child communicate his or her anxieties. Chronic pain, tiredness and past experiences are some of the factors which may occupy much of the child's mind. Relieving painful symptoms and improving the quality of life will help the child to regain a feeling of well being.

Dyspnoea, which may be experienced by the child with lung metasteses, is probably one of the most distressing sights for parents and carers to witness. The use of opiate drugs is invaluable as the child, whilst conscious, is unaware of his or her struggle for breath. There is no obvious respiratory depression where dyspnoea exists and opiates are used. Persistant coughs are often relieved with the use of Methadone. Antibiotics may be appropriate to treat chest infections where the child's general well-being will be improved. Where the child is unconscious this may be questionable. Oxygen therapy may be indicated to help distressed breathing and ensuring an adequate supply is essential. Helping the family cope with this situation asks for empathy and understanding.

It is possible to administer co-analgesic drugs in conjunction with opiates via a syringe driver. Figure 9.7 gives some examples of antiemetics, sedatives, bronchodilators and antispasmodics which can safely be mixed with Diamorphine, so relieving the child of further oral or intramuscular medication.

Fits, caused by cerebral metasteses, are not uncommon and can be difficult to manage. They are distressing for families to see and naturally cause great anxiety. Occasionally these can easily be controlled at home, utilising oral anticonvulsants or rectal diazepam. They remain, however, one of the commonest reasons for a child returning to hospital for care or control of symptoms.

Radiotherapy and chemotherapy both have a place in palliative care. Bone pain caused by tumour infiltration and painful pressure symptoms caused by tumour bulk can be effectively treated by a single fraction or a short course of radiotherapy.

ANTIEMETICS
   Haloperidol (Haldol, Serenace)
   Metoclopramide (Maxolon)
   Cyclizine (Valoid)

SEDATIVES
   Hyoscine (Scopolamine)
   Haloperidol

BRONCHODILATOR
   Salbutamol (Ventolin)

ANTISPASMODIC
   Hyoscine

EXCESSIVE NOISY SECRETIONS
   Hyoscine

Fig. 9.7   Drugs currently used in syringe drivers compatible with Diamorphine.

Intrathecal drugs, for example Methotrexate, Hydrocortisone and Cytosine are used when children who have raised intracranial pressure symptoms, caused by leukaemic cell infiltration, are experiencing severe headaches. Both forms of therapy necessitate a return to hospital for a brief period, which may be upsetting for the child – one must be sure the benefits outweigh the necessary procedures.

Where nerve pain is localised and unresponsive to drug therapy, nerve blocks using local or phenol anaesthetic agents or long-term epidural anaesthesia may all have a role. Experienced anaesthetists who have a special interest in pain control, usually in symptom control clinics within hospitals, will advise and employ the most appropriate method of nerve block. Opiate drugs can often be reduced after this treatment and sometimes be stopped. The experience of using nerve blocks in children is very limited.

Transcutaneous electrical nerve stimulation (TENS) (Meyerson, 1983; see also p. 45) is not widely used for palliation of nerve symptoms in children. It may be useful as a non-invasive procedure but, as it involves self-control by the patient and its effect on pain is often brief, it is probably more suitable for a teenager experiencing intermittent nerve pain, to whom its method and effect can more fully be explained.

The use of blood products may enhance the quality of life and treat distressing symptoms in some children. Transfusions of packed cells may be given to a child who is generally well, but anaemia is resulting in tiredness and weakness. Platelets should be infused where thrombocytopenia is resulting in distressing or persistant bleeds. To see overt bleeding is upsetting and causes great anxiety for parents and children, measures should be ensured that this is treated actively.

Nutritional needs

There is a natural need for parents to provide food, warmth and comfort for their children, and it can be difficult for them to accept their sick child's lack of interest or appetite for food. The progression of disease, sore mouth or gums and alteration of taste sensation caused by chemotherapy are some factors which will increase the childs reluctance to eat. Some children may 'pick' at small amounts of food then decide they have had sufficient, others will have 'fads' where one food is requested constantly. Feeling they are not providing sufficiently for the child can cause much anxiety for parents. Food may be an issue on which they can focus their attention when they feel they can do little else to help.

It takes time and gentle encouragement from carers to establish realistic expectations of their childs needs. The ambulant, active child may be encouraged with high calorie drinks or icepops, and a low dose of corticosteroids may stimulate his or her appetite. The child who is less mobile, or sleeping for lengthy periods, will have different intake needs. His or her condition will determine when fluids alone may be sufficient.

Children and teenagers themselves may express their own desire to eat, and worry about their lack of appetite. Their nutritional intake may have been a focus of attention throughout their treatment. Special attention to their needs and calorie supplements to food or drinks can alleviate some of their anxiety.

Oral care

The pain and discomfort which is experienced where the child has a dry or sore mouth, ulcers, gingivitis or candida will enhance his or her reluctance to eat. Particular attention to oral hygiene should be made and any ulcers or infections treated. Soft toothbrushes will help where gums have a tendency to bleed and measures such as tranexamic acid mouth washes may also be useful. Mouth washes containing a locally-acting analgesic, for example Difflam (Riker Laboratories) may help the child to eat when a 'numbing' effect has been achieved.

Oral care packs, or soaked gauze wrapped around fingers should be used to cleanse the mouth when the child is unable to do so.

When the child is drinking, fruit juices will encourage the mouth to feel fresh and will encourage salivation

Skin care

As children become progressively weaker and less mobile, care of the skin is important. A small child is easily lifted and position changed, but this can be difficult for parents of older children and teenagers, or where the child is unconscious. Advice on techniques for lifting or rolling the child will be appreciated. They may also need help with bathing.

If the child is thin and wasted, the use of a sheepskin is indicated. Ripple mattresses may be useful in some instances.

It is much less common to see fungating lesions in a child than in adults, but where this is the case, the appropriate cleansing agents and dressings should be used. Pressure sores may be a problem and specific care to these areas must be given.

Parents are usually very willing to participate in caring for their child's physical needs, and advice is often welcomed from nursing carers.

Responding to ongoing needs

The therapeutic effect of maintaining as normal a family-life style as possible should not be underestimated. Children enjoy playing with other children, or having stories read to them in quieter moments. Their attention can be diverted as their symptoms become controlled. When they feel well, it may be appropriate that they return to school for all or part of a day. When this is not possible, friends and teachers should be encouraged to visit and to include them in their daily life.

As the child becomes weaker, their room may become a central place for family and friends. Where there is space, a downstairs room may be converted into the child's bedroom, so that he or she is not isolated from daily events. Being able to participate in games or conversation may help distract the child and re-establish a sense of wellbeing.

Equipment

Parents have identified a particular area where help in practical terms is welcomed when caring for their child at home (Kohler and Radford, 1985). The provision of home nursing equipment has occasionally proved difficult, but community nurses are expert in mobilising available resources. The most commonly required items include sheepskins, bedpans and urinals, commodes, backrests and bedcradles, wheelchairs or buggies and syringe drivers. Most oncology units have a small supply of equipment which is available for home use. One item which we have found some parents have appreciated is a baby-listening device which can be moved from room to room. This allows the parents to leave the child knowing they will hear him or her should they be needed.

Employment

Caring for a child who is dying is the most stressful time for any parent. It imposes enormous physical and psychological strains on the individual and is a time when most of those in employment feel the need to be at home, to participate in care and share the time left together as a family. Many employers are sympathetic but there may be a need for a sick note to be obtained from an understanding general practitioner during this difficult time.

Finance

Caring for a sick child at home over what may be a prolonged period of time is expensive. Whilst this may seem of lesser importance, real financial hardship can be experienced where there are increased heating and telephone bills and loss of earnings if parents are at home.

It may be possible to obtain an attendance allowance from the DSS, although application of the criteria may seem to be variable. Charitable organisations will often give direct financial assistance, the most well known are the Malcolm Sargent Cancer Fund for children, the Joseph Rowntree Family Fund and the Leukaemia Care Society. (Addresses are given on p. 277.)

It is important that the family is aware of all allowances and grants available to them.

Contact, communication and liaison

Throughout this chapter the need for on-going contact and communication between carers has been stressed. Where disciplinary boundaries and roles are minimised and the channels of communication established early and then maintained, then optimal care for the child and family can be provided. The 'shared-care' management approach is most effective where there is continuing flexibility, good communication and close cooperation between oncology units and community teams (see Fig. 9.8).

Death

Caring for a child who is dying is an emotionally and physically exhausting time. The 'anticipatory mourning' of parents from the time the child no longer receives active

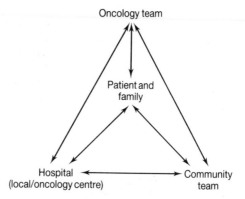

Fig. 9.8   Flexibility, cooperation and communication.

therapy encompasses knowledge of their impending loss with hope, that it will not happen, and despair that it is inevitable (Futterman and Hoffman, 1973). Families grieve at what is inevitable, then may reconcile themselves with thoughts of what their child has meant, and given to others. The emotional detachment from the child as death becomes imminent is a recognition of the inevitability of death, that their child's life will end soon, with no hopes of a future. The final stage, described by Futterman, is of 'memorialisation' where parents develop a mental picture of their dying child, which may be idealised and not actual, but a picture which will remain with them.

The duration of palliative care of children with cancer is variable, usually lasting weeks or short months. Where this time is prolonged, the time of waiting by parents may be fraught with other emotions. Parents have described how they mentally plan what will happen at the time of death, their plans for the funeral and what will happen afterwards. But when death does not happen immediately they may feel guilty for 'wishing it would end' and empty of sadness or 'lost'. The waiting may seem endless. Others may feel a comfort in knowing that it would all end, that they could prepare for life again, with a different normality (Kubler-Ross, 1969). The need for parents to know what will happen when their child dies has been well described (Martinson, 1980; Kohler and Radford, 1985). 'How will it happen', 'Will I know when the time comes?' are common questions. They fear that it will be traumatic, a struggle or that it will be sudden with no time to prepare themselves and their family. The medical issues relating to the progression of disease and its effects should have already been addressed, but parents may want to know what happens when someone actually dies. It has been found helpful to have someone explain the physical changes, changes in skin colour and of breathing patterns (Martinson, 1980). These are the issues which many fear and for which most are unprepared. At the time of death, some parents may ask that a nurse or doctor is with them.

It may also be appropriate to describe the practical measures which need to be taken: the certification of death by a doctor, the registering (an event which may be traumatic) and the arrangements to be made with funeral directors for burial or cremation. Some units may have a prepared booklet or letter which describes the procedures to be undertaken.

The wishes and needs of parents, at the time of death, remain very individual and must be respected. Some will want the formal procedures to begin immediately. Others may want to keep their child at home, to wash and dress them, cuddle them or sleep, holding them. They should be encouraged to do whatever they feel is right for them, to say their own goodbyes.

For siblings, to be able to be with their dead brother or sister and touch them or give them presents and to see that death is not frightening or a mystery may help to allay their fears or fantasies, and so not feel excluded from the adults grief.

Bereavement

The death of one's child has been described as the 'ultimate loss' (Wilson, 1988). It is a loss of part of one's-self, of an individual and of hopes and dreams for the future. No one expects their child or grandchild to lie before they do. Many emotions may be experienced during the months and years after the death by an individual, but it may be more helpful to describe the tasks of mourning which must be accomplished before any person can adjust to their personal bereavement (See Chapter 13).

● *To accept the reality of their loss* Families may initially experience feelings of relief, and release from the stresses of their child's illness. This is often followed by numbness and shock, as they begin the formalities of funeral arrangements and of informing relatives and friends. The practicalities serve to reinforce the issue of the child's death, and allows for a time of saying goodbye and shared emotions.

● *To experience the pain of grief* The aching and longing for their child will be intense. Many parents describe their need to hold, hug and cuddle their child but there is an emptiness which can only partly be filled by holding their other children. No one can replace their child who has died. The pain of grief can express itself in physical symptoms; anxiety and panic, breathlessness, lack of energy, insomnia and loss of appetite are just some of the symptoms described. Some will describe themselves as 'going mad'. They need the reassurance that their grief and feelings are being acknowledged and that these feelings are normal, that it will pass with time and to be encouraged to talk about themselves and their child.

● *To adjust to an environment in which their child is missing* This task is one that cannot be completed early or easily. The daily reminders of their loss are with families constantly: favourite music or television programmes, the child's school friends growing up, an empty chair at a table, birthdays and anniversaries all enhance the grief which is never far away. One of the most difficult questions parents have to answer is 'How many children do you have?' Do they give a long explanation of why there are now two children, not three, or just say 'I have two children', and experience all the feelings of sadness and guilt at denying their dead child's existence. The process of adjusting to a new normality of family life may take years to accomplish.

● *To withdraw emotional energy and reinvest it in other relationships* The need to take up, and enjoy, life again may seem impossible. Parents may cling to the memory of their child, anguish when they feel unable to picture his or her face or to remember his or her voice, and to feel they can never truly enjoy life again. The differing needs of other family members can be difficult cope with, when grief can be expressed in so many different ways. To smile or laugh may seem disloyal and parents feel guilty when they realise a period has passed when they have not thought about the child. Talking about the child, remembering happy times and being able to acknowledge and share emotions are part of the healing process. As time passes they are able to enjoy life again without displacing their memories.

It seems natural that one should try to protect children from the sadness around, but we must recognise that they too have lost a family member, and must also grieve. At a time when they need the closeness of their family most, it may be that other members are not able to fully respond, that their own grief is too intense. Research has shown that when a child has been cared for in his or her own home, families cope better as a unit because they have shared the experience (Lauer *et al.*, 1989). There is less guilt and they feel more able to share their sorrow with the rest of the family. This had led to a more positive and cohesive attitude for the future as a family.

Children will also express their sorrow in many ways. They too are individuals whose feelings must be acknowledged. They may be anxious or worried about being left alone, their security being threatened or about their own health – Are they too going to die? Insomnia, fear of the dark or nightmares and sleepwalking are not uncommon, neither is a regression to more childish behaviour, tantrums and bedwetting. Parents have sometimes said that their other child may never talk about his or her sibling. 'It's as if he never existed, he only wants his toys to play with'. They may recognise the need to keep something of the child who has died, but not so easily recognise other behavioural problems as being related to the sibling's personal bereavement and grief.

Children must be encouraged to share their feelings, to know that it is alright to cry, to be angry or sad. When parents try to hide their own sadness, children feel they too must deny it. They may feel responsible, that death has happened because of something they said or did, or less important and unloved, as attention has surrounded their dying sibling for so long. They need the reassurance and closeness of their family to know that they are loved for themselves and that their feelings are important too.

School teachers and friends are a major part of a child's life. The death of a classmate affects them all. Some children may be reluctant to return to school after their sibling has died. On return they may be easily distracted, disruptive, withdrawn or display what seems to be inappropriate emotions, all of which may be signs of inner distress and grief. A sympathetic teacher and close peer group can give the child support and security to talk about his or her feelings, or just be there when the child feels alone.

Bereavement following the death of a child is longer than after the death of an adult. One study reported that more than 20% of families were experiencing most intense grief at two years after their child's death (Corr *et al.*, 1985). Another 25% said their grief was most intense in the one year to eighteen months period. In many cases, the grief of siblings was experienced for longer periods than that of their parents.

It can be difficult for carers to know how best they can support families through this time. It is the practise of most oncology units to arrange for someone who has been closely involved with the family to attend the funeral. Families do appreciate the presence of someone who has helped them care for their child and who is showing that the child also meant something to themselves.

Maintaining contact by telephone calls and visits is essential. Strong bonds develop between carers and the family as they share a unique experience. Families lose much of the regular contact and input from those around in the months after the death and need to share their feelings with those most closely involved. Where contact is not maintained, families experience a 'double loss', they need to feel that they and their child are still part of our thoughts and that they and their child are still part of our thoughts and that we do care.

More obvious times when contact should be made are birthdays and anniversaries of the death. These are very personal dates which belong only to their dead child, and are usually seen as a great hurdle to be got over. Christmas is another difficult time where there are mixed emotions of the need to have a day which the other children will enjoy and yet be able to grieve for the child who is not there. Families will have many individual ways of spending these days, acknowledgement by carers that the anniversaries are important may help them feel less isolated.

Families are invited to come back to the oncology unit, usually a few weeks after the death, to talk to the physician who cared for their child. Most will welcome the opportunity to be able to talk about their child's illness, treatment and death. There may be many questions to be asked, some will come with lists prepared as they did whilst their child was receiving treatment. The impact of actually returning to the hospital should not be underestimated, it can be very traumatic to pass all the places they so often took their child. For some an alternative office may need to be found, to enable them to take the first steps of returning. They are encouraged to repeat the visit as often as they feel the need and have questions to be asked. Many will visit 'socially' for coffee and a chat, by which they are able to maintain their links.

Families will often focus their attention and energies into fund raising for the parents groups and hospitals, finding a positivity in working for the benefit of other families. Some units may have groups for bereaved parents where they can meet others and share their experiences with people who can truly say 'I know how you feel'. Others may find locally run groups such as 'Compassionate Friends' helpful.

The reactions of other family members or friends can be difficult for parents to cope with. They may meet unhelpful comments, avoidance in the street, refusal to mention the child's name or meet people who are unaware of their loss. Parents reactions will differ to each situation, relating to how they are, feeling at any one time.

It is helpful for those visiting to show that they care and to allow parents to talk about the child as freely as they want. Parents need the reassurance that they did everything they could for their child. Over time, visits and contact will naturally lessen, but even after many months, if carers should think about the family for any reason and wonder how they are, a telephone call will always be welcomed.

Caring for ourselves
To have a child die in ones community is a rare occurrence, even more so when that child is dying from a malignant disease. The experience is a very personal one, where we may question our own feelings about death and its meaning. We may relate the child and parents to our own families and how we would cope with such a situation. In sharing some of their anxieties and fears we often feel inadequate and awkward. But it is in this sharing that carers have much to offer. It can be difficult

when one feels one must be offering practical advice and performing tasks but the majority of help that we can give is by being with the family, establishing trust and being ready just to listen.

Resources are available from the oncology units to help manage specific problems which may be encountered and we must seek to strengthen these links. In working as a team, our own feelings of isolation lessen. During the palliative care and after the death of the child, it is important that we can also talk about our experience and our loss. It does help to share it with others both in our immediate unit and with others who have been involved in the care. Despite the sadness of the situation it can be a very positive and rewarding time.

Acknowledgements

Acknowledgements are due to Dr C. C. Bailey, Dr I. J. Lewis, Mrs P. Fidler, and the UKCCSG for permission to reproduce Fig. 9.1.

References

ARMSTRONG, G. and MARTINSON, I. (1980). Death, dying and terminal care: dying at home. In *Psychological Aspects of Childhood Cancer*, J. Kellerman (Ed.), p. 306. Charles C. Thomas, Springfield IL.

BLUM, R. W. (1984). The dying adolescent. In *Chronic Illness and Disabilities in Childhood and Adolescence*, R. W. Blum (Ed.) Grune and Stratton, New York.

BURNE, S. R., DOMENICA, FRANCES and BAUM. J. D. (1984). Helen House – a hospice for children: analysis of the first year. *British Medical Journal*, **289**, 1665–8.

CHAMBERS, E. J., OAKHILL, A., CORNISH, J. M. and CURNICK, S. (1989). Terminal care at home for children with cancer. *British Medical Journal*, **298**, 937–40.

CLARKE, J. and COX, E. (1988). Heparinisation of Hickman catheters. *Nursing Times and Nursing Mirror*, **84**, 51–3.

CORR, C. A., MARTINSON, I. M. and DYER, K. L. (1985). Parental bereavement. In *Hospice Approaches to Pediatric Care*, C. A. Corr and D. M. Corr (Eds). Springer Publishing Co., New York.

CROW, L. and CROW, A. (1965). *Adolescent Development and Adjustment*, second edition. McGraw-Hill, New York.

ELAND, J. M. (1985). The role of the nurse in children's pain. In *Perspectives on Pain*, L. A. Copp (Ed.). Churchill Livingstone, London.

FUTTERMAN, E. J. and HOFFMAN, I. (1973). Crisis and adaptation in families of fatally ill children. In *The Child in His Family: The Impact of Disease and Death*, E. J. Anthony and C. Koupernick (Eds). Wiley, New York.

HOLLINGSWORTH, S. (1987). Getting on line. *Nursing Times*, **83(29)**, 61–2.

JERRET, M. and EVANS, K. (1986). Children's pain vocabulary. *Journal of Advanced Nursing*, **11**, 403–8.

JOHANSEN, B. B. (1988). Care of the dying adolescent and the bereaved family. *Loss, Grief, Care*, **2(3/4)**, 59–67.

KOHLER, J. A. and RADFORD, M. (1985). Terminal care for children dying of cancer – quantity and quality of life. *British Medical Journal*, **291**, 115–16.

KOOCHER, G. P. and O'MALLEY, J. E. (1981). *The Damocles Syndrome*. McGraw-Hill, New York.

KUBLER-ROSS, E. (1969). Parent care. In *Living with Death and Dying*, pp. 95–159. Souvenir Press.

LAUER, M. E., MULHERN, R. K., SCHELL, M. J. and CAMITTA, B. M. (1989). Long-term follow up of parental adjustment following a child's death at home or hospital. *Cancer*, March 1, 988–93.

LEWANDOWSKI, W. and JONES, S. L. (1988). The family with cancer – nursing interventions throughout the course of living with cancer. *Cancer Nursing*, **11(6)**, 313–21.

MCCALLUM, L. and CARR-GREGG, M. (1987). Adolescents with Cancer. *The Australian Nurses Journal*, **16(7)**, 39–43.

MAUNUKSELA, G. L. and KOLPELA, R. (1986). Double-blind evaluation of a Lignocaine-Pilocaine cream (E.M.L.A.) in children – effect on pain associated with venous cannulation. *British Journal of A* , **5(8)**, 1242–5.

MARTINSON, I. M. (1980). Dying children at home. *Nursing Times, Occasional Paper*, **76(29)**, 129–32.

MARTINSON, I., MOLDOW, D. GAY, ARMSTRONG, G. D., HENRY, W. F., NESBITT, B. E. and KERSEY, J. H. (1986). Home care for children dying of cancer. *Research in Nursing and Health*, **9**, 11–16.

MARTINSON, I., NESBITT, M. and KERSEY, Y. (1984). Home care for the child with cancer. In *Childhood Cancer*, A. E. Christ and K. Flomenhaft (Eds). Plenum, New York.

MEYERSON, B. A. (1983). Electrosimulation procedures – effects, presumed rationale and possible mechanisms. *Advances in Pain Research*, **5**, 405–534. Raven Press.

MISER, A. W. and MISER, J. S. (1989). The treatment of cancer pain in children. *Paediatric Clinics of North America*, **36(4)**, 979–98.

NORMAN, R. and BENNET, M. (1986). Care of the dying child at home, a unique co-operative relationship. *Australian Journal of Advanced Nursing*, **3(4)**, 3–17.

NORTHOUSE, L. (1984). The impact of cancer on the family – an overview. *International Journal of Psychiatry and Medicine*, **14**, 215–43.

O'BRIAN, M. E. (1983). An identification of needs of family members of terminally ill patients in a hospital setting. *Military Medicine*, **148**, 712–16.

OAKHILL, A. (1988). Terminal care. In *The Supportive Care of the Child with Cancer*, pp. 238–57. Wright Publishers.

Office of Population Census and Surveys (1987). *Monthly Statistics: Cause.* HMSO, London.

PAPADATOU, D. (1989). Caring for dying adolescents. *Nursing Times*, **85(18)**, 28–31.

REAPE, D. (1990). Children and pain (pain perceptions). *Nursing Standard*, **4(16)**, 33–6.

SPEECHLEY, V. (1986). Intravenous therapy: peripheral/central lines. *Nursing: add-on Journal of Clinical Nursing*, **3(3)**, 95–100.

SPINETTA, J. and DEASEY-SPINETTA, P. (1981). *Living with Childhood Cancer*. C. V. Mosby, St Louis.

SPINETTA, J. J., RIGLER, D. and KARON, M. (1974). Personal space as a measure of a dying child's sense of isolation. *Journal of Consultant Clinical Psychology*, **42**,751–7.

STEIN, A. FORREST, G. C., WOOLLEY, H. and BAUM, J.D. (1989). Life threatening illness and hospice care. *Archives of Disease in Childhood*, **64**, 697–702.

STRAUSS, M. (1968). *Familiar Medical Quotations*. Little Brown & Co., Boston.

WILSON, D. C. (1985). Developing a Hospice program for children. In *Hospice Approaches to Paediatric Care*, C. A. Corr and D. M. Corr (Eds). Springer Publishing Co., New York.

WILSON, D. C. (1988). The Ultimate Loss: the dying child. *Loss, Grief, Care*, **2**(3/4), 125–30.

Further reading

DENT, ANN (19). *A Child is Dying – Care of the Family in Illness and Bereavement*. Professional Pack. Macmillan Education Centre.

ERKERT, H. (19). *Childhood Cancer : Understanding and Coping*. Gordon and Breach Science.

OAKHILL, A. (1988). *The Supportive Care of the Child with Cancer*. Wright Publishers.

10

Awareness of psychological needs

Morna C. Rutherford and W. Dawn Foxley

'Understanding human needs is half the job of meeting them.'

Adlais Stevenson

Psychological needs are many and varied, reflecting the uniqueness of the individual. As a consequence it would be a formidable task to describe those idiosyncratic needs within the confines of one chapter. A more appropriate approach is to describe the similar reactions people can have in particular circumstances. It is the aim of this chapter to explore these circumstances and reactions. The remit is the psychological needs of people with cancer and their families during the palliative phase of care.

Basic human needs

Heron's (1977) model provides a useful starting point for understanding the outcome of people's reaction to psychological disruption. He suggests three areas of human need.

- The need to love and be loved
- The need to understand and be understood
- The need to choose and be chosen

An individual who has all personal needs met suffuses characteristics such as enthusiasm, confidence and creativity. Alternatively, neglect of personal needs may cause personal distress (Fig. 10.1). It is possible to consider the distress of people with cancer and their families within the context of this model.

The need to love and to be loved

Heron (1977, p. 2) notes that 'the need is satisfied in mutual loving – a shared celebration of individual strengths and differences'. This sharing enables freedom to fulfil other needs and release creative capacity. The need to love and to be loved exists for both patient and family, but the chance of fulfilment can be eroded by the destructive power of cancer.

For the patient, the need to give and receive love may be marred by changes in self-concept. This affects the ability to relate to self which in turn disrupts the ability to relate to others. Perception of self involves awareness of the whole self and will change as self-awareness alters. For example, following diagnosis, the patient may immediately see him or herself in a different way. After being told her diagnosis, one patient said, 'I feel really strange – like I'm not myself anymore. I know I'm the same person I was yesterday, but I feel all jumbled up inside now.' This example shows how difficult it is to relate to a new self-awareness.

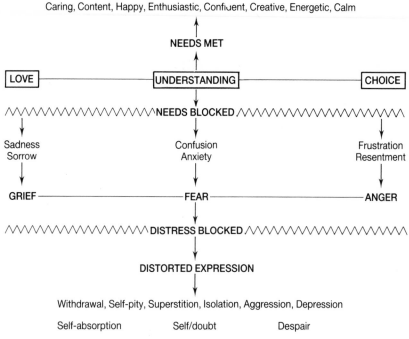

Caring, Content, Happy, Enthusiastic, Confiuent, Creative, Energetic, Calm

NEEDS MET

LOVE ———————————— UNDERSTANDING ———————————— CHOICE

NEEDS BLOCKED

Sadness   Confusion   Frustration
Sorrow   Anxiety   Resentment

GRIEF ———————————————— FEAR ———————————————— ANGER

DISTRESS BLOCKED

DISTORTED EXPRESSION

Withdrawal, Self-pity, Superstition, Isolation, Aggression, Depression

Self-absorption   Self/doubt   Despair

Fig. 10.1   Dynamics of personal needs. (Modified from Heron, 1977.)

Visible physical changes can impinge upon self-concept in a more direct way by providing tangible evidence of change: for example, the surgical removal of a limb. Even body changes which are not outwardly evident can affect self-concept. Another patient described her cancer as a 'Medusa'. Her fear and horror were expressed by this image.

Change in self-concept and fear of the cancer can lead a patient to lose confidence in self and subsequently withdraw from others. Obvious examples are malodorous or disfiguring cancers, change in body function through stoma formation, weight loss or gain, and hair loss. However, uncontrolled symptoms such as pain or sickness can also cause distancing, both physical and psychological, when the need to give and receive love is greatest. The opportunity or ability to love or even be intimate is blocked, resulting in sadness, sorrow and grief.

Just as changes in self-concept affect the way a person relates to him or herself, these changes can in turn affect relationships with others. Griffiths (1989, p. 36) describes how a disfigured person will 'test out' his or her changed appearance. Self-concept often relies on the opinions of people who matter, and a disfigured person will inevitably scrutinise the reactions of family or friends to enable self-adjustment. Families are then doubly saddled with the vulnerability of their loved one and their own reactions also to the changes which affect them.

For families, intimacy with the patient is affected by difficulty in knowing how to relate under changed circumstances. For example, families may avoid handling the person with cancer for fear of causing harm, and if the person with cancer is confused, agitated or drowsy, families may be unable to receive the love they need. It is, therefore, important to make sense of these changes and to find a way of living with them.

The need to understand and be understood

The need for understanding occurs at a practical level and also a personal level for both patient and family. The practical level includes management of functional problems with speech, hearing or language. For example, the use of language and its interpretation may be different for both nurse and patient. At a personal level, it is possible that the patient may not know how to ask for information. The patient has a need to understand the changes which are occurring and, in order to grasp personal meaning, must firstly be understood by the people from whom information is being sought. Wells (1986, p. 22) states that assumptions are made too often about the ability of the patient to understand. Even if in full command of the facts, the question 'Why me?' is only too familiar. The resulting cycle of confusion and anxiety may give way to insurmountable fear. Rapid or unpredictable changes can be difficult for both patients and their families to comprehend.

Family members also need to understand and be understood: care may revolve solely around the patient, and family members can feel that nobody is listening to or understanding them. Anxiety within the family is common, especially when considering future implications of the disease process. Lugton (1989b, p. 50) describes anticipatory anxiety in families coping with dying. She states that it is not so much the prospect of death that makes people afraid, but anxiety about the imagined effects of cancer. Experiencing fear, anxiety and confusion can be overwhelming and further remove people from having control over their circumstances. Exercising choice may help regain some sense of this control.

The need to choose and be chosen

The person with cancer can find him or herself 'forced' into a position of dependancy and professionals often appear to be in control of the whole process of care, producing resentment and anger. Porter (1988) describes how doctors decide who is eligible for the sick role: they label the sickness, decide on treatment, decide on how the sick person should act and they decide on what will happen after treatment. The patient has no real choice about his or her cancer and its effects, and treatments determined by the type of cancer are usually inflexible. In addition, patients may find that they are no longer able to partake in their usual role in life through limitations such as fatigue and decreased mobility which are imposed on the patient by the disease and/or treatment. Other people may no longer seek the patient's participation in normal daily activities for fear of putting a burden on the patient's failing strength, and so the person with cancer finds he or she is no longer chosen to share in normal life events, resulting in a feeling of 'uselessness'.

Family members are affected also by the inability to make choices. In addition they may not be chosen to give any care to the person they love. Nurses may presume to 'know better', take over the practical side of caring, and families can feel totally inadequate and helpless in offering any vestige of caring left to them.

Clearly, the changes involved in the palliative stage of care can disrupt all three personal needs, profoundly affecting both patient and family. Implications for nurses lie in the awareness of the need to enable the giving and receiving of love, understanding and choice so empowering patients and their families with the ability to be more in control and also providing opportunities for greater intimacy and connection.

Further awareness of the reactions of patients and families can be achieved through conceptualising the process involved when change occurs. Change involves transition from the known to the unknown, resulting in a discontinuation of a certain aspect of that person's life. This is particularly relevant to the diagnosis of cancer as many changes occur and are implied. For example, change in self-concept, role and status may be insidious but nevertheless dramatic, and thoughts of premature death are often inevitable following knowledge of cancer.

Responses to transition

Becoming aware of a potentially life-threatening illness initiates particular responses which are individual but may also form a pattern. There is a cycle of reactions which form a framework for understanding the dynamics of transition. It is important, however, to note that some people stick at one stage and do not progress through the whole process systematically. Hopson and Adams (1976, pp. 9–15) and Hopson (1982, pp. 124–6) describe a map of self-esteem changes during transition (Fig. 10.2).

Immobilisation

The first stage of immobilisation reflects the shock involved in response to inevitable disruption of life style. The person may feel 'paralysed' or 'numb' and be unable to think, understand or manage his or her life. When the person with cancer is told the diagnosis, the degree of shock will depend on how much he or she has already suspected. Some people will state that they knew there was 'something far wrong'. Nevertheless, having this knowledge verbally confirmed can still result in shock reaction. The degree of shock will also depend on how the information is conveyed. One patient asked how bad her cancer was, and was told, 'Bad! – don't you know it's terminal?' Utterly devastated, this patient withdrew from the world for several weeks, refusing to communicate with anyone. The family can also suffer shock,

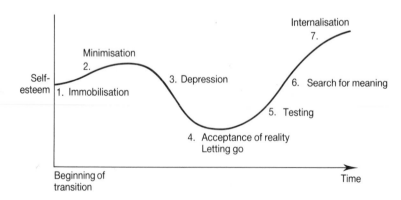

Fig. 10.2   Self-esteem during transitions. (From Hopson and Adams, 1976, p. 13.)

which is related to fear of the eventual obliteration of a joint future with their loved one. Shock takes time to 'settle' and movement into the second stage depends on coping strategies and available support.

Minimisation

One way of moving out of immobilisation is to deny that change has occurred. Some people might say 'It's not possible', 'It can't be happening', 'I don't believe it'. Denial is a coping defence which protects the person from awareness of fear and anxiety. O'Connor (1984, p. 118) states that 'denial of the reality of one's death protects the psyche from the harshness and pain of giving up life.' Denial allows time for meaning to penetrate and for potential strengths to amass, and some people never move beyond this phase. They may take tentative steps onward but the perceived reality of their situation may be so frightening that denial of reality is in effect preventing their emotional disintegration. Nonetheless, continuing changes can erode this defence. The patient may refuse to change his or her life-style, yet there may be little option when the ability to function becomes increasingly limited. The family also may refuse to change, yet awareness of the patient's struggle with life may be impossible to ignore. A deep inner tension results and profound anxiety is often evident.

Anxiety may proceed to confusion, fear and anger. Confusion can be heard when a person says, 'I just don't know how this could have happened'. Fear can be fragmented into fear of the implications of illness and loss, including worry about distressing symptoms and loss of control.

The injustice of loss may be responded to by anger. This anger can be displaced on to symbols of power, such as the medical profession: the person with cancer may feel that this institution has let him or her down and rage is often an expression of this powerful experience. Outrage can be extremely frightening for both the person and for those close at hand. It is dangerous, however, to suppress this anger, as distorted expression may result in malice, aggression or despair (see Fig. 10.1, p. 174). Expressing anger can release tensions, engender creativity and increase insight, but it does not change the situation per se. Realisation of this may give rise to 'bargaining' (Kubler-Ross, 1969, pp. 72–4), which is a belief that there will be a chance of reward for 'good behaviour'. For example, a person may bargain that giving up smoking will extend life, and if the person believes fully in this bargain, then hope is possible.

Depression

Through time the person experiencing transition may be unable to avoid the realities of change and a spiral of depression can ensue. (Lamb and Woods, 1981, p. 137) state that the disease process and treatment sometimes causes patients to 'doubt their humanness and the value of living'.

Depression is a difficult concept to define as it can range from sadness to a tangible, heavy 'blackness' which is overwhelming. Some people may express the way they are feeling in terms of regret at missed opportunities, or in terms of hopelessness or powerlessness to change things. Symptoms of depression, such as chronic fatigue, lack of concentration and sleep disturbances, compound the sense of loss of control over circumstances. Transitional depression is inevitably linked to

```
        Cancer      Treatment      Expectation of Death
            ↘            ↓                 ↙

              L O S S   O F :

Parts of body – e.g. limb, breast, organ
Body function, capacity to function – e.g. mobility, continence, speech
Self-image – e.g. body shape, perception of shape, skin colour
Self-esteem – value of self.
Choice and options – ability for control and independence
Opportunities – chances for achievement
Role as effective member of family – e.g. 'bread winner', parent
Role as effective member of society – standing in community
Status
Loved ones, places, things, projects – precious things
Enjoyment
Memories (for dying person)
Time

              LOSS OF LIFE AND FUTURE

Anger, Envy, Grief, Guilt, Confusion, Anxiety, Embarrassment, Fear
```

Fig. 10.3   Areas of loss and change.

loss. Figure 10.3 lists some losses and changes for a dying person and the family. Mourning of these losses is expressed through grief which can connect with other emotions such as anger, fear and guilt.

As this stage moves towards the bottom of the transition curve (see Fig. 10.2), the depression will reach its lowest point. A feeling of impasse may develop where, at one and the same time, there is a pervasive sense that life may continue to feel this bad, and increasing awareness that there is no going back. A fear of going on may be tied to a suspicion that life may indeed become even worse.

Acceptance of reality

There is movement into this fourth stage as the person begins to look at what comes ahead and gradually unhook from the past and 'how things used to be'. Kubler-Ross (1969, p. 100) describes this phase of acceptance as being 'almost void of feelings'. This is a deep point in the person's life where he or she realises that life has changed and, in order to come to terms with the change, the person must 'let go' of the past.

Testing

Now there is the opportunity to 'test out' this new way of being in life. Even if a person is dying and is, for example, adjusting to paraplegia, that person may still want to see what can be achieved within the imposed limitations. Personal energy becomes available as the trap of depression is 'discarded'. This is a new reality which is being examined and many 'ups and downs' can be encountered at this stage, releasing emotions such as irritation and agitation. There may even be a sense of 'slipping back' towards depression as plans are frustrated.

Search for meaning

Nevertheless, a shift towards trying to understand the whole process helps to increase self-esteem. When a person is facing death, it may seem that everything is lost. However, if this sixth stage in transition is reached, future goals and impending death converge, and finding meaning becomes a significant step towards self-fulfilment. One patient said, 'It's OK to die. I feel a whole new world is opening up to me'.

Internalisation

When meaning is incorporated into life, then growth is possible. Hopson and Adams (1976, p. 5) describe this potential as 'opportunity value' which offers the possibility of increased self-esteem. An example of this can be found in another patient who became severely limited by depression which followed the diagnosis of his cancer. With counselling (see Chapter 15) and the support of his family, he worked through this depressive phase and eventually decided he would 'make the most' of his remaining life. He discovered enough energy to work in his garden hut and use his planning abilities to design kitchen implements for his wife. He described this energy as the freedom to be creative.

Few people move through the transition process in a systematic manner. The progress of cancer and treatment involves many uncertainties and personal variables. Attitude, values and coping are about individual ways of being, and although people have the potential for growth, not every person will achieve it. The transition map (see Fig. 10.2, p. 176) emphasises the importance of completing and moving through each stage in order to achieve increased self-esteem. Awareness of the process involved throughout transition will enable nurses to clarify their concepts in relation to care.

Relationships

So far, this chapter has explored disruption of personal needs and sequential reactions to transition. It is important to consider the effect of cancer and treatment on the individual. However, palliative care will miss an essential dimension of care if professionals involved do not consider the implications and effect of cancer and treatment upon *relationships* within the family. Clearly, if each person within the family is at a different stage in their own transition process, they will have different needs, and may not have the capacity to help each other, yet the *need* to help usually exists. Hospitalisation, treatment, or the disease process itself, may mean separation of family members for the first time in their lives. Distressing symptoms such as pain or confusion can disrupt the close family bonds built in times of health. Within a family there is a need to continue sharing, yet this need is confronted with the need to protect each other. Protection often takes the form of withholding information which may cause pain. A conspiracy ensues which is difficult to maintain and the family may repress their own grief in order to present a controlled front. This causes severe tension which drives people who love each other further apart.

Family members who have not been close to each other for many years may experience complex emotions including guilt, desperation and relief, resulting in arguments and further disruption. This can be confusing to the nurse who may find it hard to appreciate the family background of turmoil and trouble.

The nurse also is forming a relationship with the patient and family, becoming an integral part of the family unit, and as such may be caught up in the tangled web of interfamily affairs. The needs of the nurse become important here, and are explored at the end of this chapter.

There is the additional dilemma of changing interdependency. Margalith (1987, p. 51) states that 'illness in one member of the family imposes demands on everyone else'. A daughter may find herself nursing her mother in a very intimate way. Inherent in this caring is the painful knowledge and meaning of loss, as this is the mother to whom she has always looked for support and nurturing. A struggling young father needs to consider child care, cooking and home management as well as maintaining a vital job when caring for his ill wife. The fight to maintain equilibrium can result in family conflict and breakdown. It is possible, however, for transformation of roles to empower hitherto unknown strengths. Patients have the potential to support their own family: this may be their last gift. It has been found that for some people the diagnosis of cancer may have a positive effect, enabling 'a couple to reassess the value of their relationship' (Lamb and Woods, 1981, p. 140).

Sexuality

Poorman (1983, p. 663) states that 'sexuality is an integral part of every human being and is lived every day of one's life. It is evident in the way one looks, believes, behaves and relates to other human beings.' Sexuality is more than a physical expression; it is all about self-concept, self-esteem, and social role, which combine to form the identity of the person. If true holistic care is to be offered to patients and families, then considering sexuality must be an integral part of that care.

The sexual urge can be very powerful. It can suppress pain and help people forget their troubles, if only for a short while. It allows a feeling of 'normality' (Buckman 1988, p. 125), a time to be valued again. However, physical effects of cancer may produce difficulties in sexual activity. Pain, fatigue and range of movement difficulties are described by Lamb and Woods (1981, p. 143) as the commonest problems. Nausea, vomiting, halitosis, bowel disturbances and discharging wounds can be added to this list. Radiotherapy, cytotoxic chemotherapy and medication affect patients externally, internally or systematically so affecting sexuality and ways of being. Surgery involving genitalia, giving vascular impairment or nerve damage is a more obvious cause of lack of sexual response. Hailey and Hardin (1988) found that patients with sex-specific cancer, for example breast or prostate, are more likely than other patients to experience sexual adjustment problems, and males are more likely than females to experience sexual problems after their illness.

Psychological needs are often associated with physical problems. If physical difficulties arise, the patient may feel unattractive or rejected. This in turn can bring feelings of guilt, anger, or frustration. Some patients try to avoid the whole issue. The resulting isolation and possible depression becomes another burden at a time when support is most needed.

Symptoms or changed appearance which make sexual contact unattractive, bring problems for the patient's partner. Alternatively, the partner may wish sexual contact but fear causing pain or trauma.

Some patients have neither the ability nor the urge for full sexual intercourse yet intimacy and human contact are desired. This is confirmed by Leiber *et al.* (1976), who found that patients with advanced cancer and their spouses experienced simultaneously an increased desire for physical closeness and a decreased desire for sexual intercourse. The importance of touch has long been recognised as essential to human development and this need continues throughout life. The value of holding hands or giving and receiving a cuddle should never be underestimated. Sims (1988, p. 59) states that 'purposeful touch can communicate security, warmth and caring and positively affect emotional self-esteem through conveying accept-ance'. Sexual health problems presented by patients and partners sometimes go unheard. It would appear that nurses do not have enough confidence to deal with these problems (Webb, 1987; Smith, 1989; Foxley, 1989). Nurse education can play an important role here. Sexual difficulties must be clearly presented in relation to biological, psychological and social aspects. If feelings in relation to sexuality can be openly discussed, then barriers, such as embarrassment and conservatism, may be dissolved. Equally important is the nurse's own self-concept in relation to personal sexuality. If this is explored in some depth, then freedom to discuss sexuality and sexual matters with patients and their partners may be enhanced. Facilitating the expression of sexuality can only add to the quality of life (Webb and O'Neill, 1988, p. 136).

Meeting needs

Needs are defined as 'circumstances requiring some course of action' (Concise Oxford Dictionary (1976, p. 729). Enhancing awareness of needs will also encom-pass ways of meeting those needs. When considering the needs of the individual facing death, Orem (1980, p. 145) describes the aims of health care as follows.

To enable individuals to

- Live as themselves
- Understand their illness and how to participate in their care
- Approach death in their own way
- Be with family, friends and health care workers in an environment of security and trust

These aims focus on empowering the patient with control over life, understanding, care, the environment and death. This calls for sensitive care rooted in acceptance, empathy and genuineness. These three conditions are the essential characteristics of a helping relationship and are explored in Chapter 15. It is important for nurses not to make assumptions about patients and their needs, but to make a real attempt to listen to and understand these needs. Facilitating choice marks the respect engendered by total patient care.

When considering how to meet the needs of the family, Hampe's (1975) study of the needs of grieving spouses in a hospital setting offers important implications for the care of *all* family members. She found their priorities as follows.

- To be with the dying person
- To be assured of the comfort of the dying person
- To be kept informed of the dying person's condition, medical plan and daily progress
- To be informed of the impending death
- To ventilate emotions
- To receive comfort and support from family members
- To receive acceptance, support and comfort from health professionals

There is a need to continue sharing life with the patient and this may require permission to be included in the care-giving. Nurses can take the initiative here to plan care *with* the patient and family. It is important to remember that within the relationship of patient and family, it is the nurse who is the newcomer. Gilley (1988, p. 122) states that 'professionals must have a great sensitivity to avoid taking over and being "better" carers than the real carer.'

Respect for the long-standing intimacy of the family's relationship will promote the natural caring capacity of patient and family. Intimacy can be facilitated by privacy, offering the patient freedom to spend time with people who are close. Even when difficult to obtain, ways of being private can be considered with the family. Once included in care, families still need support and comfort, so that they do not feel abandoned.

Reassurance of the comfort of the dying person is only possible if great care is taken to control symptoms and explain progression. Attention to detail, such as the environment and the appearance of the patient, is also extremely important. Hampe (1975, p. 117) states that spouses associated the cleanliness of hospital rooms with the comfort of their mates.

Lugton (1989a, p. 29) looked at the support of relatives in a hospice setting. She found that despite welcomed support, one third of families still found difficulty initiating contact with staff and obtaining the information needed. It is important to create the opportunity for families to ask their questions. Certain disturbing symptoms such as personality change, agitation and breathing difficulties need to be explained clearly. Too much detail, however, can be overwhelming, and the importance of responding with sensitivity to the questions asked becomes funda-mental. Preparation for the future is reflected in the need for concise and timely information. Bond (1982, p. 965) observed that it is not always 'what' is said but 'how' it is said that influences satisfaction.

The process of realisation is filled with many emotions which, if contained, result in destorted expression (see Fig. 10.1). Hampe (1975) found that spouses recog-nised their need to *express* the emotions evoked by increased understanding of circumstances. The nurse can fulfil a valuable role in providing support, privacy and space for those needing to cry, show anger or express fear. In a secure environment and with support, it may be possible for families to start 'letting go' of the person who is near death.

Children

The needs of children and adolescents in the family may be overlooked. It is just as important for a child or teenager to participate in care, to be assured of the comfort of the dying person and to be allowed the opportunity to prepare for change. Unfortunately, well-meaning protection can separate a child from understanding. A vivid imagination will fill gaps and may produce disproportionate anxiety and fear. Margalith (1987, p. 51) notes that the child's resultant behaviour will exacerbate an already stressful situation. Stedeford's study (1984, p. 32) suggests that the most important factors are the parents' attitude to death, their openness with the children and the amount of support they receive from the extended family. Henley (1986, p. 17) offers guidelines for good practice in caring for dying patients. She states that, '. . . It is most important that children should not be cut off from their dying parent.' Encouraging mutual support within the family will facilitate this. Including children in the care-giving and offering the opportunity to ask questions is absolutely vital.

The nurse

Care is a multi-dimensional process which involves the feelings of the nurse as well as those she or he cares for. The person the nurse is caring for is usually a stranger, yet the nurse is involved in a very intimate way. Care-giving can unsuspectingly take a nurse closest to her or his own vulnerability.

Elkind (1982) examined female hospital nurses' views about cancer. Her study suggests that nurses share the fear of cancer felt by women generally. Corner (1988, p. 641) reviewed studies on nurses' attitudes towards cancer. These studies indicate that 'health carers have negative attitudes towards cancer and that behaviour towards the cancer sufferer may be affected as a result.' Maguire (1985) discusses how psychological care can be blocked by nurses own attitudes, vulnerabilities and fears. This results in distancing tactics and avoidance. Alternatively, Reisetter and Thomas (1986) conclude the possibility that a professional nurse provides nursing care independent of attitudes held.

Individualised care demands a willingness to respect a person's evident needs and to be aware of unseen needs, involving care of the *whole* person. In order to respond *fully* to the wide variety of needs present, the nurse must be aware of the factors which impede his or her ability to care. These factors exist within the client, within the nurse, within their relationship and within the environment. Figure 10.4 illustrates some of these difficulties within the caring process.

The diagnosis of cancer, treatment of the illness and course of the disease create a process of change which requires continual re-examination and readjustment for all involved, including the nurse. Clearly, meeting psychological needs is extremely difficult to achieve. Assessment of needs is thwarted by the danger of stigma,

Client	Nurse	Relationship/ Communication	Environment
Physical distress	Expectations	Conspiracy	Lack of privacy
Fear	Assumptions	Ambiguity	Distractions
Guilt	Stereotyping	Dishonesty	Interruptions
Denial	Need for power	Inability to hear	Lack of time
Anger	Need for recognition	Inappropriate language	Lack of opportunity
Embarrassment	Need to be liked	Inappropriate speed of	Noise
Anxiety	Need to be helpful	information	Unattractive setting
Depression	Professional role	Inappropriate amount of	
Withdrawal	Pride	information	
Pride	Prejudice	Lack of clarity	
Expectations	Personal limitations	Beliefs	
Assumptions	Identification	Culture	
Self-doubt	Disguised reactions		
	Fear		
	Embarrassment		
	Self-doubt		
	Pity		
	Distaste		

DISTANCING-AVOIDANCE
DEFENSIVENESS
INABILITY TO COMPREHEND
MISINTERPRETATION

Fig. 10.4   Barriers to psychological care.

interpretation and poor communication, and planning and management of care is hampered by rigid practices and mismatched priorities. Reviewing the structure of care demands imagination, innovation and team work which includes patients and families. Introducing a flexibility which reflects needs may be risky for a nurse who needs to exercise control, but it is through *sharing* control that balanced care can begin. Support in nursing is essential here to enhance the value of the nurse. Support is discussed further in Chapters 15 and 16. Respecting the choices and the humanity of all people involved is the key. If nurses and patients can discard their assigned roles and find ways of relating to each other as people, then a true depth of caring will emerge.

Before she died, a student nurse reflected on the nursing care she was receiving: 'I know, you feel insecure, don't know what to say, don't know what to do. But please believe me, if you care, you can't go wrong. Just admit that you care . . . I have lots I wish we could talk about. It really would not take much more of your time because you are in here quite a bit anyway. If only we could be honest, both admit of our fears, touch one another. If you really care, would you lose so much of your valuable professionalism if you even cried with me? Just person to person? Then, it might not be so hard to die . . . in a hospital. . . . with friends close by.'

Anon, 1970. Reproduced with permission of the *American Journal of Nursing*.

Acknowledgements

See Chapter 15, p. 252.

References

ANON (1970). Death in the First Person. *American Journal of Nursing*, **70(2)**, 336.
BOND, S. (1982). Communicating with families of cancer patients: the relatives and doctors. *Nursing Times*, June 9, 962–5.
BUCKMAN, R. (1988). *I don't know what to say*. Macmillan, London.
CORNER, J. L. (1988). Assessment of nurses' attitudes towards cancer: critical review of research methods. *Journal of Advanced Nursing*, **13**, 640–8.
ELKIND, A. K. (1982). Nurses' views about cancer. *Journal of Advanced Nursing*, **7(1)**, 43–50.
FOXLEY, W. D. (1989). *Sexuality, Nurses and Cancer Patients*. Unpublished Paper.
GILLEY, J. (1988). Intimacy and terminal care. *Journal of the Royal College of General Practitioners*, **38**, 121–2.
GRIFFITHS, E. (1989). More than skin deep. *Nursing Times*, **85(40)**, 34–6.
HAILEY, B. J. and HARDIN, K. N. (1988). Perceptions of seriously ill patients: does diagnosis make a difference? *Patient Education and Counselling*, **12**, 259–65.
HAMPE, S. O. (1975). Needs of the grieving spouse in a hospital setting. *Nursing Research*, **24(2)**, 113–20.
HENLEY, A. (1986). *Good Practice in Hospital Care For Dying Patients*. Kings Fund, London.
HERON, J. (1977). *Catharsis in Human Development*. Human Potential Research Project, University of Surrey.
HOPSON, B. and ADAMS, J. (1976). Towards an understanding of transition: defining some boundaries of transition dynamics. In *Transition – Understanding and Managing Personal Change*. J. Adams, J. Hayes and B. Hopkins (Eds), pp. 3–25. Martin Robertson, London.
HOPSON, B. (1982). Transition: understanding and managing personal change. In *Psychology and People*. A. J. Chapman and A. Gale (Eds), pp. 120–45. Macmillan, London.
KUBLER-ROSS, E. (1969). *On Death and Dying*. Souvenir Press, London.

LAMB, M. A. and WOODS, N. F. (1981). Sexuality and the cancer patient. *Cancer Nursing*, **4(2)**, 137–44.

LEIBER, L. *et al.* (1976). The communication of affection between cancer patients and their spouses. *Psychosomatic Medicine*, **38(6)**, 379–89.

LUGTON, J. (1989a). Communicating in the hospice. *Nursing Times*, **85(16)**, 28–30.

LUGTON, J. (1989b). Identifying anxieties. *Nursing Times*, **85(17)**, 50–1.

MAGUIRE, P. (1985). Barriers to psychological care of the dying. *British Medical Journal*, **291**, 1711–13.

MARGALITH, I. (1987). Holding the family together. *Nursing Times*, **83(38)**, 51–3.

O'CONNOR, N. (1984). *Letting Go with Love: The Grieving Process*. La Mariposa Press, Arizona.

OREM, D. E. (1980). *Nursing: Concepts of Practice*, second edition. McGraw Hill, New York.

POORMAN, S. (1983). Human sexuality and nursing practice. In Principles and Practice and Psychiatric Nursing, second edition, G. W. Stuart and S. J. Sundeen (Eds), pp. 661–86. Mosby, Missouri.

PORTER, S. Siding with the system. *Nursing Times*, **84(41)**, 30–1.

REISETTER, H. A. and THOMAS, B. (1968). Nursing care of the dying: its relationship to selected nurse characteristics. *International Journal of Nursing Studies*, **23(1)**, 39–50.

SIMS, S. (1988). The significance of touch in palliative care. *Palliative Medicine*, 2, 58–61.

SMITH, D. B. (1989). Sexual rehabilitation of the cancer patient. *Cancer Nursing*, **12(1)**, 10–15.

STEDEFORD, A. (1984). *Facing Death*. Heinemann Medical, London.

WEBB, C. (1987). Nurses knowledge and attitudes about sexuality: report of a study. *Nurse Education Today*, **7(5)**, 209–14.

WEBB, C. and O'NEILL, J. (1988). Sexuality and cancer. In *Oncology for Nurses and Health Care Professionals*, P. Webb (Ed.), Vol. 2, 119–37. Harper and Row, London.

WELLS, R. (1986). The great conspiracy. *Nursing Times*, May 21, 22–5.

Further reading

CHAPMAN, A. J. and GALE, A. (Eds) (1982). *Psychology and People*. Macmillan Press, London.

CHARLES-EDWARDS, A. (1983). *The Nursing Care of the Dying Patient*. Beaconsfield, England.

KUBLER-ROSS, E. (1975). *Death: The Final Stage of Growth*. Simon and Schuster, New York.

LUGTON, J. (1987). *Communicating with Dying People and their Relatives*. Austen Cornish, London.

PARKES, C. M. (1978). Psychological aspects. In *The Management of Terminal Disease*, C. M. Saunders (Ed.), pp. 44–64. Edward Arnold, London.

STEDEFORD, A. (1984). *Facing Death*. William Heinemann Medical, London.

11

Spiritual care

The Reverend David Stoter

'For everything there is a season, and a time for every matter under heaven –
– a time to be born and a time to die,
– a time to weep and a time to laugh,
– a time to mourn and a time to dance,
– a time to keep and a time to lose,
– a time to love and a time to hate,
– a time to keep silence and a time to speak'

Ecclesiastes: Chap 3. v 1–7

The nature of spiritual care

Spiritual care is one of the most overlooked aspects of palliative care, probably because it is so often ill-defined and misunderstood, and for many of us fraught with unanswered questions and difficulties. Because of the many surrounding misconceptions some professionals tend to 'back off' and 'leave it to the clergy'. Nurses may ignore it apart from recording the patient's stated religion as part of the Nursing Process record (Faulkener, 1985). So often spiritual care is seen as religious care for the few who request it and therefore becomes dismissed as a footnote, just for the report. While it is important to recognise and meet the needs of those from all cultures and creeds, to see spiritual care only as religious care trivialises and diminishes its true nature. This perception may lead to paying lip service to meeting spiritual needs but in reality giving it a low priority.

It is not only those of us who are involved in the day to day aspects of practical care who find this a difficult subject. Surprisingly, in research studies considering the care of the dying person there are very few references clarifying the nature of spiritual care, although our own hospice movement has its roots in Christian foundations. (Owen *et al.*, 1989). This omission has been recognised during an international conference of experts at Yale University, when they faced difficulties in searching for a definition on the nature of Spiritual Care (Wald, 1986).

What is spiritual care?

The uncertainties mentioned above make it important to clarify the positive aspects of spiritual care from the beginning of our explorations. Spiritual care involves valuing individuals for themselves, each person having his or her own values and beliefs with the absolute right to be an individual needing affirmation of the person they are, and acceptance of their personal views and attitudes to life. Every person is a spiritual being having a spiritual dimension, only a few however have a specific religious dimension.

Spirituality includes the whole range of the person's life experiences, their successes and failures, joys and sorrows, strength and weaknesses. It embraces background, culture, work experience, home and social life – everything in fact that makes for the uniqueness of the person, with a unique capacity to respond to life events and situations. If this view is broadened to take in a partner or family group it follows that they form a unique couple or family group and the patient actually exists within that setting with thoughts, hopes, fears, beliefs or doubts and expectations all influenced by, and individual to, that group. Just as in physical care each factor is taken into account – and not just a simplistic symptom response – so in spiritual care it is important not to look into symptom control alone, but to respond to the situation as a whole for that person or family.

This means acceptance of that individual in totality, and affirmation of each person just as they are wherever we find them. It means accepting their range of beliefs, doubts, fears and anxieties as valid expressions of where they are, and affirming them with no preconditions of our own. This is a sound starting point from which to approach spiritual care, which is a gift of love with no preconditions, reflecting as it does the highest forms of human love, and for some a belief in God's love and acceptance of each of us as we are.

This then is our positive approach and starting point – that everyone has a spiritual dimension, and we need to differentiate between this and a religious dimension; that each individual is unique with personal values and needs, and each responds to a situation and to care in an individual way. This was summed up in a nicely defined statement at the above mentioned conference at Yale – 'it is the patient who defines the territory (for spiritual care) not the caregiver' (Fiefel, 1986). What is important is to recognise the potential of the spiritual dimension as a healing force for the whole person, body, mind and spirit.

The spiritual needs of the individual

Before looking at ways of offering spiritual care appropriate to each individual it helps to identify what the specific needs are, rather than embarking on a programme from our own perspective. The starting premise that each individual has a spiritual dimension, with certain values and beliefs that are unique, indicates that it is difficult to give an easy overall definition of spiritual need. However, we can say that it will vary between individuals, and that needs manifest themselves in several ways. Sometimes they are openly expressed, at others felt and not expressed. They are also relative to other conditions and, as such, may change at different times (Bradshaw, 1972).

It is, therefore, important to avoid sweeping value judgements and making assumptions about what people 'need' and thinking that there are set answers to questions asked. The discussion on spiritual care highlights the general factors which can help in meeting needs, such as recognising that there is a universal need for affirmation and unconditional acceptance, and a need for an opportunity to discover the way forward in a safe and caring environment, acknowledging that everyone is at a different stage on a personal spiritual or life journey.

The religious aspects of spiritual care

An important component of spiritual care is religious care, which needs to be related specifically to the individual's preferences and needs. For this purpose some knowledge of different denominations and of other religions and their practices is necessary to bring understanding of their complexities. Religious needs are discussed further in Chapter 12. Although it is widely recognised that there are obvious differences when considering other faiths, it is important to note that there are denominational differences not only within the Christian faith but within all religions. Even within a particular denomination, Christian or other, there is a wide spectrum of beliefs and attitudes with a diversity of practices. It is important to recognise that although some 'immigrants' remain orthodox within their culture/faith origins, others absorb from western living and education and thereby express more complicated transcultural needs. Therefore, if religious/cultural care is to be approached with sensitivity, it is important to understand these perspectives and find out what is acceptable and comfortable for the individual patient or family.

In the multiracial and multicultural society of today the range of religious beliefs may present a confusing variety of different approaches and practices, and it is helpful to have some information available on the wards or units for reference. For example a list of denominations and other faiths outlining attitudes, practices or specific needs would be useful, together with local contacts who can be approached for information if required. Frequently in large hospitals the Chaplain's Department will act as a resource base for reference purposes. A practical example may illustrate the reason for the need to understand these differences. Nursing staff in a Special Care Baby Unit were concerned when they found a small dagger under the sheet of a baby in an incubator. They were considering calling in the social worker to follow up a perceived threat of non-accidental injury until they were reassured by the information that a dagger is one of the five religious symbols with significant meaning for Sikhs, and as such was placed close to the child's body.

There are several reference books available giving clear descriptive accounts of specific beliefs and practices, which will give the carer valuable insights into religious and cultural preferences relating to food, privacy, worship, and especially to death. An understanding of any of these can make an important contribution to the patient's general well being and quality of life (McGilloway and Myco, 1985; Neuberger, 1987).

Who gives spiritual care?

The comment has already been made that some professionals see spiritual care as the responsibility of the clergy or religious people alone, but when viewed in its true dimension it becomes clear that it involves the whole team and not any one person. However, sometimes one particular person may emerge or be selected by the patient or family as the key person to facilitate their own support, and with whom they feel comfortable. The contribution of the family should also be recognised, together with the need for the back up support of the rest of the team and any necessary specialist input.

The implications for the care giver will be considered more fully later, but at this point it should be noted that often the nurse, because of the nature of the work involved and time spent with the patient, is responsible for the majority of spiritual care. The nurse has a very special relationship with the patient and family making possible an input of spiritual care of the highest quality, especially if there is a willingness to remain open in the relationship and not try to give predetermined answers. Although the observations made in this chapter are addressed primarily to nurses, the principles considered are applicable to any professional involved with palliative care.

Some approaches to spiritual care

Spiritual care poses many questions where few answers are on offer, which may make it seem a threatening aspect of care. It deals with the kind of questions often appearing with the onset of serious illness – questions which need to be explored for each individual in a safe environment starting from where the person is in their own belief and experience, and allowing the discovery of answers when the time is right. Questions are raised like 'Why?' 'Why me?' 'What have I done?' 'What has he or she done to deserve this?' 'What is happening to me?' 'Is there life after death – if so what is it like?' 'Is there a God – if so what is he like?

Other expressions often heard are 'I've done nothing worthwhile with my life', 'Who will remember me when I'm gone?' or 'Why should anyone care about me?' To these questions or statements there are no direct answers or responses which can be handed out in the way pills or medicine are given for specific ailments. An even more complex situation may appear when the patient has a different religious origin from the professional carer, or more difficult still has no faith at all, or views death as oblivion, or has a particular faith when the carer has none or considerable doubts.

A useful starting point is to begin by listening and receiving the questions and doubts as they are presented, and allowing the person to BE who they are, as they are. This is the base line from which to move forward – just to be alongside, in a non-threatening, non-authoritarian relationship which is not demanding or invasive of the patient's personal world of belief. This may present difficulties for some nurses as it is a relationship which requires some departure from the more traditional nursing role of 'delivering care'. It is important to be sensitive however, to the fact that the patient may not wish to enter into any relationship other than the professional one.

The 'history taking' approach using a question and answer method can have a depersonalising effect, giving a preconceived stereotyped photo-fit picture leading to false assumptions about the kind of care to offer. Such direct questions may be intrusive and a more 'oblique approach' is often more rewarding. For example, instead of using a question like 'Have you any children?', a more suitable approach could be to make a comment like 'That's a lovely picture of your family', an approach which may open up a relaxed conversation giving a sense of warmth and trust.

It is natural and desirable to talk about family life and this may well lead on to the patient sharing details about themselves, their families, fears, preferences and beliefs. The essential ingredient is for the patient to become aware that someone is willing to share their humanity. This should not be used, however, as an opportunity for the professional to work out personal problems in this relationship, or project personal needs onto the patient.

The patient may need to 'test out' the nurse to see if he or she has been really 'heard'. For many, once they are assured of being heard the opportunity comes for release of fears and doubts and the 'felt' anxieties and needs are openly 'expressed' as the patient takes the nurse into the darker areas of experience. Some may need to focus on impending death, and its nature, and projection into what it is like to be dead. These are powerful areas of pain and distress which are related to the unknown. Other frequent fears relate to burial, cremation, or being in a coffin; fears are often associated with dying alone, losing control of oneself or suffering pain, or anxieties about the family. Another common fear is associated with forms of loss, in terms of dignity or personal identity, loss of role, or loss of control over personal destiny. All of these are powerful fears especially for the younger patient, where loss of body image may be particularly important. Some of these fears may well find an echo in the carer.

The professional carer in the team

Personal skills needed

It is very clear that the nurse or any professional carer does need to have good listening skills to enable the patient to share these painful areas fully. Such a relationship can create a very exposed situation for the nurse, particularly when there is an expression of despair, as the patient enters into and shares the darkness. The situation may well be so threatening that the temptation is to stop the process to avoid becoming completely lost and deal with one or more aspects through a problem solving model. This feels safer but is less helpful to the patient, who is looking for someone to be with them on the journey as far as they feel able to go – to stay close without judgement or ready answers that could trivialise the situation and need. The professional carer may experience a strong temptation to reinforce their own security by comforting the patient through trite sayings such as 'Don't be frightened' or 'Don't worry, we will look after you'.

This may be a particular area of difficulty for those trying to express comfort in religious terms. It is easier to do something positive to fulfil the nursing role by attempting to bring hope or relief of pain and distress, at a time when the patient is aware of the situation which has to be faced but wants to express it to someone who can hear and accept the rawness and weakness of pain and darkness. It is helpful to know that others do not have the answers to death and dying and that professionals have their own fears and uncertainties about these issues.

The response of the carer then is not in words, but to stay and listen, to hear, and to be eyes and ears to the person expressing the pain as they enter the darkness. With this accompanying hand and presence in the shared experience they may be enabled to express the depth of their distress. Having been heard and accepted in the deepest place of darkness or despair they may find their hopelessness begins to lift as they discover that they feel heard in that most threatening place of all, and now know that in future it is safe to share at depth with that person. This may be followed by a change in perspective as a glimmer of hope comes. An example of a similar kind of experience familiar to most of us is when travelling through a long tunnel where the darkness deepens and becomes more oppressive as we approach the centre. After that point the darkness is always behind and whenever we look ahead we are looking towards the light which, even if it is only a glimmer at first, is getting brighter all the time. The carer needs to accept that this glimmer may be very faint and may remain so.

Part of the process which brings relief to the patient is being given permission to express these feelings without being told they are silly or there is an easy way out. It is not the professional's role to give hope but to enable the patient to discover a meaningful hope for themselves. This may well be the point at which the patient knows the despair is understood and accepted but this insight is something which cannot easily be put into words. It is tempting for the carer to respond by saying 'I understand how you feel' which is never helpful or true – it is the receiving of the shared experience which brings reassurance where words may trivialise the moment. When the patient feels understood they may quietly say 'I'm glad you understand'. Perhaps this listening process is best summarised in the words of Dr Cicely Saunders – for her the phrase 'watch with me' epitomised her approach to spiritual care in hospice work, and she wrote, 'Watch with me, means above all, just "Be there".' (Saunders, 1965).

Skills of cooperation in the team

The whole process and relationship for the nurse in this experience is rather like being strapped into a roller coaster at a funfair. The harness needs to be fixed at the beginning of the ride and the passenger must stay harnessed until the end of the journey and not try to get out. Trying to side step or solve the problem is like an attempt to remove the harness, and to fail to reach the end of the journey. The professional needs to 'fix the harness' and stay in until the end. This may present practical difficulties in terms of continuity of care and is a problem that needs acknowledgement, and hence the importance of teamwork and support. It is important for most people to have one key worker whom they can trust – very few can reveal themselves at this depth with more than one or two people. It is not always advisable or necessary for more than one person to hear the whole life story, and this means there is a need to develop trust between members of the team, and more senior staff may need the humility to value the contribution of less experienced members of the team. No one person can be effective for everyone at all times.

A difficult issue may arise for the team where confidentiality is concerned. By definition the sharing of deep feelings should be recognised as confidential as it is threatening for the patient to feel that his or her personal revelations are common knowledge. There is a fine line to be negotiated between sharing confidences within the team or holding them absolute. Some kind of contract or agreement may be necessary with the patient and the family where information needs to be shared for very good reasons. This is a very important area for the professional who needs to be aware of personal limitations and when to call in the specialist or a more experienced person, and at the same time to show a sense of discrimination about what can be shared.

There may well be a need for the professional to seek back-up and support in coping with personal insecurities and moving forward in a difficult relationship. It is important for a nurse not to pull out but to know where such support can be found and to have ready access to it, also that help is available to identify the problem areas and enable a return to the situation with renewed insight and confidence to see it through, while exploring new territories. It is preferable for a person with specialist skills or more experience to work with the carer, supporting and helping them to carry on rather than taking over the key role, which might have the effect of 'de-skilling' that member of staff in future helping relationships. It is sometimes necessary for a Chaplain or other professional to come in for some aspects of the work which may remain confidential to them. Even in these cases it is important that the nurse retains a continuing responsibility for spiritual care.

The whole area of adequate preparation and available support for staff working in these areas of palliative care is one of utmost importance as it will ultimately affect the quality of care given. These issues will be discussed more fully later in the chapter. Professionals in this field need to be aware of their personal limitations and of the importance of receiving help in resolving these areas of difficulty and sharing their own pain, anger, doubt and helplessness.

The caring team

The patient in the family

In considering the provision of spiritual care it is central to the observations made thus far that the patient is not just the recipient of care offered, but rather a full member of the caring team. (Owen, 1989). The traditional terminology of talking about the delivery of care mitigates against the approach which involves the patient fully in all discussions about progress, nursing, medical and spiritual care. A more usual approach acceptable today sees the individual person within the setting of the family and environment, and as a partner or fully involved member of the decision making team. Thus it is an integral part of spiritual care to help the whole family to feel involved and accepted and to enable them also to question and express fears both with the professional and/or with the patient, which will facilitate open communications within the family.

Unresolved anxieties can create barriers and lead to negative communication – it is important that the legacy left for the family is a good one and not destroyed by premature disengagement or inappropriately expressed anger. Anger expressed at the appropriate time is unlikely to be remembered with bitterness after the death is over. Feelings openly expressed within the family maybe painful at the time, but if accepted in love and openness are likely to be resolved. On the other hand, where the patient feels alone and separated and unable to express feelings openly with the family or with a sympathetic professional, feelings of isolation may follow which may well be expressed in anger and bitterness.

The professional's role

The professional's role is therefore one of enabling and not of taking over. The patient and family need to remain in control of the relationship with one or two provisos. Firstly, it is unwise to enter a conspiracy to deceive which may often be set up in the early stages of illness when the family is shocked and vulnerable – such a conspiracy may well close the ability to relate openly, and disable family communication from the time of diagnosis or prognosis. Secondly, the patient needs to relate to the nurse in two different ways, both feeling confident there is a professional/clinical control present for patient safety, and recognising that, in the spiritual dimension, the patient has the control.

Also the patient and family have the right to establish the parameters of what they are willing to receive and in whatever style and cultural form they desire. They have a right to have their own religious faith or no faith at all, to be individual or unorthodox in approach.

It is important to remember that no one has the right to set out to impose upon another their own way of thinking in this situation. It is one thing to attempt to share our faith with others by knocking on people's doors or preaching from a pulpit, but in these situations we cannot compel people to open their doors or listen to us, so we have no right to expect them to listen just because they are captive in bed and reliant on us for care. If we establish good caring relationships it is highly probable that the patient will ask for our opinions and will then be open to listen – we can then share, because, and as long as, we are invited to do so. We also have the responsibility to provide care for patients of every race, culture and creed – these principles are an integral part of the International Code of Nursing Ethics.

One area in which the nurse may be helpful and have an educative role is in enabling the family to understand what the patient needs, helping them to see how inappropriate it is to deceive, and how this deception closes communication possibilities. It may help if they understand that many patients do know there is a strong possibility that death may not be far off and may not find it easy to express this knowledge in words. (See Chapter 14 on Communication and Chapter 15 on Counselling for further discussion.)

Some important issues for the professional

One issue which may present difficulty is accepting that some patients remain angry and never appear to come through to acceptance of their situation even with constant encouragement and support. This may be more apparent in the hospice approach to care where patients sometimes find the intensely caring atmosphere inhibits their need to express anger forcefully. Nurses need to beware of the danger of matriarchialism in palliative care – of over protecting the individual from his or her stronger feelings by a 'cosseting' approach. While acknowledging the enormous contribution of the Hospice Movement (both past and present), for some people the gentle accepting aspect of their philosophy may present difficulties, when the patient feels unable to express the intensity of emotions and personal experience in an uninhibited way. Professional carers need to be aware of and sensitive to the sharp face of spiritual response, and the whole area of pain and harsh reality of loneliness in suffering as exemplified in the experience of Jesus in Gethsemane before his crucifixion (Luke, Ch. 22, verses 39–46).

Kindness and gentleness have a very positive input for some patients, and for most patients for some of the time. But many need harsh reality to be met with naked realism. It is most unsatisfying to thump a soft pillow when angry or thrown anger at a 'pillow like' person. Professional carers need to accept the patient's right to die angry, or to die not accepting their illness or death – they have a right to continue to fight or to give up. The carer has no right to dictate how or when they shall die, but simply to affirm their right to be themselves.

Guilt for the professional

There is often much guilt created for professionals in palliative care, generated by the fact that they cannot give clear answers. This is especially so where it has not been possible to relieve pain or distress, or where there is not a demonstrable acceptance of the situation. Because of how we are it takes a great deal of maturity to realise that the expression of uncontrolled tears, anger or naked fear is an affirmation of our skills in providing spiritual care and not the reverse which is a negative and more traditional interpretation. These emotions need to be translated into a model which is acceptable to the patient. In the acceptance of the naked emotions, frequently healing and a sense of peace may well follow. There are some for whom these emotions will remain fraught up to the time of death and that is not to be seen as failure on the part of the professional.

Another difficult area arises for some concerning the individual's right to receive the kind of religious or cultural faith care in whatever manner, and from whom they wish to receive it, irrespective of how that may appear to the carer. This means that, at times, the nurse may need to bring in someone to give a form of care which is felt to be 'wrong'. This may mean calling in a priest or representative of another faith or religion. (One obvious exception to this is if someone is asking for some action which is against the law of the land.) There is a need for true humility in all carers, to acknowledge that while they know what they think truth is, others may well see things differently and have a right to do so.

Sometimes misunderstandings arise where lay and professional people use the same words to express different meanings, resulting in confusion. It is important to avoid the use of jargon which is not really applicable in the field of spiritual care.

Another helpful area of preparation is for the professional carer to be assisted to identify and clarify his or her personal beliefs. This will encourage a sensitivity to the patient's uncertainties and explorations and also increase awareness of any possible prejudices arising from a particular personal perspective or belief.

Support in the professional role

There are many ways of offering support through existing networks within a particular organisation. These may include group settings or one to one relationships, in which the feelings of helplessness and questions arising in the palliative care situation may be explored in a non-threatening and non-authoritarian environment. Here the individual is in turn acknowledged, accepted and given care in his or her own personal pain or doubt. In some places programmes of self awareness and self development are available through educational channels and these are enhanced if they can be accompanied by adequate 'on the spot' back up and debriefing in the work place where real life experiences occur. Such programmes are valuable in helping individuals to be aware of their own personal humanity and therefore better able to accept the frailties of others and to become less afraid of failure.

While there may appear to be constant factors within the body of truth, if people look carefully back through their lives, truth is not a static commodity, but it develops and evolves, and most people have a broader and different perception of life and faith from that which they held ten years ago. While the core of a person's understanding of truth may remain essentially unchanged, their perception of truth develops when they make new discoveries on the journey through life. If it does not change they are not engaging with life in the world around them or growing within their own knowledge/faith/belief.

Preparation for the professional role

In looking at these aspects of spiritual care it is apparent that it requires a certain level of maturity and experience in situations which, at times, may feel threatening to the carer. This calls for a degree of adequate preparation and support provision that presents a major area for consideration, which cannot be fully explored here. However, it is worth indicating some ways in which carers can be prepared or equip themselves for this kind of work. It is helpful to build up as wide a personal knowledge as possible about various different religions, cultural and denominational groups, and to understand the thinking of agnostics, atheists and humanists (McGilloway and Myco, 1985). (See also Chapter 12.) This will help in meeting with the patient on a basis of mutual understanding. A knowledge of local resources and culture is also important so that one can learn to communicate effectively with the patient and family.

The team is an important source of support, where it engenders an atmosphere of trust and openness which acknowledges the threatening nature of the work and values each member's contribution. It should be remembered too that increasingly Chaplains are involved in providing care right across the whole spectrum of care and many make a specific contribution to staff support as well as to patient and family care.

Summary

Good spiritual care then is never heavy or intrusive, but natural, human and warm. Above all else it is acceptance by a very human being of another very human being within a safe, affirming and loving environment. Although there are common responses and ingredients within the process of dying and bereavement (Kubler-Ross, 1969; Carr, 1982), and models of care are excellent for understanding the process of dying and grieving, they can be dangerous if used in a prescriptive manner to push or steer people along their journey. Each pathway to death and each personal grief is essentially individual and a unique experience for that person and therefore cannot be standardised in any way (Clench and Neville, 1982). The recognisable stages may not all be present or they may appear all at the same time or in different sequence. Therefore these models, while a useful aid to acknowledging the process, cannot be seen as a definitive statement (Sims, 1988). Good spiritual care demands a close empathy – a closeness and ability to touch and hold appropriately and one of the greatest skills is to use and value silence.

'Never speak unless you think you can improve upon the silence'

Archbishop Michael Ramsey

References

BRADSHAW, W. J. (1972). The concept of need. *New Society*, **30**, 640–3.

BURNARD, P. (1990). Learning to care for the spirit. *Nursing Standard*, **4(18)**, 38.

CARR, A. T. (1982). Dying and bereavement. In *Psychology for Nurses*, J. Hall (Ed.). The British Psychological Society and Macmillan Press.

CLENCH, P. and NEVILLE, M. (1982). *Introducing Nursing.* Series 1, **34**, 1475.

FAULKENER, A. (1985). *Nursing. A Creative Approach.* Bailliere Tindall, Eastbourne.

FIEFEL, H. (1986). Foreward. In *In Quest of the Spiritual Component of Care for the Terminally Ill.* Proceedings of a Colloquium, Yale, USA.

KUBLER-ROSS, E. (1969). *On Death and Dying.* Macmillan, New York.

MCGILLOWAY, O. and MYCO, F. (1985). *Nursing and Spiritual Care.* Lippincott Nursing Series. Harper & Row, London.

MORRISON, R. (1989). Spiritual Health Care and the Nurse. *Nursing Standard*, **4(13)**, 28.

NEUBERGER, J. (1987). *Caring for Dying People of Different Faiths.* Lisa Sainsbury Foundation Series, Austin Cornish.

OWEN, G. M. *et al.* (1989). *A Study of the Marie Curie Nursing Service.* The dying person, pp. 14–16. Marie Curie Memorial Foundation, London.

SAUNDERS, C. (1965). Watch with me. *Nursing Times*, **61**, 48.

SIMS, S. (1988). Cancer and ageing. *Nursing Times*, **84(27)**, 26–8.

12

Religious needs of the dying patient

Bill Kenny

'The Great Learning is rooted . . . in being still, in coming to rest in a perfect equilibrium'

Confucius

All religious faiths have one common dimension; they always deal with the major events of the life-cycle such as marriage, the birth of children and death. While religious faiths have many different forms and also vary enormously in the extent to which they impinge on everyday life, they all contain special rites or rituals dealing with these events.

Some simple knowledge of different religious traditions can be especially helpful when caring for people who are dying. When equipped with such knowledge health care professionals are better prepared to help people face the task of dying with the greatest degree of acceptance or equanimity possible. Our own understanding of our patients' religious feeling may often add something very important to its significance: when we offer someone our understanding of their religious faith, we may actually increase the degree of comfort that the faith can give them.

This chapter deals with some relevant features of the major religions that nurses and other health professionals may expect to meet in an increasingly multi-racial society: its content is best understood by additional reference to Chapter 11 on Spiritual Care.

Religious needs and the nursing task

To introduce this subject it might be useful to notice some very important aspects of any declared religious belief. Firstly, people following religious faiths vary a good deal in their *attachment* to their declared religions: some are *deeply committed* while others are very *casual* (or even nominal) adherents. Nurses can never be sure that a person who declares him or herself as 'Church of England' on the hospital admission form has actually been to church since the day he or she was baptised as an infant. The same may be true of other kinds of declaration, since many people feel obliged to say something about 'their' religion on admission to hospital, rather than claim to have none. For this reason alone, the health professional should always be wary of making easy assumptions about the *personal meaning* of religious faith; we should remember that faith *is* always personal, that any faith is always worthy of respect (even when we may disagree with its teachings), and that all *appearances* of faith (or its absence) can be deceptive.

Since most people are judged by their behaviours, unless great care is taken a person's feelings about religion may easily be wrongly assessed. When religious faith seems deeply held and obvious, for instance, health professionals may feel that they can help provide facilities for its observance fairly easily. This may be a false assumption however. One significant aspect of many religious traditions is that they help people feel a separate and perhaps special kind of *identity* that distinguishes them from others. This can manifest itself in a variety of behaviours (by patients and relatives) that cannot be otherwise easily understood. Since by far the commonest difficulty that health professionals face is to deal with patients whose declared religion is one of which they have no personal knowledge at all, some recognition of the idea of special identity defined by religious observances can be an extremely telling factor in a patient's judgments about the standard of care he or she receives.

Good nursing will try to attend to the needs of people whose faiths pervade all aspects of living: certain religious practices can determine the types of food, clothing, work, arrangements for hygiene and leisure activities that people keeping the faith can accept. In such cases there is no essential difference between sacred and secular activities. Then, virtually *all* daily activities have some religious significance. A patient with this kind of religious background will make judgments about good nursing care that are influenced by the extent to which he or she feels the religious aspects of his or her lifestyle are understood.

Alternatively, sometimes people can be deeply (and seriously) religious in some traditions, without any obvious demonstrations of their faith. Some religions do make very clear divisions between secular life and sacred practice. The correct religious observances for them may be confined to set times in the day, week or year carried out in complete privacy, and there may be few other behavioural clues to suggest how deeply held religious faith may be. To offer good care here, the carer may have to be exceptionally alert to a person's behaviour, constantly looking for clues as to whether or not this kind of person's basic needs for privacy and quiet are being met adequately.

Lastly, in thinking about people who seem to have little interest in religious expression, we should remember that many people facing death find that half-forgotten religious questions suddenly become significant again. These questions may sometimes have *frightening* as well as *comforting* aspects. Since most religious ideas are acquired in childhood, and because they may not have been developed or considered since that time, there may be a real need for some people to re-evaluate or to reaffirm something of their declared faith despite having ignored it for a lifetime. Nursing that recognises this kind of problem is clearly very sensitive and thoughtful, and may have considerable significance to a patient and his or her relatives.

Because of their constant contact with patients and their families, nurses may be key figures in ensuring that their patients receive religious support that is really appropriate for them. Nurses relationships with patients are such that the sparse information contained in admission forms can be expanded into insightful assessments of patients needs for religious care. To be able to do this well nurses may need to acquire a little specialised knowledge and some particular sensitivities. A good deal can be achieved, however, by remembering that it is always *difficult* for patients to practice their religions in hospitals.

Religious observances always need some form of privacy, some dedicated time in terms of opportunities for them, and may also need some special facilities. Good nursing care can usually provide the first two of these and may often be able to arrange for the provision of the third, by making some fairly simple arrangements.

Maintaining contact with hospital chaplains, and collection of literature on the requirements of major religions which is easily accessible to all staff who might need it, are two very practical things that nurses can do to meet the needs of patients. Above all else, however, it is nurses' traditional abilities for open-mindedness and their observational skills that create the greatest possibilities for ensuring that religious needs of patients are met. This is why nursing can make such a singular contribution to a neglected aspect of care for the dying patient.

Varieties of religious practice

In the same way that different levels of commitment are hidden within the simple statements in records, it is also clear that two people whose recorded religion is the same may practice different *versions* of the religion. All major religions have different branches whose practices may differ markedly from one another. In the short accounts of major religions that follow, only the themes common to all branches are mentioned. To learn more it will be necessary for readers to seek out and consult an appropriate leader from the religious tradition about which information is required.

Buddhism

Buddhist teaching is a prescription for ethical behaviour and spiritual well-being that informs all aspects of everyday living. Buddhists are not theistic; they do not believe in a personalised God but revere the Buddha as an example of right living. Buddha nature is said to exist in every person and is released by prayer, purification, meditation and virtuous conduct.

Buddhists respect all forms of life and follow a pathway of compassion for every living creature, of service to others and of generosity. All Buddhists believe in reincarnation and choose to live in a way which they believe affects the subsequent lives that may follow this one. Aspects of right living in the Buddhist tradition include practising selflessness, not killing, fasting at appointed times and developing unfailing compassion.

Buddhists are opposed to abortion, euthanasia and contraception that acts after conception. They do not usually object to transplants or transfusions. Diets vary according to climate but many Buddhists are vegetarian. Fasting days occur on New Moon and Full Moon days. Festival days take place on Buddha's birthday and death day, his enlightenment, his first Sermon and others. On such days Buddhists eat at the regular times, which means before 12 noon and not afterwards. A quiet place for meditation and prayer is a helpful facility for Buddhist patients: they will advise on the times when such a place is most helpful to them.

A Buddhist priest should be informed as soon as a Buddhist dies. The priest will say prayers over the body and will conduct a burial service, advising on its appropriate timing after the death. Since there are several schools of Buddhism, most Buddhist patients and their families will be happy to advise on a priest who should be contacted when they are admitted to hospital.

Major Asian religions: Hinduism and Sikhism

Hygiene is exceptionally important in Asian religions. All Asians will need water for washing in the same room as the WC itself. They will require a container of water if a bedpan has to be used and Hindus prefer free flowing water for washing (for example a shower), rather than sitting in baths.

Asian women are very modest. They will prefer a female doctor and female nurses, will be uncomfortable in mixed wards and will need great care with hospital clothing, for example gowns, because of over-exposure of the body. Some men may prefer male doctors and male nurses.

Hindus

Hindu men have three names, a personal name first, a complimentary name second and a family name third. The family name equates to the surname, the personal name to the 'Christian' or 'given' name. Hindu women have a personal name and a family name.

Hinduism is an old religion with thousands of gods and goddesses who are thought by some to be different manifestations of one God. Hindu deities are hierarchic with three supreme gods – Brahma the creator, Shiva the destroyer and Vishnu the preserver. Hinduism is divided into many sects and according to Neuberger (1987) the majority of Hindus in Britain are Vishnavites, worshipping Vishnu principally and his incarnations as Rama and Krishna. Hindu religious literature includes the Vedas, the Upanishads and the Bhagavad Gita. Hinduism was responsible for the caste system which, although now illegal in India, may have some remnants in relationships among older Hindus. Brahmins (the priestly castle) were the highest order and Haridjans (Untouchables) the lowest. Menstruating women and mourners are temporarily untouchable during the purifications required of them at these times.

There is no standard form of Hindu worship. Attendance at the Temple ranging in frequency from twice daily to once weekly may be required however, dependent on sect. Worship may consist of meditation, prayer and Yoga exercise. Central to all Hinduism is the belief in progressive spiritual development as life itself progresses so that early attachment to worldly necessities gradually gives way to loosening of physical and emotional ties to worldly things. Ultimately Hindus wait for death as freedom from the world and unification of the spirit with God. The idea of Karma is also central to Hindu thought: Karma indicates the extent of spiritual progression and return to earth in various life forms may be necessary (in higher or lower forms) for further spiritual development, dependent on conduct in the present life. In hospital patients will usually require privacy for meditation and prayer: this should allow them to be completely alone if they require it. They will also need space to keep small idols or pictures of gods, charms and flowers related to their worship.

Hinduism has its own science of life and medicine, Ayurveda, which recommends practices for sleep, diet, defaecation, exercise, sexual activity and personal hygiene. Illness is believed to be a function of the life led and final illness may cause a Hindu patient to be concerned that his life was faulty and somehow causal of the illness. Death, however, may hold little fear because Hindus believe that death leads to oneness with God.

Hindu thought and Ayurvedic medicine require that patients will need special facilities for washing and for their diets. Washing the body requires running water, and is part of purification rituals, but additionally washing the hands and rinsing the mouth are needed before and after eating. Diet is often vegetarian, has a total ban on beef which includes any suspected contamination of other foods by beef in any way at all. Many patients will prefer their food to be brought from home rather than risk breaking food taboos in a hospital setting. Fasting is common, especially among women and great care is necessary to overcome the religious need for fasting in circumstances where it might be dangerous to health.

Last offices for Hindus must be performed by Hindu priests, Brahmins. They will assist dying patients with acts of worship and will reinforce Hindu ideas about the meaning of death. Cremation is always required after death: Ganges water will be needed for the ceremony but priests will provide this. There are no taboos about handling bodies by non-Hindus following death.

Sikhs

Unlike Hinduism, the Sikh religion is monotheistic. It has no priesthood and is essentially organised by and identified with a Sikh *community*. The centre of religious activity is the temple or gurdwara. Sikhism has a strong tradition of hospitality (towards other Sikhs and non-Sikhs alike) and has no caste system. Sikhs follow the teachings of the 16th century spiritual leader, Guru Nanakh: these emphasise the importance of a virtuous life, and individual relationships with God. Sikhism stresses virtuous involvement with the world, stresses family, friends, community and service, instead of the ascetic practices and unworldliness of Hinduism. Both religions share beliefs in reincarnation, and cycles of birth and rebirth through which each soul must progress before perfection is achieved and unification with God is attained. Karma is also a feature of Sikhism, leading to belief in living a good life and so affecting the progression of the soul.

Sikhs have visible symbols of their faith which are extremely important to them. These are uncut hair (in both men and women) which men cover in a turban, a comb which must be retained at all times even when not worn in the hair, a steel bangle worn on the right wrist (except for left-handed Sikhs who wear it on the left), a symbolic dagger which is worn at *all* times and special shorts which are nowadays a symbol of modesty and sexual morality. Great care must be taken by nurses in dealing with any of these symbols: it may be exceptionally difficult to remove any of them from a patient *for any reason.*

Some food restriction are observed by Sikhs. Meat must be killed in the halal way (see p. 204) approved by Moslems, and some Sikhs will eat neither beef (following the Hindu tradition) or pork (following Islam). Many Sikhs are vegetarian and some will not eat eggs. Alcohol is forbidden and tobacco is found distasteful.

The Sikh holy book is the Guru Granth Sahib, written in Punjabi but in a special alphabet. Sikhs who are dying are likely to feel extremely cut off from their temple because it is the focus for all Sikh life. The local temple will usually send people round to a hospital to sit with a dying person if here is no family. Sikhs also have a tradition of private prayer which involves rising early to shower and to pray for one or two hours before breakfast. Privacy is greatly appreciated and assistance with washing before prayer, when the patient needs this help, will be welcomed.

A dying Sikh's family will prefer to remain with him or her and the family may wish to be responsible for last offices. After death, nurses should not attend to the body other than by closing the eyes and wrapping the body in a plain sheet without religious emblems of any sort. The family will prepare the body for cremation by washing and dressing it. Cremation should take place as soon as possible after death.

There is an important point to note about Sikh names. All Sikh men have the middle name or title Singh, and all women the middle name or title Kaur. The order of names is as in Hinduism: personal name, Singh or Kaur (both of which are honorific titles) and then the family name. Sikhs prefer to be known by their personal name and the honorific name, which is why all Sikh men seem to be called 'Mr Singh'. Their wives are not 'Mrs Singh' but 'Mrs Kaur'. The correct name for identification purposes in official records is, however, the last or family name.

Islam

The religion based on the teachings of the prophet Mohammed is called Islam. Its followers are called *Moslems* or *Muslims*: they may come from all over the world but the majority come from Arab countries, from Bangladesh, Pakistan and North Africa. Because Islam is so widespread, Moslems may speak a variety of languages including Arabic, Urdu, Punjabi and Gujerati. Moslems believe that Mohammed was the last in a long line of prophets which included Moses, David, John the Baptist and Jesus.

According to Islam, Mohammed completed the work of his predecessors. Islam teaches that Mohammed was a mortal man, not a mediator between men and God but was a special teacher of the message that everyone is called to the service of the One God, Allah and should try to live perfectly according to God's Holy Book the Koran (Quran). There are five religious duties imposed on Muslims, the five pillars of Islam. These are having faith in God, daily prayer, fasting during Ramadan (see below), giving alms to the poor and making a pilgrimage (hajj) to Mecca.

All Moslems say prayers five times each day. The times for prayer are, after dawn, noon, mid-afternoon, just after sunset and at night. The observance of these prayer times is affected by variations in daylight hours in Britain: so that the prayer day is extended in summer and compressed in winter. Moslems must wash before prayer, and prayers must be said on clean ground (or on a mat) while facing Mecca. Shoes are removed and the head covered before prayer begins. Friday is the holy day for Moslems: all males over 12 will go to the mosque. Women will either be provided with a private room in the mosque, or will stay at home for their prayers.

Washing the body is of great importance in devotions. Facilities to wash in running water are imperative and may create some difficulty for a bed-ridden patient, even though seriously ill people are technically exempt from these obligations. Moslems must also wash after urination or defaecation and cannot pray unless they do so. A Moslem patient may wish to be given a jug from which water can be poured in order to wash after using a bed-pan.

Modesty is exceptionally important to Moslems. Women's clothes traditionally conceal the shape of the body and Moslem women will expect to remain fully clothed even at night. Moslem men are also very modest: they are always clothed from waist to knee even in the presence of other men. Older Moslems, including men, may insist on keeping their heads covered at all times. Moslems will expect to be cared for by nurses and doctors of the same sex as themselves.

Moslems eat Halal food, meat from animals killed by a Moslem over which prayers are said. Pork meat and blood are forbidden and all types of alcohol are prohibited. This may include alcohol in drug preparations. Fasting occurs during the month of Ramadan (which occurs at different times each year, because the Islamic calendar is lunar) and may have special significance for a person who is dying because the observance of Ramadan will be an opportunity for personal reconciliation with God. During Ramadan food may be taken only before dawn and after sunset. Neuberger (1987) notes that even very ill people may insist on fasting and that the fast requires nothing to be taken into the body during fasting hours. This may include drugs and may therefore cause problems with pain control regimes.

Moslems believe in life after death, so that death may be accepted by relatives as only a temporary separation. The family will offer prayers for a dying patient and the dying person should be placed with his or her face turned towards Mecca. The local mosque will provide someone to pray over a dying person if there is no family. After death, the body should be buried as quickly as possible, and the body should not be touched by hospital staff. If touching by a non-Moslem is essential, disposable gloves should be worn to avoid actual contact. A family member (or perhaps someone from the local mosque) will attend to the body. Post-mortem examination should be avoided if legally possible: organs should be buried inside the body.

Judaism

Judaism considers that there is one universal God with whom Jews have a particular and personal relationship. Jewish religion and culture are closely mixed together. After centuries of dispersal from their land of origin, Israel, Jews have spread throughout the world and may be indistinguishable in appearance, dress and behaviour from any other member of their present home country. Nonetheless, many Jews feel that they have a separate cultural tradition which unites them with all Jews in other countries and transcends national boundaries. Religious practice is one important aspect of this tradition. Judaism is based on the Torah or Pentateuch (the five books of Moses) of the Old Testament. Orthodox Jews believe that God literally handed the Torah to Moses on Mount Sinai and dictated the Ten Commandments to him. Progressive (reform or liberal Jews) believe that the Torah is divinely inspired and was written down by different people at different times. The principal religious precepts of Judaism are to worship one God, to carry out the ten commandments and to practise charity and tolerance towards other human beings.

All Jews derive comfort from keeping the Sabbath (from nightfall on Friday when candles are lit, to the sighting of three stars on a Saturday night) and observing the Passover. Orthodox Jews regard the Sabbath as a day of rest: they will not write, travel (except to the Synagogue), work, cook or switch on electrical appliances during the Sabbath. The Passover, a celebration of Jewish freedom from Egyptian slavery, requires special food, unleavened bread, bitter herbs, cinnamon, apples and wine.

The centre of worship is the synagogue where services take place on Friday evenings and Saturday mornings. Orthodox congregations may hold discussion groups on the holy books, led by Rabbis, on Saturday afternoons. Other important Jewish religious festivals are Yom-Kippur, the day of atonement, usually falling in late September or October, when 24 hour fasting is required, and the Jewish New Year. Yom-Kippur is regarded by many Jews as the holiest day of the year and, if health permits, most would prefer to keep the day quietly in prayer and a mood of penitence, to set the path for the year to follow.

Jews are subject to many dietary restrictions. All meat must be kosher (fit) from animals killed in a humane way (with as much blood as possible drained from the animal) and prepared by soaking and salting by specially trained personnel. Pork is absolutely forbidden, as are shellfish, and most Jews will have considerable qualms about mixing milk and meat at the same meal. The ban on this mixing includes a requirement to keep utensils for milk and meat completely separate.

There are no last rites in Judaism. Orthodox Jews claim to believe in an after-life and the physical resurrection of the dead, but there are wide variations in actual belief. A dying person may, however, ask to see a Rabbi who may offer prayers including the Shema Yisrael, the first line of which the patient may be encouraged to speak – 'Hear O Israel, the Lord is our God, the Lord is one'. Judaism expressly forbids any form of euthanasia but allows the withdrawal of treatment when death is near, and so also obviously allows the control of pain and severe discomfort.

After death, the body is traditionally left for eight minutes or so with a feather over the mouth and nostrils to ensure that breathing has ceased. The body is prepared by washing and dressed in a shroud before being placed in a coffin. Mutilation of the body is not permitted except when post-mortem examination is necessary. The funeral usually takes place within 24 hours; cremation is forbidden. Family mourning of seven days is required in Judaism, during which time prayers are said and mourners visit the household.

Christianity

Christians of all denominations believe that Jesus was the human embodiment of a loving, just and personal God. As the Son of God in human form, Jesus has set all Christians an example of God's mercy in action and has provided a remedy for human sin through the personal sacrifice of the Crucifixion. The triumph of Jesus over death, through his resurrection from the grave, and ascension to heaven to be with God is the symbol of all Christian hope.

Virtually all Christians believe in an after-life, although their visions of this may vary considerably. Christians of a fundamentalist persuasion believe both in Heaven, a place of perfect existence in which God is revealed clearly, and also in Hell, a place of darkness and torment in which the souls of unredeemed sinners are cut off from God eternally. More 'liberal' but committed Christians may have different and less polarised views of the after-life. All Christian theologies, however, teach that a new spiritual birth comes about by accepting Jesus into one's life, as Saviour and example. All Christian denominations celebrate the festivals of Christmas, the birth of Jesus, and Easter, the death and resurrection of Jesus, although some traditions celebrate the festivals on slightly different dates from others.

There are some important differences in required last offices and burial rites between different Christian denominations. Roman Catholic Christians who are dying will wish to make confession (if they are able) and to have a priest administer 'the sacrament of the sick', sometimes known as 'last rites'. The priest annoints the patient with oil, prays to God to ease suffering, and administers absolution – a statement of God's forgiveness for past sins. After death Roman Catholic families may prefer that the deceased person's hands are placed in an attitude of prayer holding a crucifix or a rosary.

There is no universal equivalent to 'last rites' in the Protestant Christian tradition; chaplains may pray with the dying patient or may administer communion if the patient is able to receive this. Some Anglican patients may however wish to receive the 'sacrament of the sick' since certain branches of the Anglican church are quite close in belief and practice to the Roman Catholic tradition.

Christians of the Orthodox tradition (Greek or Russian) may be comforted by having a small icon near them, in addition to the more usual prayer book, Bible and crucifix of other branches of Chrsitianity. An Orthodox priest will be welcome to the dying person and may hear a last confession, anoint the patient with oil and given communion. There are no special difficulties about handling the body after death. Orthodox Christians are usually buried rather than cremated and there may be a formal lying-in-state in their church so that family and friends may pay their last respects.

The nurse's own religious views

Like anyone else, nurses and other health care professionals may hold religious views themselves or may have none. In one sense the meeting of patients religious needs asks the greatest degree of professionalism possible from nurses, because it may be necessary for them to set aside their own religious views in favour of those of their patients.

Where nurses own views are deeply meaningful and important to them, they may be tempted (reasonably enough) to offer them as a source of comfort to people in distress. Perhaps this should be guarded against. The argument throughout this chapter has been that, in offering care to dying people, the patient's own religious views are what matter most, simply because it is always difficult for a person from one religious tradition to understand the personal meaning of a different tradition. To this idea might be added, the thought that death is in some sense a summation of life: if religious belief has been any part of that life then the opportunity to deal with unresolved questions about belief is extremely important. By doing this well, a dying patient may find that the whole of his or her life suddenly makes perfect sense.

Robert Pirsig in his book *Zen and the Art of Motor Cycle Maintenance* expresses this thought clearly when he says, 'Sometimes when you look at where you're at and look back at where you've come from, a kind of pattern seems to emerge. Sometimes you can use the pattern of the past to see more clearly where you're going to next'. Good nursing that attends to the religious needs of patients can certainly help this kind of process along. To do this well is surely to see holistic nursing in action.

References

NEUBERGER, J. (1987). *Caring for Dying People of Different Faiths*. Lisa Sainsbury Foundation Series, Austin Cornish London.

Further reading

Our Ministry and Other Faiths: a Booklet for Hospital Chaplains (1983). CIO Publishing, London.

13

Bereavement

Jenny Penson

'A man's dying is more the survivor's affair than his own.'

Thomas Mann (1875–1955)

The experience of being bereaved and the grieving that follows the loss of someone loved is as old as life – and death – itself. Bereavement is a natural phenomenon regardless of whether it is discussed in terms of attachment and separation (Bowlby, 1981) or as a process (Parkes, 1972), as a series of tasks (Worden 1984). Bereavement affects people of any age, and all social classes.

It was the philosopher Ivan Illich (Illich, 1976) who first alerted us to the possible dangers of the 'medicalisation' of life events. By using this term, Illich means that the management of natural events like birth and death may be taken over by the medical and nursing professions, causing power and control to be taken away from the individuals experiencing them. It seems possible, therefore that the significance of bereavement can be overstressed in terms of morbidity and mortality and, by providing professionally-run bereavement services, wrongly begin to treat this natural event as an illness.

It seems to be part of the philosophy of our times that our health and well-being are considered to be our own responsibilities. This may lead people to think that everyone should be able to cope with bereavement by drawing on skills that they have used in the past. If this were so, there would be no need for outside interventions of any kind. The corollary to this view is to ask the question, 'Is providing supportive care simply a matter of common-sense?' It may then be argued that Tender Loving Care may be all that is needed. If helpers have been bereaved themselves (and almost everyone has experienced loss in their lives), this might constitute sufficient preparation for them to be able to reach out to others. Additionally it might properly be asked, 'If the helper means well, would not all *be* well?'

Perhaps not. Some balance between these opinions may be required. Lack of knowledge and skills can make any helper feel inadequate. Lack of self-awareness might cause helpers to be over-protective or over-sentimental in their approach.

The aims of this chapter therefore, are to add to the knowledge that most nurses have about bereavement and hopefully to stimulate some reflection by helpers. This is necessary because it is part of the philosophy of palliative care to provide comfort and skilled support to patients' relatives whenever this is needed.

The definition of bereavement which I find most helpful is, 'to be robbed of something valued'. This indicates that something or someone has been wrongfully and forcibly taken away from you – wrongfully and forcibly in the mind of the bereaved. The key concept for understanding bereavement is therefore *loss*. Caplan (1964) suggests that the emotions felt after losing someone you love may be similar to those felt in other kinds of losses. In their work, nurses become aware of the feelings of loss which many patients experience as a result of their illness or its treatment. Examples are the loss of familiar body-image felt by patients after a colostomy or mastectomy, or as the result of the reduction in weight that can occur in cancer. The loss of a limb through amputation is a further example. When you are bereaved you have lost a part, perhaps a very substantial part, of yourself.

In your professional life you will have felt sorrow at the death of a patient you have known and liked for some time, someone whose age or personal situation perhaps reminded you of your own. These kinds of deaths touch us all – but still from a distance. If you have lost someone deeply loved, for whatever reason, then you know that this is a devastating event, shattering confidence in the future and changing your life forever. You feel you will never be the same person again and may not want to be. To explain these events the nature of grieving can be looked at from two perspectives. The first is that of Parkes who sees bereavement and grieving as a *process* which he describes as the 'cost of commitment' (Parkes, 1972). The second is that of Worden who sees bereavement as a *series of tasks* to be completed (Worden, 1984).

Bereavement as a process

According to Parkes (1972), bereavement is a process that has four distinct phases occurring in order. Each phase is characterised by particular emotional states and each must be experienced before the bereaved person can move on to the next. Parkes' phases are:

- Experiencing the pain of grief
- Experiencing fear, guilt, anger and resentment
- Experiencing apathy, aimlessness and sadness
- The emergence of hope and moves in new directions.

Phase 1: The pain of grief

For everyone who experiences the death of a loved one, there is first of all a sense of shock, and this may be felt even when the death has been long expected. This initial shock and numbness may last for several days allowing relatives to cope, often very efficiently, with all the necessary practicalities of bereavement and may help to carry them through the ordeal of the funeral.

It is not until the numbing effects of shock have started to wear off that the bereaved person begins to feel the physical intensity of their loss. Only then can they begin the long process of coming to terms with it. Mind and body are not two separate entities and so each influences the other. Grief may therefore be felt as a very physical pain, and newly bereaved people frequently complain of symptoms such as chest tightness, palpitations, shortness of breath, loss of appetite and insomnia. Bereaved relatives may also experience physical symptoms similar to those of the person who died.

The pain of grief may also be experienced as a sense of isolation and loneliness. Often this begins with nursing the ill person at home, which may involve drastic changes to life-style and the need for commitment to caring throughout the 24 hours of the day, even though help may be available within the community. If the patient is in hospital then life revolves around long daily visits. There is usually a need for carers also to take on the obligations and chores normally performed by the patient. The demands from the practicalities of living together with the emotional toll taken by the caring situation tend to separate the bereaved person from other people even before the death of the loved one occurs.

Phase 2: Fear, guilt, anger and resentment

These are strong emotions and it may be a relief for them to be expressed. They are not as Lindemann (1944) has put it, 'uniquely wicked': they are also not uncommon. Fear may be felt as insecurity or a longing to escape from reality. It may also show itself as undue anxiety over apparent trivialities, fussiness over small details or in actual panic attacks. These happen when fear and anxiety overwhelm the individual and may occur in specific situations such as waiting at a bus stop or walking around a supermarket.

Most bereaved people appear to have a need to express guilt. They may wish for instance that they had expressed their feelings more openly when the loved one was living or had encouraged them to fulfil their ambitions or interests more strongly. With long term illness such as cancer, many people express guilt for not interpreting early signs of the disease as potentially serious.

Guilt may also be felt at ceasing to mourn. A Volunteer Bereavement Visitor (herself a widow) expressed this well: 'I don't want him to go, and as long as I feel the pain he will stay alive for me. And when the hurting stops, death becomes final. So many cling to pain. Maybe time, hopefully, will erase that'.

Anger may be directed at different targets. Doctors and, to a lesser extent, nurses may sometimes be blamed; this may not be inappropriate if it is remembered that their primary function is seen as being to cure patients. If a patient dies there has been a failure to cure and death has been, in a sense, allowed to happen. It is understandable therefore that anger directed at the caring professions tends to centre on wards and departments where a relative first begins to realise, or is told directly, that a patient has died or is not going to be cured.

Another common target for anger is God. Many bereaved people make such statements as 'He was such a good man', 'She was just an innocent child', which indicate the feeling that God has let the deceased person down in some way, or has not kept his side of the bargain. Even people who profess a formal religious faith may experience such doubts.

Phase 3: Apathy, aimlessness and sadness

The disengagement from the usual patterns of daily life that often takes place before the death of a loved one can lead to feelings of apathy. Plans are impossible to make, the future seems uncertain or even frightening and the effort required to get through the day seems futile.

Often nurses may find that relatives cannot help but dwell on all the sad events which led up to the patient's death; they remember in every detail every aspect of the illness and treatment. It may take many months before a bereaved person is able to work through this phase sufficiently to be able to put it aside. Only then do they seem able to go further back to happier times (if these did indeed exist) and begin to find pleasure and comfort in these memories which still remain poignant. If this sadness is labelled as depression, the idea that these feelings are abnormal or an illness may be inadvertently encouraged, rather than a justified reaction which inevitably accompanies the bereavement process.

Phase 4: Gradual hope and moves in new directions

After the negativity of the other three stages, the last one has a positive message. Sometimes this revelation comes quite suddenly to the bereaved person, more often it is a very gradual part of the process. Either way there is, for most people, some kind of turning point. Lewis (1961) who mourned the death of his wife eloquently described this experience: '. . . something quite unexpected has happened. It came this morning early. My heart was lighter than it had been for weeks . . . suddenly at the very moment when so far I mourned her least, I remembered her best. It was as if the lifting of the sorrow removed a barrier'.

Bereavement as a series of tasks

The process approach to bereavement has been criticised as being too passive. An alternative view is offered by Worden (1984) which sees bereavement as a series of tasks and implies that the bereaved person can influence their progress through it. The task based approach is linked to Freud's concept of grief-work and assumes that if emotional energy is deliberately invested in each task and if the bereaved person can be helped to face up to them, then grieving will be completed more fully and with less complication. Worden's tasks are as follows.

- To accept the reality of the loss
- To experience pain and grief
- To adjust to a new environment
- To withdraw emotional energy from the deceased and invest it in other relationships

Task 1   To accept the reality of the loss

It is not until the bereaved person has faced up to the fact that the dead person can never return, in this life at least, that they can begin the task of adjustment. It is suggested that in our society we do not help the accomplishment of this task, because, for example, we avoid referring to the fact that the person has died. Many euphemisms are used to avoid the word 'death' and, instead, things like 'passed over', 'gone across', 'gone to heaven' are said. Therefore the bereaved should be encouraged to talk about what has happened and to express how they are feeling.

Task 2   To experience pain and grief

This is very painful and so it is understandable that the very intensity of these feelings make others want to distract the bereaved person. Gorer (1965) suggests that the expression of grief is stigmatised in our society as a being morbid and unhealthy. We need to listen.

Task 3 To adjust to a new environment

The environment is suddenly strange and new because the deceased person is missing from it. All the roles that the deceased person played are unfilled. For example, the newly bereaved mother of young children who has lost her husband has also lost her companion, lover, child-minder, accountant, driver and drain-cleaner! It can be salutary to reflect for a moment on the number of roles performed in your life by the person closest to you.

But whatever these roles are, they incude one universal role, that of 'audience'. We all use those closest to us as an audience for our ideas, a sounding board for our plans, hopes and dreams and to reflect back to us the kind of person that we are. Here again we can see that when we lose someone close to us, we lose part of ourselves.

Task 4 To withdraw emotional energy and reinvest it in other relationships

This is linked to Freud's (1957) statement that 'the function of mourning is to detach the survivor's memories and hopes from the dead person'. Freud sees this work as difficult and slow, a painful inner process of letting go. This is considered to be the most difficult task, as people feel that by doing this work they will be dishonouring the dead person in some way. There is often a feeling that to make moves towards a new way of life is betraying all that was most important to the individual before.

Having considered two perspectives of what may be experienced as 'normal' patterns of bereavement, the possible role of the nurse in bereavement care will now be looked at. The nature of nursing means that it is often the nurse who is closest to the patient and his or her family.

The role of the nurse

There are two main aspects to the nursing role in relation to bereavement and grieving. These are *assessment and detection of abnormal grieving* and *helping*.

Assessment and detection of abnormal grieving

In assessment the nurse needs knowledge of normal patterns of grieving as a starting point. A further aspect of this knowledge is familiarity with the timescale involved in normal grieving (Fig. 13.1). The importance of this is that abnormal grieving may be detected when unusual delay occurs in either a phase of grieving or when that phase is unduly prolonged.

The nurse's observations of non-verbal as well as verbal communication in the grieving person are important aspects of emotional assessment. Additionally the nurse may also observe the person's appearance, his or her environment and the apparent networks of support that are available. Each type of observation can give clues to the emotional state of the bereaved person and can signal the presence of abnormal grieving. Although these observations are important and helpful, nurses

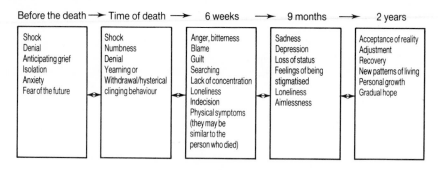

Fig. 13.1   The bereavement process: an approximate timescale.

should not underestimate the equal importance of their own intuitive feeings when assessing. Experience may sometimes be the best guide of all.

Certain factors may indicate people who may be particularly at risk of grieving abnormally. There is no single indicator of abnormal grieving but several factors should be taken into account. People affected by multiple factors may usefully be thought of as being at greater risk. Table 13.1 provides a useful guide.

Table 13.1   Factors which may indicate abnormal grieving.

- Previous mental illness, especially depression.

- A history that indicates unresolved grief from a previous loss. Intense grief reaction in apparently inappropriate circumstances may indicate this.

- A delay in expressing feelings of grief by whatever means – by sheer effort of will, or by prolonged use of tranquillisers or anti-depressants. Avoidance of any death-related rituals, customs or activities related to the deceased.

- Extreme expressions of self-blame and guilt, including a need for atonement. Self-blame may be expressed as low self-esteem and in extreme cases as self-destructive impulses.

- Over-idealisation of the loved one, feeling that the person who died was perfect and that they are still directing one's life. This may be a form of denial when the individual cannot contemplate having an independent existence.

- Preserving the environment of the deceased just as it was when they were alive and so creating a shrine. Regarding every belonging and association as sacred for prolonged periods (e.g. for more than a year). However this does not mean that keeping some clothes, mementoes or a special place in the home is abnormal. Many people keep a special corner of the house (or garden), often with a photograph as a permanent reminder.

- A hypochondriacal fear of the illness the dead person suffered from. This may not surface until an anniversary or when an indivdual reaches the same age. This hypochondriasis is of course overlayed on the generalised fear of cancer that is common in our society.

- Very radical and sudden change in lifestyle, especially if it excludes lifelong friends and usual activities. Hasty substitution of another close relationship without grieving the loss of the previous one. A move to a new and unknown part of the country.

The nurse as helper and resource

Nurses often say nowadays, that they are 'counselling' their bereaved clients. I prefer the term 'helping'. Helping people in grief is a wider function than counselling and may include many aspects of the traditional nursing role. Nursing is a holistic profession and nursing care should always attend to physical needs as well as attempting to meet emotional needs. Helping could include offering physical care when it is required, should attempt to prevent illness always, and may include aspects of health education. So when the nurse takes on the role of helper to a bereaved person what should his or her objectives be? What outcomes are intended? Are these likely to be the same or different from what the bereaved person is hoping for?

To be an effective helper to the bereaved person it is probably necessary to have evolved some kind of personal philosophy of living and to have a developed sense of self-awareness. Speck (1978) makes the point that the professional helper may face particular problems in 'having the confidence to remain human' rather than hiding behind a role. This statement may apply especially to nurses.

It is important for any helper to ensure that the bereaved person understands what the purposes of any supportive visit might be. In dealing with the emotional aspects of bereavement these purposes might include the following.

● To search for meaning in what has happened. Frankl (1963), describing his experiences as an inmate in Auschwitz, quotes Nietszche, 'He who has the why to live can bear with almost any how'. All bereaved people need time to make some kind of sense of their loss or at least to rationalise it in some way.

● To express and let go of feelings, which includes being able to cry but also to be able to stop. There is much talked about the possible value of encouraging the expression of emotion but, as Parkes and Weiss (1983) point out, it is often more difficult to restore emotional stability after this kind of release.

● To help the bereaved person share memories of the person they loved and of their life together. It often seems that the bereaved person avoids doing this with family and friends in order to protect them from their emotional reaction to it or because they are actively discouraged from doing so. People may avoid this because they feel embarrassed or over-protective. This is often to do with their own defences.

● To have the ability to make and confirm any necessary decisions. Newly bereaved people may respond to this major change by feeling that they should make other changes. It would appear from the work of Holmes and Rahe (1967) and others that is may be unwise for other avoidable changes to take place at least within a year of the loss. Stability can also be achieved by keeping other 'anchors' in place by maintaining as near as usual a routine as before. Predicting the times when the bereaved person may feel particularly vulnerable, such as Sundays, Bank Holidays and dates which are of particular significance to the individual, and planning ways of coping with them can also be helpful.

● To restore or maintain physical health and fitness. This is often overlooked, even by nurses, yet it is known that standards of physical fitness are related to the individual's ability to cope with stresses of many kinds. Information about such aspects as healthy eating, exercise plans and relaxation techniques, provided that this is geared to consideration of the individual's life-style, can be very welcome. These may also meet the need for security by communicating the message that the bereaved individual is a valued person in their own right who should be taking care of themselves.

In helping, the nurse acts as a resource to the bereaved person by his/her knowledge of what is available in the community in which the bereaved person lives. This may include self-help groups and support systems of many kinds as well as the availability of statutory and voluntary services offering practical help. The nurse's knowledge of appropriate literature and its availability (including locations like public libraries and Adult Education Centres) may be a very positive factor in promoting self-help activity in clients.

One aspect of the Health Education function in nursing that has benefited bereaved clients has been the use of a diary in which to record feelings and memories and in which to chart progress. Some people are very encouraged to help others in similar situations, or are even to teach professionals by completing diaries in note-book or other forms. The feeling that negative experiences can be turned to usefulness is an important aspect of the recovery process. Sharing experiences for the benefit of professionals allows clients to express a kind of gratitude and to give something back for the help they received themselves.

Nurses are of course, members of a health care team. It is not essential that nurses deal with all aspects of care by themselves. This may be especially important when abnormal grieving is suspected: appropriate and early referral to the family doctor (since most bereaved clients will be at home) is a particularly necessary service to offer.

The bereaved nurse

One of the groups of bereaved people who Parkes (1972) identifies as being 'At Risk' in bereavement are those which he refers to as Image-Conscious Individuals. By this he means those who are accustomed to being helpers. Nurses are helpers and givers of care and may find it difficult to show vulnerability by asking for help for themselves. The nursing profession tends to value coping very highly. Others may have the expectation that nurses can accept and cope with any crisis and so may not consider it appropriate or necessary to offer help.

Crawley (1984) who founded CHAT, the Royal College of Nursing Counselling Service for nurses, discovered that many had problems in adjusting to bereavement because their family perceived them as being the one who was able to support them. Therefore, the nurse's own grieving was often delayed until the family's own grief had been resolved.

In nursing people who are dying, sometimes over a considerable period of time, the nurse may have become close to the patient and feel a sense of loss at the patient's death. The nurse may require support from colleagues at this time. Mechanisms for coping with stress are discussed further in Chapter 16.

Conclusions

Parkes (1986) sums up the inherent problem of attempting to help bereaved people:

'Pain is inevitable in such a case and cannot be avoided. It stems from the fact that neither the helper nor the bereaved can give each other what they want. The helper cannot bring back the person who died and the bereaved cannot gratify the helper by feeling helped. No wonder both seem dissatisfied with the encounter'.

The long-terms goal of providing some kind of bereavement support has been put forward by Mathers (1976):

'The pain of bereavement is the price we have to pay for loving; so that though it is costly it is not too dear, since the experience of losing what you have loved and grieving over it, is a challenge to learn more about yourself, to become more mature, more healthy and truly human.'

These two views reflect the negative and the positive aspects of caring for bereaved people. Both are true. Wherever death takes place, it is nearly always the nurse who supports those most affected by the loss. If both aspects of the problem of caring are born in mind, it is clear that the nursing skills of assessing and helping and the nurse's ability to act as a resource can be of great potential value to the grieving family. The balance between over-medicalisation of bereavement and the neglect that comes from dealing with its problems only on the basis of common-sense is perhaps one of the greatest strengths that nursing can offer to this group of clients.

References

BOWLBY, J. (1981). *Attachment and Loss: Volume 3.* Penguin Books, Harmondsworth.
CAPLAN, G. (1964). *Principles of Preventive Psychiatry.* Basic Books, New York.
CRAWLEY, P. (1984). Coping with the death of a close relative. *Nursing Standard,* 25th October.
FRANKL, V. (1963). *Man's Search for Meaning.* Beacon Press, New York.
FREUD, S. (1957). *Mourning and Melancholia.* Hogarth Press, London.
GORER, G. (1965). *Death, grief and mourning in Contemporary Britain.* Cresset Books, London.
HOLMES, T. H. and RAHE, R. H. (1967). The social readjustment rating scale. *Journal of Psychosomatic Research,* Vol II, 213–18.
ILLICH, I. (1976). *Limits to Medicine: Medical Nemesis.* Penguin, Harmondsworth.
LEWIS, C. S. (1961). *A Grief Observed.* Faber & Faber, London.
LINDEMANN, E. (1944). Symptomatology and management of acute grief. *American Journal of Psychiatry,* 108–51.
MATHERS, J. (1976). In *Health Education: Perspectives and Choices,* I. Sutherland (Ed.). Allen & Unwin Ltd, London.
PARKES, C. M. (1972). *Bereavement: Studies of grief in Adult Life.* Penguin, Harmondsworth.
PARKES, C. M. (1986). *Bereavement: Studies of grief in Adult Life,* second edition. Penguin, Harmondsworth.

PARKES, C. M. and WEISS, R. (1983). *Recovery from Bereavement.* Basic Books Inc., New York.
WORDEN, W. J. (1984). *Grief Counselling and Grief Therapy.* Tavistock, London.

Further reading

LAKE, T. (1984). *Living with Grief.* Sheldon Press, London.
MARRIS, P. (1986). *Loss and Change.* Routledge and Kegan Paul, London.
PENSON, J. (1990). *Bereavement: a Guide for Nurses.* Lippincott Nursing Series. Harper and Row, London.
PENSON, J. (1990). Teaching Bereavement Care, *Bereavement Care,* **9,** no. 2; 22–24.
RAPHAEL, B. (1983). *The Anatomy of Bereavement.* Hutchinson, London.
STEARNS, A. K. (1987). *Living through Personal Crisis.* Sheldon Press, London.
STROEBE, W. and STROEBE, M. S. (1987). *Bereavement and Health.* Cambridge University Press, Cambridge.
VIOST, J. (1986). *Necessary Losses.* Simon and Schuster, New York.
WILSON-BARNETT, J. and RAIMAN, J. (1988). *Nursing Issues and Research in Terminal Care.* John Wiley & Sons, London.

14

Communication

Sally Anstey

'Much unhappiness has come into the world because of bewilderment and things left unsaid'

Dostoevsky

Introduction

For the purpose of this chapter it is presumed that the reader will have a prior working knowledge of the basic skills of verbal and non-verbal communication. The purpose of this section is to build on to these general communication abilities particular skills tailored to meet the needs of individuals and their families receiving active palliative care.

Research background

Why is a research background important? It is important to discuss past research for a variety of reasons. Nursing interventions and interactions should be made in response to evidence from scientific research, rather than on the basis of the maxim 'We will do it like this because we have always done so'. Research also highlights the inadequacies of nurse training, and consequently of the nurse's role in effective communication in the area of death and dying. Stedeford (1984) states that 'poor communication about illness causes more suffering than any other problem except unrelieved pain'.

Communication and professionals

Over many years a growing body of literature, highlighting the difficulties faced by professionals in communicating with people who have life-threatening diseases, especially cancer, has been produced. It has been recognised that patients can evoke reactions in professionals that lead to various forms of direct or indirect avoidance, so that their communication and psychological needs are never appreciated or dealt with. The most intense avoidance responses are probably triggered by the circumstances of dying and death (Barton, 1972), and are, in part, influenced by individuals' own prior experiences of death which directly affect their attitudes and feelings.

A study by Maguire (1985) has suggested that many doctors and nurses consistently use distancing tactics with dying patients; this occurred when observations were made of their interactions in real, simulated or role play situations. The tactics were described as being used to protect the professional emotionally but, in practice, served to discourage patients from disclosing their psychological concerns, thus detracting from effective care in this area.

Studies concerning nurses specifically are rare, but Fielding and Llewellyn (1987) confirm that they also have difficulty in communicating with patients, especially those who are emotionally distressed or dying. These authors point to the importance of organisation issues, in that communicating with patients and relatives is often perceived to be of little value, and consequently left to the most junior member of staff. Such issues may explain the findings that nurses are more likely to respond to the expressions of physical rather than emotional distress, even when they perceive the latter. There is also recent evidence implying that although nurses may have knowledge relating to psychosocial aspects of care, they do not necessarily use this in their interactions with patients, which still tend to be largely task orientated (Peterson, 1988).

Touch and other non-verbal skills are an important facet of communication, but are sorely neglected in the training of nursing staff. Moy (1981) suggests that few nurses receive any formal instruction on the subject, but states that their ideas about touch in particular develop through gradual professional self awareness. Most qualified nurses questioned said that the main intention of using touch was to convey caring; the commonest response to it was that the patients or relatives further expressed feelings, or that there was an increase in verbal responses (Aguilera, 1967; Langland and Panniccucci, 1982).

Communication and patients

Many studies highlight the difficulty for professionals to communicate effectively with dying patients and their families. There is also disturbing evidence that the poor quality of communication adversely affects the psychological wellbeing of patients. Brewin (1977) discusses the importance of good communication in improving patients morale and reducing their fear, and Stedeford (1981) identified considerable suffering resulting from poor communication, with patients generally wanting more information than they had been given. There is also evidence that confirms the importance of the attitude of professional carers: Francis and Morris (1969) state that patients are more satisfied when professionals are warm, concerned and empathetic, but not necessarily more skilled practically.

Communication and training

The teaching of professionals, particularly nurses, in communication skills specifi-cally appropriate to the area of palliative care is now undertaken by many hospices or hospice-type organisations in Great Britain. Parkes and Parkes (1984) compared individuals who had died at St. Christopher's Hospice with others who had died in general hospitals in the same part of London and found no difference in pain, symptoms and general distress between the two groups. This was in contrast to a similar study conducted ten years earlier where hospice care was found to be universally superior. The change was attributed by the authors to the teaching work undertaken by the hospice to hospital personnel in the intervening years. Reisetter and Thomas (1986), in a Canadian study of hospital nurses, support the view that post-qualification education in the field of death and dying can improve the quality of palliative care provided.

Difficulties which affect effective communication

In the palliative care setting, the nurse, by the very nature of his or her role – be it in hospital or the community – has a direct, continuous and intimate relationship with the patient and their carers. Nurses' satisfaction with the quality of their care is related to the perceived openness or ease of communciation with the patient and family (Wilkinson, 1988). However most recognise that there are many barriers to good communication which should be explored, as they directly affect care/performance. The following is not intended as an exhaustive list and is not in order of importance

- *External* difficulties e.g. organisational issues
- *Internal* difficulties e.g. personal fears and anxieties
- Difficulties imposed by the *ambiguities* in the nurses role
- Difficulties imposed by the *multidisciplinary team*

External difficulties

Time
Nurses' time is seen as precious and there is a perception of constantly racing against the clock to provide patient care. In some instances it is non-nursing duties: for example in hospital, answering the telephone, ordering stock, accompanying *all* the doctors on *all* ward round that takes their time; in the community it is paperwork, inadequately completed transfer documents, auditing of visits/journey times and the grey area of social care versus clinical care. When time is short it is the physical needs of patients that are dealt with and their communication needs which are neglected. GRASP (Grace Reynolds application and study of Peto) (Hiscocks, 1990) data on nursing workload in South Glamorgan Health Authority corroborates these findings. There is a widely held myth that communication, in whatever form, takes a large amount of time. Perhaps this is, in part, due to the fact that when communication does occur it is often in response to a crisis, when there is much about which the patient needs to talk. However, communciation should be seen as an on-going process, and as such it may be regular short bursts of support or encouragement which meet some needs and ease distress. One gesture of physical touch – a cuddle or hand held should not be underestimated as its therapeutic benefits are highly valued by patients. It is the 'quality' not the 'quantity' that counts.

Pressure from superiors and/or peers
The patient's physical needs, for example washing and the skilled tasks, performed for patients are perceived to be of paramount importance and are recognised by superiors as 'real work'.

Communicating with patients and relatives is seen as an easy option (which of course is not true); a sign of laziness and not part of the nurse's job. Such explicit disapproval and pressure from colleagues, peers and superiors influences practice, since it is important to be accepted as part of the team. Superiors influence professionally, complete appraisal forms and directly affect the nurse's career.

It is learning in the ward environment which has been suggested to be most influential and junior nurses learning from role models in that environment are provided with a guide to determining future practice. But in most instances practical tasks are shown and very rarely communication skills.

Nurse training
There is a wide disparity between the training school and the ward environment (see earlier research section. In particular, training in the care of the dying patient is inadequate with regard to psychological and communication aspects. Talking to dying patients and their families is a frightening area of care to embark upon especially if it is untaught, viewed as unacceptable and unsupported. It may also be assumed that if something is a proper subject then it will be taught as part of the curriculum; its exclusion implies that nurses do not need to venture into that area of practice.

Organisation of ward work
The use of the nursing process, nursing models and theories and patient allocation, has implications for nurses in that they are held individually responsible for the holistic aspects of patient care. Often the most junior members of staff are involved in the care of the dying as it is regarded as 'basic nursing' whereas the more experienced staff are involved with those requiring potentially life-saving or technical skills. The stresses involved for junior staff who are unsupported, untrained and feeling vulnerable mitigate against them. Communicating ineffectively ultimately makes them less satisfied with their performance, but also renders them less likely to try to provide this facet of care.

Sanitisation of death (as first described by Buckman, 1988)
We live in a society where dying is not seen as an acceptable part of living, it is not acknowledge or discussed in a natural way but seen as something alien or taboo. So, when a person is dying, the denial of death creates a barrier between them and the rest of society, isolating them when they most need support. The causes of this may include the following.

- The loss of the extended family with more people dying in hospital. Fry (1983) presents national figures on site of death including sudden deaths
    25% occur at home
    64% in hospital
    4% in hospices
    7% elsewhere
When cancer deaths alone are considered Fry estimates that seven out of twenty (35%) occur at home – thus when death does occur, more often than not it is partially hidden in an institutional environment. This enables the nurse to avoid the prospect of death, viewing it as clinical and distant.

- Medicalisation: medicine is seen as being 'high tech' with the emphasis on keeping alive and having power to stave off death, so the care of the dying may, in part, be seen as a failure of health care.

- Society's acceptance of a materialistic way of life placing more emphasis on possessions than the way life is lived, quantity not quality.

● Most people have never seen anyone dead or dying and so are afraid of the unknown; the horror of the unseen often being worse than the reality.

Internal difficulties

Internal difficulties are related to the health professionals' own personal fears and anxieties.

● Personal fears of illness and death are linked, in part, to the sanitisation of death discussed earlier, in that talking about death and dying is seen as a social taboo and beyond the realms of the carer's personal experience. In addition, psychologists suggest that some individuals become doctors or nurses to exorcise their own fears of death and dying by perceiving that they have a direct responsibility 'to keep individuals alive at all costs' – power over life and death. By avoidance of close contact with people who are dying they do not have to confront the threat of their own mortality and consequently are not threatened.

● Fear of being seen as responsible for the patients situation or being blamed for the patient's impending death. The implication being that perhaps the doctor or nurse did not try hard enough or possess appropriate skill or expertise to 'cure' them. This is linked to the general public's view of the omnipotence of the medical and nursing professions.

● Fear of the consequences of our interactions. Firstly, precipitating a reaction in the patient or relative, especially if it is emotional. What do we do if the patient breaks down and cries or gets angry, abusive and shouts? This fear of an emotional reaction and being labelled as 'the nurse who upsets patients' may make people wary of embarking on some areas of communication.

Secondly, there is the fear of expressing their own emotions. Nurses are taught to behave in a professional manner, remaining detached and uninvolved, hiding behind their uniform but, in reality, becoming distressed when having to hide this. For patients it is sometimes supportive and helpful if nurses show that they care about the patient's situation or distress, but not that they are accepting the blame for it.

● Anxiety about not knowing the answers: admitting we don't know is seen very much as failure since medicine is expected to be an exact science. But in palliative care 'don't know' is an honest response as the situation of death and dying is not clearly predictable. How long have I left to live? What will my dying be like? These are common questions, for which inappropriate reassurance and an exact time limit are not helpful responses as they are not likey to be accurate. Often the questioner needs the nurse to listen to how they feel, what they think and what their problems are – rather than to provide them with the answers.

● Over-identification with the patient or their relatives by being reminded of a member of the nurse's own family or a past bereavement. It is important for nurses to accept limitations in the care which they provide, they cannot be 'all things to all men' and they need to remain effective, not overwhelmed by past and current emotions. There is no disgrace in admitting that a situation is causing anguish and asking to be relieved of caring for a particular individual: it takes courage but is important for the nurse's own welfare and to ensure high quality care that the nurse is unlikely to be able to give in such a situation.

● Relationship difficulties in nurses' professional lives are not unknown. In palliative care, there is the need to establish a relationship more quickly than normal and, by necessity, it is more personal and less formal – if the relationship does not appear to be working on either side there is no harm in withdrawing and handing over to a colleague. Ultimately, there is more harm to all parties in persevering and not establishing an effective quality caring relationship.

● For all nurses there are particular areas of care that they find rewarding and those they find either difficult or unsatisfying. It is important, therefore, to recognise that some nurses, for a variety of reasons, are not comfortable in caring for the dying, and consequently should not be forced to become involved at a level they find difficult or distressing. This however is not a blanket absolution in allowing individuals to opt out of palliative care totally, as it unfortunately forms a very large body of nurses' work, but should encourage awareness of the problem by colleagues.

Ambiguities in the nurse's role

The changing role of the nurse
In the United Kingdom the pressures internally and externally on nursing to redefine its roles and spheres of influence are increasing with the proposals of the English National Board for Nursing, Midwifery and Health Visiting (1989) for Project 2000 relating to nurse training, those of the United Kingdom Central Council for Nursing, Midwifery and Health Visiting (1989; 1990) for post-registration education (the Post-Registration Education and Practice Project, PREPP), and the shifting emphasis from the treatment of disease to the promotion of health.

COMMUNITY
For community nurses the implementation of General Practitioner's contracts, the Government's Community Care White Paper, the suggestions of role re-alignment, numbers of practice nurses, nurse prescribing, and the extended role of the nurse with its ambiguities cause increased anxiety. On the positive side, the extended role of the community care assistant may release more time for the community nurse and his or her team to spend on skilled nursing care, including holistic palliative care. The evolution of the role of the Macmillan Nurse from providing '5 star' clinical care to a small number of patients to the provision of education to enable primary carers to provide effective palliative care to the majority of patients dying from advanced cancer, has implications for the wider teaching of communication and other relevant skills.

HOSPITAL
There have been vast changes of the role of the nurse within the hospital setting: the moves from task to patient allocation; the adoption of nursing models; the nursing process with individualised patient care; nursing development units; team and primary nursing; the change in roles for the enrolled nurse and auxiliary within the

emerging multi-level health care assistant. All these changes have implications for the evolution of the nurse's role. Individualised patient care has implications for improving communication skills at all levels – it is more difficult for a nurse to respond to the patient's questions by saying 'I will go and ask Sister' for each nurse has the individual responsibility to deal with the situation. This is particularly so in team and primary nursing, where the Ward Sister acts as teacher and facilitator rather than overall clinical manager and care provider.

ADVOCACY

The growing acknowledgement of advocacy as an integral part of the nurses role is especially relevant for care of the dying patient and family. In this particular sense, advocacy implies respecting the human rights of patients including the promotion and protection of their autonomy. The ultimate implication of this includes the patient's right to participate in decisions which affect them, either directly, or by using the nurse as a 'go-between' in their interactions with other members of the health care team, or between their family and friends.

ACTIVE VERSUS PASSIVE COMMUNICATION

Nurses have no obligation to involve themselves at *every* level of communication with their patients. In Palliative Care communication needs can include the following.

- 'Normal' communication on a wide variety of subjects, e.g. gossip/jokes
- Relating to diagnosis and prognosis
- Specific problem areas relating to the process of dying

It is apparent that patients will select who they feel is appropriate to deal with a particular subject area. If chosen, nurses have to make the decision as to whether to become actively or passively involved. Active involvement implies that the nurse is prepared to support the patient and their family throughout the time of living with a terminal disease, the actual dying process, and the immediate bereavement period, caring for the myriad of communication needs. Passive involvement implies that the nurse feels, for whatever reasons, that communication needs are not their direct responsibility and, as a consequence, may avoid the issues entirely, but must actively pass on that aspect of care to other members of the caring team.

The multidisciplinary team

Who is the multidisciplinary team?
Anyone who has involvement with the patient and their family should be included as a member of the team, whether it be the porters or ancillary staff, the receptionist, consultant or nurse, social worker, occupational therapist, physiotherapist – each has a unique contribution to make and should be valued and supported as such.

For true multidisciplinary palliative care to be effective there needs to be an overlap between the roles of team members. Distinct differences serve only to act as barriers in providing holistic care. It is important to acknowledge that the patient and their family are part of the team – in the sphere of palliation there are few clear cut best choices of care, the implication being that where possible the individual's own wishes are important treatment indicators. However, to include the patient in decision making requires clear and open communication among all members of the health team.

Role ambiguity

Often within the multidisciplinary team it is perceived that there is a doctor–nurse clique which isolates others and serves to undermine/negate their contribution; also within nursing there is the qualified/unqualified gap with qualified staff appearing to forget the trauma of death as a student nurse experiences it.

Further difficulties occur when either the policy for talking to patients or relatives is unclear or there is an authoritarian relationship with medical staff in the multidisciplinary team whereby interactions and communications are subordinate to the senior doctor's wishes. In the USA and some other countries, the patient's right to know is enshrined in law, however, in the UK it is still (theoretically) possible for senior doctors to forbid others to communicate about certain matters, particularly prognosis and dying, thus denying the nurses active contribution in these areas.

If the nurse's role among team members is regarded as equal, then the patient's interests are well served by a collaborative relationship. This is especially apparent if not all team members are informed or there is no documentation as to the information given to terminally ill patients and their relatives about their illness. Obviously this situation makes further support uncertain and interactions unnecessarily problematic.

At present what is happening in terms of the relationship primarily between doctor and nurse, is that the nurse offers active input into the partnership. Sometimes that input is accepted, sometimes sought and encouraged, and sometimes discounted. This relationship is certainly one step onward from the traditional authoritative model. However, it is still a long way from open communication, which is necessary to meet the needs of the patient and family. Ideally, the collaborative model of multidisciplinary care does offer such open communication and is demonstrated by mutual decision making and respect for the integrity of all parties involved, patients, relatives and team members.

Field (1984), in his observational studies, states that it is still doctors who control the information nurses are allowed to give patients and relatives about diagnosis and prognosis. Wilkinson (1988) identified stressful incidents as perceived by nurses and found 'nurse/doctor conflicts' to be the most stressful. These were rated far higher than the second and fourth on her list of stressors, which were the 'inability to communicate effectively with the patient' and 'difficulties with communicating with and supporting relatives'.

However it cannot be overlooked that, in some instances, the responsibility for lack of communication may lie with the patient and/or relatives.

Team needs

Mutual advice, support and encouragement are among the benefits of good teamwork. Health professionals are often very isolated in their care of the dying, so team meetings and case conferences work as an effective bolster to improve performance, providing they are not excessively formal, monopolised by one or two members, or under the authoritarian influence of the medical staff. To be effective they should be based on the mutual respect of all parties and work as a forum for improving patient care, updating education by increasing knowledge and skills in palliation, and increasing support by fostering self-disclosure and openness in discussing difficulties, triumphs and auditing of care.

Within the team concept it is important to recognise that it is unlikely that one person can cope with all the communication needs of the dying patient and family, hence sharing the situation improves support for the patients and relatives as well as for the team members. Occasionally there are communication needs within the multidisciplinary team. Some individuals need to act as arbiters, mutual supporters, ethicists or teachers, so that the team can learn and grow as a result of the care they are providing.

Patients and their families, as members of the team, have a part to play in aiding health professionals to communicate with them and each other; they are excellent teachers, often guiding the professional through difficult situations. Patients sometimes find it easier to talk with health care professionals about particular emotional concerns. An example of the Nurse and Doctor sharing a 'breaking bad news' consultation is beneficial on many levels. It identifies weaknesses; improves skills through role modelling, provides mutual support during a difficult encounter; and enables one person to act as observer of verbal and non-verbal cues relating to distress, incomprehension, to perhaps translate the medical jargon, or to intervene if the consultation becomes problematic.

How to communicate:
General guidelines for effective communication in palliative care

Setting the scene

Aim
To optimise the non-verbal quality of the communication, by appearing to take account of the vulnerability of the patient's relative's situation, preparing them for a difficult conversation, and returning some control of the interaction to them. This 'setting of the scene' should enable the professional to feel more comfortable (by using practical guidelines) with what follows and prepare them in switching to communication mode.

How to do it
The health care professional needs to pay attention to the following.

- **Environment** Creating a sense of privacy and quiet, e.g. drawing the curtains or using an office, preferably without a telephone.
Non-verbal behaviour
    — Appearing unhurried, that time is not a problem (even though it probably is).
    — The professional positioning him or herself well by sitting down, being on the same level or slightly lower than the patient with a comfortable distance between them, not too close or too far away.
    — Ensuring that the patient is physically comfortable, e.g. not in pain or actively vomiting, otherwise these symptoms will act as a barrier to effective communication.

— Enabling the patient to be adequately dressed so that they do not feel intimidated.

Getting started

Particular skills – open questions

Aim
The purposes of this type of question are

• To find out how the individual is really feeling, not to confirm what the professional thinks he or she is feeling. In particular, what they are feeling at the time/moment of the conversation.

• To ensure that both professional and patient are on the same 'wavelength'.

• To discover if it is an appropriate time to embark on a deeper type of conversation: Is the patient pain free? Is the patient expecting visitors?

• To determine whether the relationship between the professional and the patient is good enough to cope with the ensuing conversation.

How to do it
• Note that there must be congruence between questions and non-verbal behaviour.

• Elicit information precisely, e.g.
'How are you feeling today?'
'How were you feeling yesterday?'

• Give the patient the opportunity to respond at a level at which they feel comfortable and in the way they choose, e.g.
'Not so well today, I seem to have a lot on my mind.'
'Surprisingly well, I really feel I'm getting so much better.'

• The patient is thus in control and guiding the subsequent conversation.

• It is important to be aware of the significance of the patient's non-verbal responses, e.g. Do they look relaxed/anxious/tearful?

How not to do it
• When using open questions the professional should not bias or prejudice responses for their own convenience or safety, e.g.
'You look really well today – how are you feeling?' Most patients would find it difficult to respond other than positively to such a question. The opposite may also be true, e.g.
'Gosh you do look exhausted – how are you sleeping?'

- Do not ask open questions
    — without setting the scene to deal with the responses
    — whilst looking at your watch or looking busy and pre-occupied
    — with a large number of other people present, mostly unknown to the patient,
e.g. whilst taking visitors around the ward
    — as 'throw away lines', e.g. asking 'How are you?' and either walking away
before the patient can reply, or pre-empting the reply by automatic responses such
as 'That's good', 'That's great'.

Asking unhelpful open questions will only serve to preclude the beneficial effect of
appropriate open questioning by the patient being uncertain as to when the
professional is willing to establish an effective communicating relationship.

Particular skills – conversation encouragers

These are techniques of facilitating conversation by enabling and encouraging the
patient to talk freely and feel comfortable with the health care professional. They are
extremely simple and may even seem obvious but are highly effective.

Aim
- To keep the communication channels open for the benefit of the patient/
relative by giving support and consequently easing their distress.

How to do it
- *Non-verbal prompters* For example nodding, smiling, touching a hand or
arm (especially when the conversation is proving painful), maintaining/encouraging
eye contact.

- *Verbal prompters*
    — Saying 'Yes', 'Yes, I see, do go on', 'hm mmm', 'Could you tell me more
about that', 'Explain what you mean', 'Help me to understand what you mean'.
    — Being comfortable with silence, not talking for the sake of talking or
interrupting prematurely, but using it as an encourager, allowing people to think or
to feel safe about their next words.

- *Repetition* Occasionally repeating the last few key words of the patient's
sentence encourages them and proves that the professional is actively listening.
However, if this skill is used too much it can sound like a learned rather than
spontaneous response.

- *Reflecting/Paraphrasing* Repeating what the patient/relative has said
using the professional's own words proves that the professional is understanding
exactly what has been said.

- *Displaying warmth and empathy* The professional can show that they
understand how the patient/relative is feeling by moving closer if they become
distressed, by showing that they are at ease with the patient's emotions and that they
will stay with the patient. The professional should not respond to anger with anger,
but should feel able to encourage the patient/relative to give vent to their feelings.

(Responding to overt emotions is difficult for most people, but fear, anger and sadness are all normal reactions. Helping people to deal with them is beneficial to their emotional wellbeing.)

- *Talking about distress*   This can, in part, help to relieve it.

- *Encouraging the patient/relative to express their thoughts and emotions*   Thoughts and emotions that are repeatedly buried may eventually do harm, by increasing distress and the sense of isolation of the individual 'being alone with their dying'.

- *If a pause/silence is prolonged*   Encouragement may be helpful by saying, for example
'What are you thinking about?'
'Would it help to share what you are thinking about?'
However, this should not be so powerful that it makes the patient feel forced to continue or precipitate withdrawal.

- *Slight hesitancy* on the part of the professional (not having the right words on the tip of your tongue) helps the patient/relative by making them feel that their situation is unique and personal and that the communication is not merely an academic exercise.

Specific areas relating to palliative care

- How much does the patient know?
- How much do they want to know?
- Sharing the news
- What next?

How much does the patient know?

This is an important part of the communication process as it enables the professional carer to establish a starting point on which to build. A patient's knowledge may not be the same as they have been *told* or what their family and friends believe they are aware of. Nurses and doctors are poor predictors of patients' levels of knowledge relating to life-threatening disease, and tend not to allow for the usual initial reaction of denial.

Professional carers have to accept at face value what the patient remembers and understands of what has been said previously relating to diagnosis and prognosis.

- Patients forget at least 40% of what they hear in an interview, and this is likely to be much higher when the news is bad.

- Patients and relatives often state that after they hear key words like 'CANCER', 'DEATH', 'NO FURTHER TREATMENT' they cannot remember anything of the conversation that follows.

- The patients choice of words about their disease (Malignant neoplasm, tumour, cancer, ulcer or growth) gives clues as to what has been said previously and how much jargon was used, how they have dealt with and interpreted the information and which word they are suggesting or insisting be used when talking to them.

- By eliciting the patient's level of knowledge it is possible to estimate the 'bad news gap' (Buckman, 1988), the gap between their expectations and reality.

- For the individual with advanced cancer their knowledge may not have been updated. Consequently they may be still expecting active, potentially curative treatment, or be angry or distressed by the lack of cure resulting from a variety of unpleasant treatments.

- It is important to understand that, in some circumstances patients and/or relatives need to apportion blame, for example to their previous professional carers. Ascertaining their level of knowledge may trigger expression of their emotions. This approach may also help in avoiding being drawn into blaming or excusing previous professional carers.

Possible useful questions
'It would be helpful if you could tell me what the doctors looking after you before have told you about your illness?'
'I see, and what do you understand by that?'
'How does that information make you feel?'
'What did it all mean to you?'
'How did that information affect you?'
'Could you tell me what you have been told about your husband's/wife's illness?'

How much do they want to know?

By returning control to the patient it is possible to get a clear idea of how much they want to know; this gives permission to proceed and discuss the bad news in accordance with their wishes.

The nurse's professional responsibility, as outlined in the Code of Professional Conduct issued by the United Kingdom Central Council for Nursing, Midwifery and Health Visiting (1984), is primarily to the patient. At their request they are entitled to full knowledge about their medical condition, being assured that such information will be treated in strictest confidence. Any imparting of such information to family/friends will only occur after their permission is obtained and, if it is their decision, such information will be withheld.

The patient may ask directly for information, be it the results of the tests or whether their condition is serious.

Check

- Are they prepared for bad news?
- Do they look relaxed, are they asking the questions calmly?
- How well do you know the patient/relative?
- Are they anxious, asking the question without being prepared for the answer?
- Do they need some support (relatives/friend present) to cope with the news?

Before answering direct questions it may be helpful to ask the patient what they *think* is likely to be going on.

'Have you had any thoughts about what is wrong?'

'What sort/type of thoughts?'

This enables the professional to gauge how seriously the patient is interpreting his or her symptoms. Some individuals do not ask for information because the possibility of their condition being serious has not occurred to them. This is especially true for the young and fit; for others, denying the seriousness may be appropriate if it reduces their anxiety.

Giving individuals an element of free choice over the information may prove beneficial. Prior to investigative procedures, or after receiving test results, they can be given control of decisions relating to their illness. Questions like 'If your condition turned out to be something serious would you like to know the full details?' can, for those who says 'Yes', give a clear indication to proceed, showing that the patient is prepared for and is requesting information. In this way the health professional is enabling the patient to share in the decision-making surrounding their illness and restoring a sense of personal autonomy.

When a patient says 'No' or 'No, I don't want to know', they should still be able to maintain their own strategies, for example denial for coping with the situation. Professionals must respect all different ways of coping. Whatever the patient's response, it is always important to maintain non-judgemental support following their decision, to be aware that communication needs may change as their disease progresses, and to be available to talk and/or listen whenever the patient is ready.

Sharing the news

The patient is in control of the news, the knowledge is theirs by right although the professional carer has the key to it. The professional's role is to be their guide and supporter through the information sharing process and beyond.

What is bad news?

Buckman (1988) states that bad news can be defined as

'any news that materially alters the patient's view of his/her future.'

In other words the 'badness' of bad news is the gap between the patients expectation of their future and the reality of the situation.

Maguire and Faulkner (1988) state that:

'You cannot soften the impact of bad news since it is still bad news however it is broken'.

The following ponts showed be remembered.

- Bad news can never sound good.
- The honesty of the message should never be changed to improve its accept-ability.
- It is important to encourage and support hope realistic to a patient's particular circumstances, and to describe palliative care as an active treatment modality in its own right.

How to approach it?

The key to breaking bad news, as stated in Maguire and Faulkner (1988) is

'to try to slow down the speed of the transition from a patient's perception of himself as being well to a realisation that he has a life threatening disease'.

This can be facilitated by the following.

- The professional carer warning the patient/relative that they are going to be given serious information. This gives the patient/relative time to psychologically prepare themselves rather than to switch off the communication channels. It also gives the communicator the opportunity to monitor non-verbal reactions as well as to respond to verbal responses, for example, Do they want to continue or have they heard enough?
- Progressing along the 'bad news staircase' over a short period of time, allowing the patient/relative to adjust slowly to more serious levels of knowledge and leading to realisation at their own pace.
- When imparting news the communicator must avoid jargon, tailoring language and information to fit individual needs and levels of comprehension.
- The use of checking, phrases like 'Does that make sense?' 'Do you understand what I am saying?' allows the communicator to check that the message is being received and understood by facilitating two way communication.
- Following the breaking of bad news, the patient's emotional and psychological well-being is influenced by the subsequent support by their family/friends and the health care team.

What next?

After the breaking or confirming of bad news it is helpful to explore the person's feelings about the 'news', to discover their immediate fears and concerns, rather than predicting their responses. Concerns about dying may be influenced by past experiences, acceptance of myths and 'old wives tales', the portrayal of death in the media, and our cultural sanitisation of death, with the desire to protect family and friends from unnecessary anguish.

Exploring feelings and concerns

Sister   'How do you feel about this news?'

Mrs P.   'Really quite shocked I think. It is frightening to have your fears confirmed. My mother died from cancer it was so horrible, she had such a bad time . . . just got so terribly thin and the pain oh . . . to see her suffer'. [Whilst saying this Mrs P. looked extremely distressed, was wringing her hands, avoiding eye contact and biting her lip].

Sister   [Picking up on the non verbal as well as verbal responses] 'That experience must have been very difficult for you, I can see you're very distressed. Would you like to talk about it further'.

In the above example the Sister displays awareness of the immediate emotional and physical concerns and gives Mrs P. permission to continue.

The following points may assist in exploring a patient's feelings and concerns.

- One block to the effective sharing of information is if the patient has a large number of concerns on their mind. It is sometimes useful to obtain a 'shopping list' of anxieties and questions before attempting to answer them: if the patient's first question is answered immediately, thoughts about further questions may distract their attention from the answer.

- Sometimes an initial question may appear quite trivial but hide deeper concerns. If deeper concerns are suspected it may be worth trying to gently question the patient further. If there is no deeper problem such gentle questioning is unlikely to cause the patient any undue distress.

- Patients may ask an apparently simple question to test the professional carer's responses, enabling the patient to decide whether or not the professional can be trusted, or will cope with their deeper concerns.

Mrs A.   (following her mastectomy)   'Do you think I'll be able to use my normal bra with the prosthesis or will it slip?'

Nurse   'I don't know, it might be alright.'

This nurse's response is unhelpful, unsupportive, uncaring and would stop or deter Mrs A. from asking this nurse any other questions.

Alternatively, the nurse might reply:

Nurse   'It seems as though you are a little worried about the prosthesis and how it will fit and will it be secure. Would it be helpful to have a look and perhaps discuss the matter further?'

This response displays a more caring attitude, that Mrs A.'s concerns are important and resolvable but also leaves room for Mrs A. to discuss more intimate concerns that she may have.

Dealing with feelings and concerns

Once the patient's feelings and concerns are established it is important to help him or her to deal with them. Some of their concerns are potentially resolvable:

Mr W.   'The thought that it is going to be painful worries me.'

Nurse   'Yes, that's understandable.'

Mr W.   'Can you do anything to help the pain?'

Nurse   'Yes, it is likely that we will be able to help with the pain. But it is important to let us know if you have any pain so that we can discuss with the doctors and get something sorted out for it.'

The nurse did not promise to eliminate the pain, as that might not be realistic bearing in mind the complex nature of pain, but offered help and support in attempting this.

Offering ongoing support

When the prognosis is poor and the patient has been told that no further treatment is possible, the patient is likely to be overwhelmed by the situation believing that nothing can be done to help him or her. In this circumstance it is realistic to indicate that palliative care can improve their quality of life, by controlling their symptoms and facilitating effective communication to help with their psychological, emotional and spiritual concerns. Indicating that support will continue through the ups and downs of the disease process and apparent non-medical concerns are acceptable areas of discussion.

It is important to remember that, when sharing bad news with the patient and/or relative, they are left with further dilemmas.
— Who else to tell? Close/extended family? Friends?
— How and how much to tell them?
— When and where to tell them?
These decisions, and the control of them, are the patient's, but they may need non-judgemental support and guidance in imparting or concealing such knowledge.

Specific problem areas

Difficult questions

Patients and relatives may ask questions that are difficult to answer, but are important to them in coping with their limited future. Consequently, the health care professional needs to explore and respond to them appropriately.

Treatment questions

'Is it worth me having any more chemotherapy?'
'Will it do any good?'
'What are my chances?'

These questions are problematic in that often there are no clear-cut answers and it is unlikely that an individual's response to any treatment can be accurately predicted.

● Never make the decision for the patient (they will blame the professional if it works out badly) and encourage them not to be overly influenced by their relatives wishes because only they will experience the effects of the treatment.

● In the short term it is easier for the nurse or healt care professional to tell someone what to do, but that is always their decision, not the patient's.

● Aim to give the patient as much information about a particular treatment as possible in a way that they can understand. This enables them to make an informed decision themselves, although no decision can be truly informed in these situations.

● Be aware that it is appropriate to give patients the pros and cons of a particular treatment, to be realistic about potential side effects as well as benefits.

● Make the patient aware that there are some questions for which 'I don't know' is the true answer.

Is it cancer?
When communicating with patients who have cancer, most people dread being asked difficult questions, in particular: 'Is it cancer?' When such a question is asked it is difficult to predict what reply is wanted.

— Does the patient want reassurance that it isn't cancer (to help them deny the reality of their situation)?
— Does the patient want the truth?
— What are the patient's reasons for asking the question? Occasionally the way the question is asked may give clues in determining the response. However, the patient may partly want to know or be undecided as to how much/what they need to know.
'I haven't got cancer have I?' 'I'm sure its cancer', 'Is it caner?' gives little idea as to how to respond; therefore it is important to elicit further information as to the way the patient wishes to proceed. Stating that you are happy to answer the question but reflecting the question back, for example 'I am happy to answer your question but it would be helpful if I could ask you why you're asking me?' is useful in:
— preparing all parties for the ensuing conversation, giving them permission to continue or withdraw;
— and checking that professional and patient/relative are on the same 'wavelength';
— that the patient wants information about their condition and situation;
— how much the patient is aware of;
— what words have been and should be used; and
— the degree of matching between the verbal and non-verbal behaviour of the patient.

Questions relating to dying and prognosis
   'Am I dying?'

'I'm going to get better aren't I?'
'I'm dying aren't I?'

These questions can be dealt with in a similar way to those relating to a diagnosis of cancer but further exploratory questions may ensue, for example 'How long have I left to live?'

● It is essential to emphasise to patients and relatives that the nurse and/or doctor cannot predict how long someone has to live.

● Remember that giving a time limit, be it weeks, months, years, is useless, unreliable and inaccurate. Patients and relatives have to learn to live with un-certainty.

● Be aware that the patient/relative may selectively recall (however careful the nurse or doctor may be) a precise time limit out of context of the conversation.

● Ensure that the patient is offered continued support for however long they have to live, and that their relatives will be supported in bereavement.

● Acknowledge that pre-existing problems can be exacerbated or diminished by a life-threatening illness, and that the health professional is unlikely to be able to solve them. Relationships, likewise, can be enhanced or deteriorate according to the responses of patients/relatives/friends/health care workers.

● For those with a limited life-expectancy, realistic goal setting with regard to planning activities is useful in maximising quality of life so that individuals learn to 'live' rather than 'die' prematurely with their illness.

● Be aware that fear of the future may stop someone enjoying the present.

'What will my dying be like?
For most people their fears and anxieties can be divided into two groups: the fear of death, and fears associated with the process of dying.

THE FEAR OF DEATH
This is a fear of the unknown, of the actual ways and means of dying; the event itself and what happens afterwards. Questions relating to these concerns are impossible to answer. Although spiritual support is helpful in easing the passage towards death, dying is inevitably a lonely business, accompanied by uncertainty and many unanswerable questions.

FEARS ASSOCIATED WITH THE PROCESS OF DYING
These fears include loss of control and dignity, fears associated with the symptoms of disease, regrets of what might have been, that is 'our potential'; how family and friends will cope. It is important to recognise that there is often a disparity between intellectual recognition and emotional responses; people may reach intellectual awareness before they reach emotional awareness.

Effective communication will enable individuals to make decisions about death, for example
— *where* one is likely to die – home/hospice/hospital – not *when*;
— legal and funeral arrangements;
— organ donation;
— decisions relating to physical symptoms and deterioration in their condition; and
— practising facing up to death by discussing dream experiences – sometimes this is a more acceptable way of exploring their own feelings and discovering other people's responses.

How can nurses help?
This is a particularly difficult area of communication as *there are no precise answers*. Support can be offered by talking, listening and touching; trying to ensure the ease of physical symptoms; but no-one can predict how someone will die, whether it be peacefully or as a result of an emergency event.

As Nurses it is difficult not to be able to give definite answers but, in this situation, 'I don't know' is the only true answer, with the assurance of continued support. If appropriate, it *is* possible to warn the patient and/or relatives of a deterioration in the patient's condition, a deterioration which is perhaps leading to death.

Difficult situations

Some emphatic relatives insist that information relating to diagnosis and prognosis should be withheld:

> 'My husband must be given the best possible treatment but must never be told what is wrong with him, he couldn't cope'.

What can be done in this situation?

● Explore the possible reasons for the request. Are the relatives anxious that the patient will not be able to cope when he or she is aware of the true situation? Do they have distressing past experiences regarding the death of friends/relatives? Have they previously been given instructions about what their relative, the patient, would like to be told?

The relatives should be assured of the following.

● Such information would never be 'blurted out' with the patient being unprepared, and such information would usually be given in response to questions from the patient. Quite often the patient has guessed the true situation and is merely wanting his or her suspicions confirmed.

● Patient's imaginings are often worse and/or more disturbing than the known; opening up fears and anxieties allows them to be confronted and, in part, resolved.

The nurse should be aware of the following.

● The relatives burden of keeping the truth from the patient is very difficult, and can cause a barrier between them at a time when openness is crucial and may leave them with a sense of guilt in the bereavement period.

- If the relatives still insist that information be withheld the nurse must emphasise that his or her primary responsibility is to the patient and that, as a professional, the nurse will not lie to the patient.

- Where possible it is important not to alienate the relatives as they are part of the caring team and may need continuing support.

Telephone communication

Breaking bad news over the telephone is particularly difficult, especially if the news is unexpected or it is the middle of the night. All relatives of seriously ill patients should be asked, as a matter of routine, if they wish to be telephoned at night. In particular if they wish to be informed of a deterioration in the patient's condition or if they wish to be present as their loved one is dying. Relatives and friends must not be made to feel obliged to behave in a particular way to please the health care professional, but should have free choice in their decisions.

Some elderly people find the telephone daunting. In these situations it may be helpful to have the telephone number of another member of the family for contact so that someone will be with the elderly person and pass on the news face to face.

The Police are trained in and used to passing on bad news and they may be able to act as go-betweens from hospital to home should the health professional be worried about a particular family. Often, if needed, the Police will accompany the relatives to hospital.

However well prepared, the news of someone's death invariably comes as a shock; the health professional must be prepared for the relatives' responses to manifest themselves in a variety of different ways, and must support the relatives as needed.

Written communication

Nursing care plans placed at the end of the patients' beds or left in patients' houses must display a congruence with their known level of knowledge, since is well known that patients and relatives will avidly read them. The campaign for freedom of information and the potential 'Access to Health Care Records Bill' will ensure a more honest relationship between health care workers, patients and relatives, facilitating more open communication by allowing patients access to their own notes.

One of the most useful questions to ask is: 'Do our notes aid communication with other health care professionals?' That is their purpose and, if they do not aid communication they should be rewritten or updated. Their primary use is as an effective medium for the giving and receiving of information on behalf of, and for the benefit of, the patient.

Conclusion

Effective communication should improve the quality of life for the patient, their family and friends and increase their satisfaction with the care received, and, as a consequence, increase the nurse's job satisfaction, lessen stress and improve

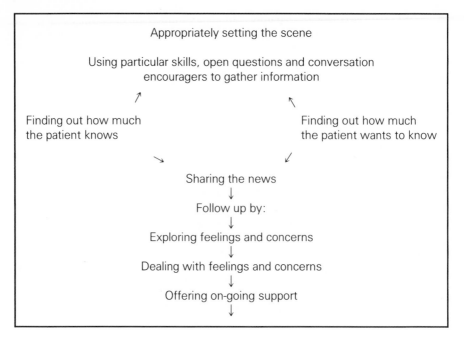

Fig. 14.1   Summary of steps aiding effective communication.

relationships within the multidisciplinary team. A summary of the steps aiding effective communication is given in Fig. 14.1.

Communication is a delicate network of interaction between patients, relatives and staff. It is hoped that this chapter proves there is no mystique about it; the skills can be learnt, mastered and effectively used, providing the carers have the confidence to try and are well supported with their interactions. For many patients, it is not only the complexity of skills, or the depth of understanding but the fact that someone cares enough to try that is important.

> 'I know you feel insecure, don't know what to say, don't know what to do. But please believe me, if you care, you can't go wrong. Just admit that you care. . . . Don't run away. . . . Wait. . . . all I want to know is that there will be someone to hold my hand when I need it. I am afraid. Death may get to be a routine with you, but it is new to me'.
>
> *Anon, 1970*

(The above words are taken from an account written by a student nurse who was dying.)

Acknowledgements

Thanks to Dr Ilora Finlay for her support and confidence in my abilities; to my multidisciplinary colleagues at Llandough Hospital, Cardiff, in particular the trained nurses on Ward E5 who identified actual and potential areas of difficulty. Especial thanks to the proof readers, Julia, Anthony and Gill who improved my grammar, spelling and punctuation and to Joyce Harding who, with infinite patience, efficiently and speedily prepared this chapter.

References

AGUILERA, D. (1967). Realtionship between physical contact and verbal interaction between nurses and patients. *Journal of Psychiatric Nursing*, **5**, 5121.

ANON (1970). Death in the first person. *American Journal of Nursing*, **70**, 336.

BARTON, D. (1972). The need for including instruction on death and dying in the medical curriculum. *Journal of Medical Education*, **47**, 169–75.

BREWIN, T. B. (1977). The cancer patient: communication and morale. *British Medical Journal*, **2**, 1623–7.

BUCKMAN, R. (1984). Breaking bad news: why is it still so difficult. *British Medical Journal*, **288**, 1597–9.

BUCKMAN, R. (1988). *I don't know what to say – how to help and support someone who is dying*. Papermac, London.

English National Board for Nursing, Midwifery and Health Visiting (1989). *Project 2000 – 'A New Preparation for Practice'; Guidelines and Criteria for Course Development and the Formulation of Collaborative Links between Approved Training Institutions within the National Health Service and Centres of Higher Education*. ENB, London.

FIELD, D. (1984). 'We didn't want him to die on his own' – nurses accounts of nursing dying patients. *Journal of Advanced Nursing*, **9**, 59–70.

FIELDING, R. G. and LLEWELLYN, S. P. (1987). Communication training in nursing may damage your health and enthusiasm: some warnings. *Journal of Advanced Nursing*, **12**, 281–90.

FRANCIS, V. and MORRIS, M. (1969). Gaps in doctor-patient communication: patients reponse to medical advice. *New England Journal of Medicine*, **280**, 535–40.

FRY, J. (1983). Deaths and dying. *Update*, 15th Dec, 1706–7.

HISCOCKS, S. (1990). Unpublished G.R.A.S.P. data. Unit 4, Llandough Hospital, Penarth, South Glamorgan.

LANGLAND, R. M. and PANNICCUCCI, C. L. (1982). Effects of touch on communication with elderly confused clients. *Journal of Gerontology Nursing*, **8**, 152–5.

MAGUIRE, P. (1985). Barriers to psychological care of the dying. *British Medical Journal*, **291**, 1711–13.

MAGUIRE, P. and FAULKNER, A. (1988). Communicate with cancer patients: 1 Handling bad news and difficult questions. *British Medical Journal*, **297**, 907–9.

MOY, C. (1981). Touch in the counselling relationship: an exploratory study *Patient Counselling and Health Education*, 3rd quarter, 89–85.

MULLIGAN, J. C. A. (1989). Dying at Home – An evaluation of a specialist home care service. Unpublished PhD thesis, University of Wales.

PARKES, C. M. and PARKES, J. (1984). Hospice versus hospital care: re-evaluation after 10 years as seen by surviving spouse. *Postgraduate Medical Journal*, **60**, 120–4.

PETERSON, M. (1988). The norms and values held by three groups of nurses concerning psychosocial nursing practice. *International Journal of Nursing Studies*, **25**, 85–103.

REISETTER, K. H. and THOMAS, B. (1986). Nursing care of the dying: its relationship to selected nurse characteristics. *International Journal of Nursing Studies*, **23**, 39–50.

STEDEFORD, A. (1981). Couples facing death. II Unsatisfactory communication. *British Medical Journal*, **283**, 1098–101.

STEDEFORD, A. (1984). *Facing death: patients, families and professionals.* Heinemann, London.

United Kingdom Central Council for Nursing, Midwifery and Health Visiting (1984). *Code of Professional Conduct for the Nurse, Midwife and Health Visitor.* UKCC, London.

United Kingdom Central Council for Nursing, Midwifery and Health Visiting (1989). *Information on Post-Registration Education and Practice Project (PREPP).* UKCC, London.

United Kingdom Central Council for Nursing, Midwifery and Health Visting (1990). *The Report of the Post-Registration Education and Practice Project.* UKCC, London.

WILKINSON, S. (1988). Identifying the major stressors in cancer nursing. In *Cancer Nursing: a revolution in care*, P. Pritchard (Ed.), pp. 68–72. Scutari, London.

Further reading

General communication skills

BURNARD, P. (1989). *Counselling Skills for Health Professionals.* Chapman and Hall, London and New York.

Specific areas of death and dying

BUCKMAN, R. (1988). *I don't know what to say – How to help and support someone who is dying.* Papermac, London.

DE BEAUVOIR, S. (1969). *A very easy death.* Penguin, London. (Last reprint, 1987).

OWENS R. G. and NAYLOR, F. (1989). *Living while dying.* Thorsons Publishers, Wellingborough.

STEDEFORD, A. (1984). *Facing death: Patients, families and professionals.* Heinemann, London.

Further viewing

'Why don't they talk to me?'. Parts 1–5. Dr Robert Buckman and Dr Peter Maguire. Available from Lindward Productions, Shepperton Studio Centre Shepperton, Middlesex.

An audio-visual communication aid – attempting to help improve skills when listening and talking to patients.

15

Applying counselling to nursing care: A person-centred perspective

Morna C. Rutherford

'So when you are listening to somebody completely, attentively, then you are listening not only to the words, but also to the feeling of what is being conveyed, to the whole of it, not part of it.'

J. Krisknamurti

Facing cancer involves many emotions. People with cancer confront the challenges of loss and change together with their families. Chapter 10 describes the dynamics of change and some of the implications of loss. Nursing practice requires a keen awareness of individual needs and the intention to care. Care, however, is shapeless without human connection and communication. As counselling provides a direct opportunity to promote this form of communion, nurses are called upon more and more to use counselling skills. The nurse who is offering the counselling is referred to here as 'the counsellor', and the person receiving counselling is called 'the client'. This chapter discusses counselling skills within the context or a Person-centred philosophy of care.

What is counselling?

The aim of counselling is to provide a safe, supportive and caring atmosphere in which the client will be enabled to find strength and direction. 'Enabling' is defined as 'empowering' a person to take certain action (*Concise Oxford Dictionary*, 1976, p. 340). Counselling is not an activity where the counsellor behaves powerfully to direct the client, but a process where he or she uses counselling skills to help the client find his or her own power.

There is no place here for the counsellor to make judgements or to try to influence the client. Advice-giving, if requested, may indeed be part of a helping relationship, but it is inappropriate within the context of counselling as defined above. Burnard (1987, p. 279) states that 'the counsellor who offers a lot of advice is asking for the client to become dependant'.

McLeod (1990, pp. 14–16) reviewed some recent research on what clients experience as helpful in counselling. It is interesting to note that 'advice from their counsellors . . . is highly valued, and the absence of advice is seen as unhelpful or uncaring.' It is necessary to know what clients mean by 'advice'. Clients may not be asking to be told what to do. Rather, they might be wanting to find out for themselves what to do through a system of problem-solving, and may need some guidance and support with this by taking one problem at a time. The locus of choice and responsibility for life lies firmly with the client, committing the counsellor with responsibility *to* clients, but not *for* them. (Mearns and Thorne, 1988, p. 29).

Counselling is a journey of self-exploration and discovery involving challenges and hurdles on the way. It is, however, the client's personal journey, and the counsellor is a chosen companion. As such, the counsellor has no right to impose values or interpretations on the client.

Emotional release is part of the healing process. It is therefore essential that the client's emotions are not ignored or smothered. Laura Allen (1990, p. 25) describes her experience of failure in counselling. When the counsellor tried to take her 'out' of her desperate crying with 'there, there, it will be alright', Laura stopped crying and became really 'stuck'. Blocking emotional release devalues the client and is certainly *not* helpful. There is no place in counselling for trying to stop the flow of emotions. Reassurance and encouragement do little to help people discover their strengths. For example, if a client expresses guilt it is basically *unhelpful* to discount the guilt by praising or 'reassuring' the client. The client's guilt will be stronger than the counsellor's platitude, and the client is still left saddled with the guilt. It is essential to acknowledge guilt in order to free the client to explore personal meaning.

In considering what is and what is not involved in counselling, it is important to mention that the counselling relationship is not an arena within which the counsellor should attempt to satisfy personal needs. Nurse (1980, p. 41) describes the need to be needed. She states that 'the counsellor who feels unimportant or unnecessary in (his or) her personal life is especially vulnerable to seeking satisfaction for (his or) herself by keeping the client bound to and dependant upon (him or) her'. This will block the counsellor's ability to facilitate the client's growth. Counselling, therefore, ties in beautifully with individualised nursing care. The reality, however, is less than ideal when nurses are limited by process, environment and personal needs. This notwithstanding, given the right conditions, it is possible for nurses to incorporate counselling into their care.

The relevance of counselling

In nursing, counselling is relevant in two sense: there is the pertinence of counselling skills in day to day communication, and the relevance also of more explicit counselling contracts. Counselling skills, such as listening and responding to another person, can be used at any time, whereas a counselling contract defines a more intense therapeutic partnership. The intention of a therapeutic partnership is well defined, with the client firstly making a choice to see a counsellor. The contract will involve a negotiation on how and where the counsellor and client will work together and how much time they will initially spend on the issue at hand. This brings in the necessity of privacy and a discussion on confidentiality which must be explicit at the outset. If potential interruptions are prevented, both counsellor and client are assured the opportunity to work together without external inhibitions. Any evident limitations need to be defined as part of the contract which now creates the potential for a trusting relationship. More than the counsellor's skills are involved in a therapeutic partnership: the relationship itself becomes a therapeutic medium. Although the contract is usually informal, it is important to review the conditions of the relationshp from time to time to check if the client's needs are being met. If the client experiences some kind of regularity in the commitment of the counsellor, then this regularity enables a safe, containing environment for the client.

The therapeutic partnership is a potentially dynamic and potent area of care.

Benefit, however, will only be achieved if the client is ready and willing to enter into a working relationship with the counsellor. Watson (1983) reviewed the data on the efficacy of psychosocial intervention programmes for patients with cancer. She found that provision of a support service for all patients is probably unnecessary. However, there should be improved methods of identifying those at risk so that selective support can then be offered with specific aims defined. Watson (1983) concludes that support may be needed over a long period.

Watson's (1983) report confirms the need to clarify the services offered to patients. Many nurses find it difficult enough to meet the basic physical needs of the people they care for. Consideration of the time and commitment needed for a counselling relationships may be beyond the scope of the nurse unless colleagues and management enable the redefinition of nursing priorities. With this support, the nurse can take the initiative in creating counselling opportunities. If time is short, the value of counselling skills should never be underestimated, as listening to and responding to a person may take just a few minutes and be all that is needed. Nevertheless, the nurse may be able to offer a more intense therapeutic relationship, if it is requested, by prioritising responsibilities so that time is created for the client's need.

This chapter will now explore counselling skills with relevance to nursing, then define a person-centred philosophy of care which enhances basic skills and creates the potential for therapeutic development.

Counselling skills

Any enabling interaction begins with counselling skills, and listening is the foundation of those skills. Burnard (1987, p. 280) states that 'to really listen to another person is the most caring act of all, and takes skill and practice.' Nurse (1980, p. 70) describes the art of listening by saying; 'In counselling it is important to listen to what is said, how it is said, and also to listen to what is being implied behind the words'. This requires intensive use of the senses: hearing, watching, touching and smelling are all media of reception. Non-verbal processes can speak far louder than words, and may tell a very different tale. An example of this is given below.

Actions speak louder than words

John is in hospital for the results of his tests. He asks to see a nurse.

John [shaking hands with the nurse]: 'Well, the doctor confirmed my suspicions. He told me the growth is cancer [voice breaks slightly]. But I don't mind [defiant stare]. I'm going to fight it if it's the last thing I do!'

The nurse notices that John's hand is clammy when she shakes it. She hears the tremor in his voice when he mentions 'cancer'. She notices him shaking slightly. She also senses a mixture of emotions behind his defiant stare.

Effective listening requires concentration and focusing on the most important issue(s) presented. In order to focus on the client, the counsellor requires to develop an internal 'stillness' (Mearns and Thorne, 1988, p. 54), which is only possible if the counsellor can mentally set aside other concerns. Gendlin (1981, p. 71) calls this 'clearing a space' and describes a method of 'distancing' the self from personal troubles. This method can be practised and learned.

Attention on the client is often facilatated by eye contact. Alternatively, some clients feel very self-conscious of constantly being held in the counsellor's gaze. The relative position of the counsellor is important in facilitating communication as some clients may need space between them and the counsellor, whereas others find closeness important: a table between the client and counsellor, for example, can feel like a barrier, and should be removed. Sensitivity to the cleint's need is built up through close awareness of his or her reactions.

If listening is the foundation of counselling skills, then clients need to know that they are heard. Acknowledging the important of the client's communication and feelings is paramount, and Hodgson (1983) describes this as one of the factors which reduces fear and anxiety.

Acknowledgement can be conveyed by touch or facial expression and both are powerful means of communication. Marilyn Butcher (1988, p. 16) describes her fear when her cancer was diagnosed. As she talked to her anaesthetist, he held her hand, and 'that non-verbal reassurance reached and soothed the small child inside me who was frightened and alone.' She went on to say, 'I have learnt a lot about myself, but the most valuable thing of all is that a hand held is worth a million words'. This was evidently really important for Marilyn. However, not every person can tolerate touch. It is important to be sensitive to intrusion or conveying unwanted sympathy, as the meaning of non-verbal responses is not always evident to the client. It can be helpful to verbally acknowledge the important issues for the client. A response the nurse might make to John following his statement in the example given above is illustrated below.

Response by counsellor

Nurse: 'I hear how important fighting the cancer is to you. I also see that you are shaking' [reaches out and touches his arm].

This example of the nurse's response to John shows verbal acknowledgement of what he is saying. The nurse also shows verbal and non-verbal sensitivity to John's feelings. John now knows that the counsellor is 'with' him and he has the opportunity to say more about how he feels. He also has the opportunity to deny his feelings if he wishes and to talk about his need to fight.

Response should flow naturally from the counsellor to the client and the counsellor should refrain from 'slipping in his (or her) interpretations' (Mearns, 1980) which might interfere with the client's process. Burnard (1987, p. 280) states that 'it is possible to pay so much attention to techniques that they impede listening and communicating', and McEvoy (1988, p. 458) supports this statement by describing failure in listening resulting from the counsellor concentrating on his or her own reply. Lamerton (1984, p. 583) suggests a way of transcending the counsellor's concern over his or her response. He states that 'there is no need to know what to say', and if the counsellor is focusing *fully* on the client, then his or her response will probably be appropriate. Lamerton (1984, p. 583) describes the 'trap' when no response comes to mind. However, this can be trusted also. If no reply is forthcoming, 'then we need not manufacture one' (Lamerton, 1984, p. 583): silence can be an important space for the client. Many counsellors feel the urge to fill this space. This urge is often precipitated by the counsellor's own discomfort. The value of silence can only be learned through experience and can be a very powerful way of 'being with' a client. However, if it feels right to do so, the counsellor may observe the silence by saying: 'We have been quiet for some time now. How does that feel?'

Respect for the client is shown by the willingness of the counsellor to proceed at the client's own pace, with patience only being possible when the client's perspective is really valued. Simsen (1988, pp. 31–3) describes the need to 'stay with the person who is testing his (or her) own beliefs or struggling with questions of fear and faith'. This supportive presence does not need to be continual over 24 hours a day, as the client will need space to discover underlying strengths. Sensitive availability to the client may be all that is required.

A person-centred approach

Person-centred counselling exists as a distinct therapeutic approach through the work of Carl Rogers. He believed that an individual has sufficient insight and resources available for personal growth. Stevens (1967, p. 29) wrote, 'everything that I needed was right inside me'. This realisation embraces a unique approach which facilitates the cleint's selfawareness and inner strengths.

Roger's general hypothesis is:

> 'If I can provide a certain type of relationship, the other person will discover within (her or) himself the capacity to use that relationship for growth, and change and personal development will occur'.

This is an enormous claim. Inherent in the claim is a belief in the potential of the individual. It is one thing for the counsellor to believe in the clinet's potential, but it is quite another thing for the client if low self-esteem has destroyed all confidence in self. The task of counselling is to empower the client with self-belief, and the power of a therapeutic relationship makes this possible. Rogers (1961, p. 33) mentioned a 'certain type of relationship'. He defines this in terms of three core conditions:

- Acceptance
- Empathy
- Realness

If the counsellor can bring all three conditions to the relationship, and if the client can experience them, then, 'constructive personal development will invariably occur', (Rogers, 1961, p. 35).

Acceptance

There may be a great deal of fear involved in revealing innermost thoughts and feelings. So many values are imposed on an individual by society and significant others, and experience shows that exposing part of oneself leaves this part open to judgement. A client certainly will not risk sharing his or her vulnerabilities if he or she does not feel safe. The counsellor can build up a client's trust through warmth, valuing and respect. Rogers (1961, p. 47) describes this acceptance as 'unconditional postive regard'. Mearns and Thorne (1988, p. 59) state that 'the counsellor who holds this attitude deeply values the humanity of (his or) her client and is not deflected in that valuing by any particular client behaviour. The attitude manifests itself in the counsellor's consistent acceptance of and enduring warmth towards (his or) her client'. It can be difficult to like a client who is angry, manipulative or withdrawn, or there may be particular aspects of the client's behaviour which are impossible to tolerate. Mearns and Thorne (1988, p. 59) suggest that 'it is possible to accept the client as a person of worth while still not liking some of the things he (or she) does'. This allows the counsellor to have unconditional warm regard for the client while still not compromising person values. Offering accepance or this calibre means that no judgements, assumptions or conditions are made on how the client 'should be'. This attitude of acceptance is rarely found in health care, yet it is one of the fundamental conditions in a person-centred relationship, making it possible for the client to begin to find personal value.

Empathy

Empathy is a process of understanding how the client thinks and feels. Any preconceptions (for example, things which have helped other people in the past, or something which has helped the counsellor) may distort true understanding of the client's world. Empathy is not how the counsellor would feel in the client's position, nor is it how other people have felt in similar situations, it is understanding how this individual client feels here and now. Empathy involves setting aside personal values and experiences, and entering into the perceptual world of the client, 'as if' it were the counsellor's own world. Rogers (1961, p. 62–3) emphasises the importance of the 'as if' quality. The counsellor needs to let go of personal philosophies and principles in order to understand fully and appreciate the client. The counsellor, however, must not let go of his or her own identity. If this does occur then the counsellor will be drawn into the client's world and will be unable to maintain the degree of separation which is required to be deeply empathic.

It is possible to learn empathic skills. The simple analogy given below may help introduce empathy.

Understanding empathy

'Let me try on your shoes so that I can feel where they pinch you. My feet are a different size and shape to yours, so I cannot feel exactly as you feel. However, I am willing to try if you are willing to let me.'

Experiencing someone else's world as they experience it is virtually impossible, yet the willingness to reach out and try can enable awareness and insight.

Communication of empathic understanding to the client is an essential part of the process of empathy. It is important for the counsellor to 'check out' what is being communicated. This can be done by focusing on an important statement from the client. The counsellor may use the phrase 'I'm hearing you saying . . .'. This is seen in the response by the counsellor given in the example on p. 249. Another kind of empathic response is illustrated below.

Reflecting on important issues

Client: 'I've been spending so much time looking after Sheila that I don't seem to have much time left for anything else, let alone the children.'

Counsellor: 'It seems like it's been really hard for you to have time for other things in your life – especially time for the children.'

This is a reflection of the client's statement, with the counsellor trying to get a sense of the client's perspective. If the counsellor's response is not quite accurate, the client has an opening to correct and 'help' the counsellor understand. In the above example, the client may well have replied: 'Well, yes, but my real concern is how to look after Sheila'. This 're-directs' the counsellor towards the client's concern, and gives the client the important opportunity to stop, clarify his position and determine his own understanding.

Reflecting on important statements may not be enough. It may be additionally important to reflect on any sense of underlying *feelings* the client may be experiencing. The counsellor above might have gone on to say: 'You seem really frustrated by that . . .'. All these responses can enable the cleint to say or feel more, if chosen. Nonetheless, the cleint may be needing more *depth* of empathy from the counsellor. The counsellor may have been able to offer that greater depth by saying: 'You seem really frustrated by that . . . but I sense something more . . . almost like a desperation?'

Truax and Carkhuff (1967, pp. 46–58) describe various degrees of empathy. These range from the inaccurate response through the reflection of surface statements and feelings to a 'depth reflection'. The depth reflection is described by Mearns and Thorne (1988, p. 42) as sensing deeper insight of which the client may not yet be aware. This may be facilitated by offering the client an opportunity to achieve this deeper sense. An example is: 'I see that you are shaking . . . I wonder if there is something more happening inside you?'

Gilley (1988, p. 12) describes 'holding together knowing and not knowing'. There is regard here for the delicacy of a human being who is seeking support, yet who needs to discover a personal path.

Sensing the client's world as he is experiencing it, draws on the intuition and imagination of the counsellor. Burnard (1989, p. 52) describes intuition as 'knowledge beyond the senses' – it is an unexplained inner ability to 'know'. Mearns and Thorne (1988, p. 53) on the other hand, suggests that it is perfectly possible to explain this intuitive ability in terms of the vast experience gained through a lifetime of personal encounters. Trusting this sensitive ability will help enhance the counsellor's response.

Realness

While working with a client, the counsellor will experience various personal feelings. Some of these feelings will emanate from personal experience while others will be in response to the client. Feelings in response to the client will occur if the counsellor is empathically 'in tune' with the client. Being 'real' involves an awareness of the feelings which are related to the client, and a willingness to express them. There is little point in smiling at a client when deep down the counsellor feels anxious or shaken by what he or she is hearing. More often than not, the client will sense the counsellor's real feelings and this can lead to a confusion which is separate from the client's own dilemma. It is difficult for a client to trust a counsellor who is not genuine.

A counsellor who is 'willing to be fully present as a real, alive, relating human being who is not concealing' (Mearns and Thorne, 1988, p. 86) will risk sharing his or her personal feelings in response to the client. Rogers (1961, p. 61) describes this way of being as 'congruence'. The counsellor is 'genuine and without "front" or façade, openly being the feelings and attitudes which at that moment are flowing in him (or her)' (Rogers 1961, p. 61).

The counsellor may be confused by what the client is saying. Within this context, 'being real' means admitting to the client that there is a lack of understanding. For example: 'I must stop you just now, as I can't seem to grasp what you mean.' This allows the possibility of clarification. More important, it brings the counsellor back into the relationship. Effective relations with clients requires this kind of honesty and openness. Furthermore, the clarification may help clients to see ways in which they have been misleading themselves.

Another example of congruence is sharing a feeling which is persistent and seems to be related to the client. For example: 'I'm feeling really tense just now, and I'm not sure why that is. It's like I'm trying so hard to reach you, but there's some "barrier" in the way.' There is no accusation here. The counsellor is simply stating a feeling by offering a reaction to the client. If there is significance to the client, he or she may be able to work with a new awareness. Has the client been putting up 'barriers' in relation to the counsellor? Is this something the client usually does in relationships? In this way, the counsellor's realness in reflecting his or her experience of the client may help the client to make self-discoveries.

Being open in response to a client is different from self-disclosure. The counsellor's experience of life is never the same as the client's. It is rarely helpful in counselling to share life experiences with the client; 'even then the focus of attention would remain on the client rather than the counsellor' (Mearns and Thorne, 1988, p. 82). An example of this is: 'My son also left home when he was that age. I felt "lost" too. However, it sounds like you felt "abandoned" somehow . . . ?'

This returns to the empathic response. Sometimes a common life experience can 'block' the counsellor's ability to be empathic. Clearly, the three conditions of acceptance, empathy and realness are entwined and work together. For example, being real enhances the empathic response which is facilitated through valuing the client. Professional distancing or aloofness blocks the whole counselling process. This may be a necessary defence for some, yet it will never facilitate a true depth of caring. It is important for the counsellor to find a safe environment in which to explore any need for self-protection. Self-awareness at this level can free many defences.

Self-awareness and support

The counsellor's self-awareness is an essential pre-requisite to effective counselling. Mearns and Thorne (1988, p. 23) state that, 'the relationship which the counsellor has with (him or) herself will, to a large extent, determine the quality of the work (he or) she is able to initiate with clients'. Self-knowledge helps distinguish between self-needs and empathic response. This knowledge is vital if the counsellor aims to enter fully into a counselling relationship. Self-awareness is enhanced and enabled by personal support and, without support, a counsellor may suffer undue stress (see Chapter 16). Alternatively, he or she may unconsciously protect him or herself by becoming complacent. Hodgson (1983, p. 65) describes complacency in staff. 'Someone who is sure he (or she) is doing everything right will not be really in touch with someone who is feeling all wrong'.

It is the counsellor's responsibility to seek support. This is an important part of personal value and work. Support through personal supervision is an invaluable way of clarifying issues, discovering resources and moving forward. Support may be also found in group situations. The members can work together to share difficulties and enable insight. Implicit in any support is the need to trust the other person or people. As in counselling, trust is aided by drawing up a working contract and discussing confidentiality.

Confidentiality

If a person discloses something meaningful to another person, then the other person is being trusted with something personal. To pass this on the others might devalue this trust. With the importance attached to communication in nursing, confidentiality poses a dilemma. Support, however, is offered through the Professional Code of Conduct for Nurses, Midwives and Health Visitors (United Kingdom Central Council for Nursing, Midwifery and Health Visiting, 1984) which clearly defines the nurse's position: 'Each registered nurse, midwife and health visitor is accountable for his or her practice, and, in the exercise of professional accountability shall:

Respect confidential information obtained in the course of professional practice and refrain from disclosing such information without the consent of the patient/client, or a person entitled to act on his/her behalf, except where disclosure is required by law or by the order of a court or is necessary in the public interest' (UKCC, 1984, p. 3).

Within the context of counselling, whatever clients discover or reveal about themselves is their own. Except under exceptional circumstances, this should never be disclosed to another party. It is up to the client whether any personal information is to be shared.

If the counsellor feels there is something important to communicate with others, then it is vital that this is discussed firstly with the client. The counsellor has no right to share anything about the client with others, unless prior permission has been given. The value of the counselling relationship is dependant on the maintenance of this confidence.

Applying counselling in nursing care

Whether the nurse sets up an agreement to see a client regularly for counselling so offering the opportunity of a therapeutic partnership, or whether he or she uses counselling skills in everyday communication, a person-centred approach offers a philosophy of care which facilitates the client's self-discovery. An example of counselling skills used with a client whom this writer has been visiting is given below. The client has given permission for this material to be reproduced. The conversation described took less than ten minutes of time, then the client moved on to discuss other matters.

Use of counselling skills

Client: [appearing really agitated] 'I just can't settle after seeing these two other women dying in the same room as me [referring to other patients] – I feel I've been forced to look at something I'm not ready for. You know, I *know* I'm going to die, and I'm not frightened of death – in fact I welcome it – but it was just *terrible* watching those women die.' [eyes wide]

Counsellor: [reaching to hold client's hand] 'I can feel you trembling and I sense your fear . . . I hear you saying that you're not frightened of death, yet I feel that there's something about dying which terrifies you'.

Client: [Silence – shaking increases] 'It's the *process* of dying – [involuntary sobs] – it's so undignified! [grips counsellor's hand tightly]

Counsellor: [silence] . . . 'I really hear the *horror* in your voice . . . Keeping your dignity seems absolutely *vital* to you'

Client: [starts to relax a little – withdraws her hand] 'It's the idea of losing control over bodily functions – I just couldn't *bear* that' [starts shaking again].

Counsellor: 'Something about losing that control which horrifies you.'

Client: [stops shaking] 'Yes – it's the thought of other people clearing up my mess – it's so *disgusting*' [draws back and screws up face].

Counsellor: 'The thought of other people clearing up your mess seems really impossible for you to *allow?*'

Client: [looking directly at counsellor] 'Oh! I could't *possibly* accept it!'

Counsellor: 'That really strikes me! – it's like it would be impossibly hard for you to let someone tend to you or care for you in a physical way'.

Client: [looks down] 'Yes, you're right, I would be so embarrassed and ashamed.'

Counsellor: [quietly] 'There's something about these feelings you have . . . and I sense you don't want me to touch you right now . . . it's like you feel you're untouchable or maybe . . . not worth caring for?'

Client: [silence and tears] 'How can I be worth caring about?'

Counsellor: [silence] '. . . You sound so desolate, almost like you feel totally rejected.'

The client went on to talk for a short time about past events where she felt rejected by her father.

This counselling session is an example of the counsellor 'keeping track' with the client and not jumping to conclusions about the client's fear. When the client said, 'I've been forced to look at something I'm not ready for', the counsellor was aware of the fear and anxiety which the client had been carrying since the deaths of the other patients. In addition, the counsellor sensed that the client probably *was* ready to look at that 'something', but that a safe and supportive relationship would be necessary to help release the client's fear. The counsellor did not even try to reassure the client about her stated concern over incontinence, realising that this reassurance would have blocked the client at this point, preventing her from exploring the significance of her disgust. The counsellor had no idea what that significance was, and worked sensitively with empathic responses, so enabling the client to reach the depth of her troubles. By openly stating the sense that the client did not want to be touched, and yet by showing willingness to stay with and not back away from the client, the counsellor empowered the client to talk freely about painful past events. Once the client reached this very difficult area in her life, the counsellor was able to 'be with' and acknowledge the client's pain, and, most important, not reject or diminish the client in any way. This embodies the person-centred philosophy, offering acceptance, empathy and real presence with the counsellor's approach. The counsellor did not try to interpret the client's troubles: the client showed that she had the capacity to understand herself in her own way and in her own time. One week later, during another visit with the counsellor, the client said briefly: 'You know, I've been thinking a lot about my father recently, and I've actually forgiven him for what he did to me. I feel a warmth for him now, and that makes me feel better'. Only the client could reach inside herself and know what it is like to offer forgiveness and experience resultant warmth.

Rogers (1961, p. 357) states that 'the farmer cannot make the germ develop and sprout from the seed: he can only supply the nurturing conditions which will permit the seed to develop its own potentialities'. Clearly, the 'nurturing conditions' of the person-centred approach can free 'the natural healing capacity within the client' (Mearns and Thorne, 1988, p. 129), so enabling potential development. This development is still possible towards the end of life.

A client with cancer who is struggling with the attendant emotions brought by change and loss may present the counsellor with feelings such as fear, grief, anger and guilt (see Chapter 10). Initially, the counsellor may feel overwhelmed by these strong emotions. This notwithstanding, Mearns and Thorne (1988, p. 104) state that 'the very activity of empathic understanding often has the effect of defusing a crisis, of slowing down the pace and relieving to some extent the crippling sense of anxiety and dread which the client may be undergoing.' Slowing down the pace is one way of enhancing the quality of time, and offers an invaluable gift to the person whose life-time is limited. Clearly, being with a client in a person-centred way is a powerful use of counselling in nursing care.

If people with cancer and members of their family can experience acceptance, depth of understanding and genuineness from Health Care Professionals, then they may be empowered by their own strengths and internal resources to live life to capacity and find meaning in the here and now. Through encountering life in all its painful dimensions, a process of discovery is launched which holds the dynamic potential for growth. Person-centred counselling can help release this potential through freeing the healing power of the individual, enabling creativity and increasing self-esteem.

Acknowledgements

Thanks go to Professor Stuart Aitken, Department of Geography, San Diego State University; Diana Guthrie, Student Advisory and Counselling Service, Univesity of Edinburgh; Elke Lambers and Dave Mearns, Co-Directors, FDI course in Person-Centred Counselling; Alison Shoemark, colleague and friend; and members of the

Scottish FDI Supervision Group. The support and insight gained from all was invaluable. Special thanks also go to Mrs Sheena Hogg for typing, and to my husband Sam for his unfailing patience and respect.

References

ALLEN, L. (1990). A Client's Experience of Failure. In *Experiences of Counselling in Action*, D. Mearns and W. Dryden (Eds), pp. 20–7. Sage, London.

BURNARD, P. (1987). Counselling: basic principles in nursing. *The Professional Nurse*, Jun. **2(9)**, 278–80.

BURNARD, P. (1989). The 'Sixth Sense'. *Nursing Times*, **85(50)**, 52–3.

BUTCHER, M. (1988). The nightmare of the dreaded diagnosis. *The Independent Newspaper*, 18 Oct., 16.

United Kingdom Central Council for Nursing, Midwifery and Health Visiting (1984). *Code of Professional Conduct for the Nurse, Midwife and Health Visitor*. UKCC, London.

GENDLIN, E. T. (1981). *Focusing.* Bantam, New York.

GILLEY, J. (1988). Intimacy and terminal care. *Journal of the Royal College of General Practitioners*, **38**, 121–2.

HODGSON, S. (1983). Enhancing patient-nurse communication. *Nursing Times*, Occasional Papers, **79(18)**, 64–5.

LAMERTON, R. (1984). Communication with the dying patient. *The Practitioner*, **228**, 581–3.

MCEVOY, P. (1988). Introducing nurses to the counselling process. *The Professional Nurse*, Aug. **3(11)**, 456–60.

MCLEOD, J. (1990). The Client's Experience of Counselling and Psychotherapy: A Review of the Research Literature. In *Experience of Counselling in Action*, D. Mearns and W. Dryden (Eds), pp. 1–19. Sage, London.

MEARNS, D. (1980). *The Person-Centred Approach to Therapy*. Unpublished paper produced for the Scottish Association for Counselling, May 31.

MEARNS, D. and THORNE, B. (1988). *Person-Centred Counselling in Action*. Sage, London.

NURSE, G. (1980). *Counselling and the Nurse*, second edition. H M & M, England.

ROGERS, C. R. (1961). *On Becoming a Person*. Constable, London.

SIMSEN, B. (1988). Nursing the spirit. *Nursing Times*, Sept. 14, **84(37)**, 31–3.

STEVENS, B. (1967). From My Life 1. In *Person to Person: The Problem of Being Human*, C. R. Rogers and B. Stevens (Eds), pp. 29–40, Souvenir Press, London.

TRUAX, C. B. and CARKHUFF, R. R (1967). *Towards Effective Counselling and Psychotherapy*, Aldine, Chicago.

WATSON, M. (1983). Psychosocial intervention with cancer patients: a review. *Psychological Medicine*, **13**, 839–46.

Further reading

AXLINE, V. M. (1964). *Dibs – In Search of Self.* Penguin Books, Harmondsworth.
BOND, M. (1986), *Stress and Self-Awareness: A Guide for Nurses.* Heinemann Nursing, London.
BURNARD, P. (1985). *Learning Human Skills.* Heinemann Nursing, London.
DRYDEN, W. (Ed.) (1984). *Individual Therapy in Britain.* Harper & Row. London.
GENDLIN, E. T. (1981). *Focusing.* Bantam, New York.
KAGAN, C., EVANS, J. and KAY, B. (1986). *A Manual of Interpersonal Skills for Nurses.* Harper & Row, London.
MEARNS, D. and DRYDEN, W. (Eds) (1990). *Experiences of Counselling in Action.* Sage, London.
MEARNS, D. and THORNE, B. (1988). *Person-Centred Counselling in Action.* Sage, London.
NURSE, G. (1980). *Counselling and the Nurse: An Introduction,* second edition. H M & H, England.
ROGERS, C. R. (1961). *On Becoming a Person.* Constable, London.
ROGERS, C. R. and STEVENS, B. (1967). *Person to Person: The Problem of Being Human.* Souvenir Press, London.
TSCHUDIN, V. (1987). *Counselling Skills for Nurses,* second edition. Bailliere Tindall, London.

16

Learning to cope with the stress of palliative care

Pat Mathers

'The ultimate measure of man is not where he stands in moments of comfort and convenience but where he stands at times of challenge and controversy'
Martin Luther King, Strength to Love, *1963*

Introduction

The participants in the caring situation of a patient with advanced cancer are the patient, the family and relatives of the patient and the nurse. Flows of communication in the form of commitment of self take place between the nurse, the family and the relatives as they endeavour to maximise the quality of remaining life for the patient and the patient tries to ease any possible distress experienced by those around him or her. To understand some of the complexity of the flows of self this chapter proposes a model in which care is identified with the energy and resource of the participants.

It is clear that the demand for energy and resource will be greatest for the nurse for it is the nurse who provides the specialist care for the patient, the family and the relatives and who also endeavours to maintain harmonious interrelationships between the participants of the model. The role of the nurse then is that of a manager who determines whether or not the caring situation is maintained in a steady state. Such a role can be draining and exhausting for the nurse and some renewal of energy and resource is essential if this steady state or homeostasis of the model is to be achieved.

The practice of relaxation and controlled breathing are two therapies whereby this replenishment can take place. They give the body and mind time to recover and tap hidden energies and strengths. Thus refreshed the nurse can return to the caring situation and renew those around him or her. Hence the chapter concludes with a description of the benefits to be derived from these two techniques of stress management.

The energy and resource model of care

The structure of the proposed conceptual model is shown in Fig. 16.1. Function in the model is based on the energy and resource flows between its participants. How it

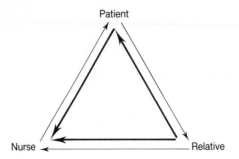

Patient

Nurse   Relative

Inner emotional exchange of energy and resource through touch, laughter, anger etc.

Outer exchange of energy and resource through communication and the coping strategies and skills of the participants.

Fig. 16.1   A conceptual model of palliative care based on the energy and resource of the participants.

reacts and behaves is dependent on the energy and resources of the participants as well as the transactions within itself and the surrounding environment (Lazarus and Launier, 1977).

Each participant, whether patient, family or nurse, will bring those resources and energies to the model which are dependent on the stresses and strains they experience in its function. These latter may be external environmental stressors that develop in the social and interpersonal relationships of the model or they may come from within the participants themselves and be concerned with the need to counter the threat to security and control over the situation (Karasek, 1979). The scenario that embraces palliative care places the nurse as the key figure in the model. The nurse's task is to act both as a source of positive energy and resource as well as the recipient of negative flows of energy and resource.

The speed of development of the model will be dependent on how quickly the ebbs and flows of energy and resource are established. Systems theory postulates that the slow development of function in a model makes for a smoother and more efficient adaptation over time (Beishon and Peters, 1972). Hence a hasty and hurried contact with the patient and his or her family in initial model development will not be conducive to the later stability of the model. Time and resource expended in building up of relationships in the early stages will reap abundant dividends in the future with respect to the equable management of the model.

The tangible nature of these ebbs and flows of energy and resource in the model is evidenced in a number of ways. The efficacy of energy transfer through touch for the restoration of flagging patient energies has been documented by McCorkle (1974), Heidt (1981), Kreiger (1986), LeMay (1986), Sims (1986; 1988) and Smith (1990). The value of laughter between nurse and patient as an antidote for negative emotions and a release of pent up emotional energy has been described by a number of authors (Martin and Lefcourt, 1983; Dillon *et al.*, 1985; Bellert, 1989). Positive feedback from the patient and family with respect to nursing care can also act as a source of renewal of the energy and resource of the nurse him or herself (Adams, 1984). Positive emotional exchange of this type can tap inner strengths and enhance the psyche of the participants of the model.

By the same token, negative flows of energy can disturb the smooth passage of the model. Such negative flows of energy take place when patients or relatives become anxious, angry or depressed. Perception of the potentially hopeless situation can trigger physiological and biochemical changes that will release resource and energy to cope with the lack of control they feel. This energy may be released slowly or it can result in random explosive outbursts of frustration and anger against those that are in the caring role. It is usually the nurse in palliative care who has to absorb these outflows of energy as well as provide those additional inputs of energy and resource to bring the model back into homeostasis.

Strong emotional energies are seen as part of the inner flows of the model and are more effective in giving the model predictability. More peripheral are those flows of energy and communication utilised through the vision and hearing of the participants. The chemical energy of the food intake of the participants is translated into the mechanical energy of the posture and movement of non-verbal communication and in the completion of tasks essential in the purely physical process of caring. Energy is used to create the sound waves for hearing which are then re-translated back into the chemical and nervous energy of the receivers of the communication. In all such transfers there is a loss of some energy so time again is an essential resource if the maximum transfer of energy is to be achieved. Concentration of the flow of energy will ensure that it is focused on the recipient and will prevent the wastage that accompanies hasty communications and care.

Also included in the outer energy flows are the coping strategies and skills of the participants themselves. These have been learned over time and represent small packets of information that can be utilised by the nurse in palliative care for the smoother function of the model. The strategy of stress monitoring in all the participants can alert the nurse to possible depletion of the energy stores of the model whilst the skills of reducing pain in the patient can add power to the model and prevent the energy drain that accompanies severe and continual pain.

Negative and stereotyped attitudes of the general public and health care professionals towards cancer (Corner, 1988) may cause each participant to undergo cycles of depression, guilt, despair and anxiety (Penson, 1979; 1984). These negative flows may cause an imbalance in the model and allow it to depart from the bounds of a carrying capacity defined by its maximum and minimum energy and resource content. The trajectory of the model will therefore be determined by the balance of positive and negative flows prevailing at any one moment in time.

The passage of the model across the time continuum is illustrated in Fig. 16.2. In homeostasis the model will move and fluctuate between the boundaries of its upper and lower limit of function (Appley and Trumbull, 1986). If the energy and resource input of one of the participants is low, perhaps due to depression, then the model may move below the lower limit of function. The danger points of C and D indicate that the model can drift into entropy unless some input of energy and resource can restore it to normal function. Similarly the sudden inputs of energy during a strong negative emotional experience such as anger can cause the model to exceed its normal levels of function at E and F and so become out of control.

It is at this point that the nurse in palliative care can be of the greatest service and

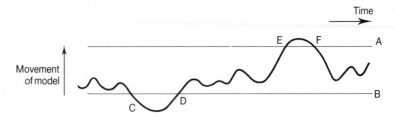

A – B   represents the carrying capacity of the model. Movement within A and B occurs when the model is in homeostasis.

C – D   Drift into entropy due to energy and resource lack of the participants.

E – F   Drift out of control due to explosive inputs of energy and resource by the participants.

Fig. 16.2   Movement of the model of palliative care over a time continuum.

help. If the model is out of control, then accessibility of staff who are willing to inform, explain and support can be of great value to all concerned (Penson, 1984). A nurse who is knowledgeable, resourceful, decisive, warm, friendly and supportive (Oskins, 1979) can do much to negate the face of anger, frustration and despair of those concerned.

Acting as a source of energy and resource for the model can be demanding and draining for the nurse and the need for renewal becomes paramount. The stresses and strains experienced by nurse who care for the terminally ill are described well by a number of authors (Kastenbaum, 1967; Knight and Field, 1981; Chiriboga *et al.*, 1983; Conboy Hill, 1986; Power and Sharp, 1988; Cathcart, 1989) and strategies for coping are identified. These strategies are both cognitive and palliative in nature (Lazarus and Folkman, 1984) but do not really describe how the nurse may rebuild his or her energy and resource supplies which have been depleted in the caring process.

To understand how this replenishment may take place, it is necessary to know how the energy and resource is released as a response to the stress engendered by being part of the model.

Responses to stress

The release of energy and resource during the early stages of the model is in response to the perception of a demand. Psychological processes are translated into physiological processes through the Autonomic Nervous System and the Endocrine System. The response to the demand is the classical stress response described by Selye (1976) and it can take place through two pathways. The short term response to stress will take place through the hypothalamo-adrenal medullary component of the Autonomic Nervous System whilst the resources for the long term response to stress are mobilised through the hypothalamo-pituitary-adrenal cortex

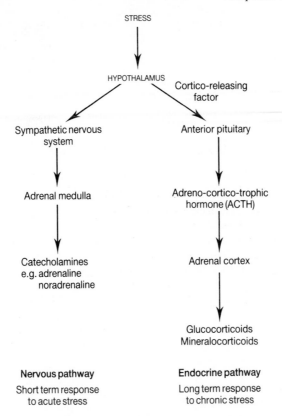

STRESS

HYPOTHALAMUS   Cortico-releasing factor

Sympathetic nervous system

Anterior pituitary

Adrenal medulla

Adreno-cortico-trophic hormone (ACTH)

Catecholamines e.g. adrenaline noradrenaline

Adrenal cortex

Glucocorticoids Mineralocorticoids

Nervous pathway
Short term response to acute stress

Endocrine pathway
Long term response to chronic stress

Fig. 16.3   The nervous and endocrine pathways of the response to stress.

axis of the Endocrine System. The pathways do not occur in isolation but probably run in parallel with each other. Which one predominates is dependent on individual perception of the situation at the time. The details of how the resources are mobilised are summarised in Fig. 16.3.

The effect of the hormonal release is to change body stores of resource and energy into forms that can be used in the immediate and long term response to the demands of the model. The changes are accompanied by certain signs and indicators of the psychological and physiological processes involved. Broadly, these indicators can be categorised into emotional, behavioural and physiological factors and some examples of these categories are shown in Table 16.1 (Derogatis *et al.*, 1974; Selye, 1976).

In a recent survey of Palliative Care Nurses on an International Conference in Cambridge emotional and behavioural indicators were predominant with physiological indicators only accounting for 17% of the recorded symptoms. This would seem to indicate that the behaviour techniques employed by the nurses were sufficient to prevent the breakthrough to the physiological spectrum. Highest on the list was the need to be alone and the urge to sleep leading to the conclusion that the nurses require time, rest and peace for a renewal of strength and purpose.

Table 16.1   Emotional, behavioural, and physiological indicators of stress.

Emotional	Behavioural	Physiological
Exhaustion	Increased activity	Nausea
Exhilaration	Decreased activity	Constipation
Depressed feelings	Urge to sleep	Urinary frequency
Uneasy or anxious	Difficult to sleep	Palpitations
General tension	Urge to eat	Tremulousness
	Loss of appetite	Weakness
		Dizziness

Hans Selye (1980) has described the finite nature of the stress response in the General Adaptation Syndrome. In the initial stages of Alarm, resources are mobilised quickly and for a time the body adapts and maintains levels of resources and energy sufficient to maintain the body in a state of homeostasis. However, high continual use of these resources without rest results in rapid depletion of body stores and the individual can soon move into a state of exhaustion. It is clear that some of the nurses in the survey were beginning to be aware of those subtle changes that occur over time for exhaustion and depressed feelings received a high priority in the recording of symptoms.

Renewal of strength

How then can the nurse in palliative care renew his or her strength and purpose and find sufficient energy to maintain the model of palliative care which has been described?

A nurse who is under stress, tired and exhausted will subconsciously communicate these feelings on to those with whom he or she interacts. In conceptual terms his or her own energy field will be narrow and withdrawn. Smooth energy flow will be blocked by muscle tension and anxious expression whilst concentration, performance and memory will be impaired. Visually this is described in Fig. 16.4 which depicts the normal smooth energy flows in health as compared to the distorted energy flow of the individual not in balance with the environment.

Relaxation and diaphragmatic breathing are two ways in which physiological homeostasis can be restored. In its wake comes the psychological homeostasis important in the maintenance of the physiological homeostasis so attained by these methods.

Relaxation

The physiology initiated through relaxation can have dramatic effects. Relaxation reduces muscle tension and lowers the level of blood lactate and hence the levels of anxiety induced by the build up of this metabolic by-product of muscle biochemistry (Pitts, 1969). Heart rate, blood pressure and respiratory rate are lowered and the

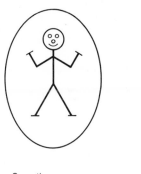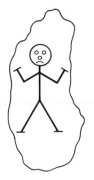

Smooth even energy field of an individual in homeostasis

Uneven, distorted and narrow energy field of an individual under stress

Fig. 16.4   The energy fields of an individual in health and homeostasis and an individual under stress.

generalised vasodilation that occurs evens the heat energy field of the person under stress. The electrical energy field is also normalised through an increase in the alpha and theta activity of the EEG and the Galvanic Skin Response (Pitts, 1969: Wallace and Benson, 1972; Luck, 1989). A summary of these changes appears in Fig. 16.5.

In progressive relaxation it is important to create optimum conditions of quiet, comfort and loose clothing. Details of the exact procedures are described by Jacobsen (1938) and Berstein and Borkovec (1973) and this would seem to be the best method to adopt. In this method each muscle group is tensed (30 seconds) and relaxed (40–60 seconds) twice.

The rationale of the method requires the recognition of tension in the muscle and the ability to remember what it feels like to release tension from the muscle. Continual monitoring of the induced relaxation is essential to ensure that muscles, once relaxed, remain relaxed.

The exercises have to be repeated each day for several weeks for maximum benefit. Eventually the process becomes faster and it is possible to reach complete relaxation in a very short time.

Breathing techniques

Relaxation combined with a breathing technique can be even more beneficial (Bailey, 1985). Each individual has their own pattern of breathing and breathing can vary with the state of mind. An anxious person tends to show a hasty and erratic pattern while intermittent gasps and sighs typify anger.

A person who is endeavouring to achieve the control of stress through breathing should aim for a slowing of the breathing pattern through slow and gentle prolonged exhalation followed by spontaneous inhalation at the end of each exhalation (Bailey, 1985). The mild hyperventilation that may occur during prolonged exhalation may

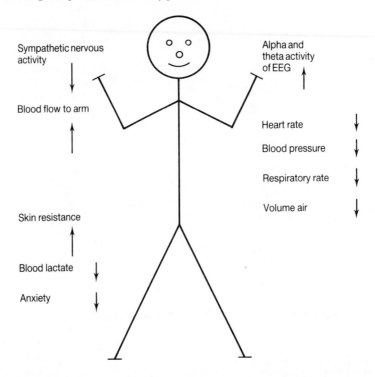

Fig. 16.5   The physiological correlates of relaxation and diaphragmatic breathing.

produce a slight tingling in the hands and feet. If this does occur then a temporary cessation of prolonged exhalation will rectify the physiological imbalance of hypocarbia.

Theoretically however, the slow breathing pattern should allow the build up of carbon dioxide to replace that which has been lost in the prolonged exhalation. In this way there should be no disturbance to the carbon dioxide and acid base balance of the body.

Breathing through the nose induces warm feelings in the body and using the diaphragm stimulates the calming parasympathetic component of the Autonomic Nervous System. Thoracic and clavicular breathing contribute to heightened states of arousal and should be avoided. Breathing from the diaphragm also increases the depth of penetration of the air into the lungs. It is the base of the lungs that has the greater blood supply and it is here that the maximum exchange between the blood and respiratory gases can take place.

Concentration on breathing patterns frees the neuronal circuitry of the brain which is concerned with the anxiety of a situation. The higher centres of the brain cause muscles to tense automatically when demands are seen to outstrip coping. If these centres are occupied with control that is required for breathing patterns then muscle relaxation will be enhanced still further (Brown, 1978).

Mind and body become balanced and tension is reduced. The sensation is one of floating and complete freedom to ride on the wings of space and time. The experience of present existence produces a sense of personal identity and oneness with self. It is perhaps in these states of relaxation that the tenets of the Eastern philosophy of Zen and the art of pseudo-enlightenment are most nearly achieved, for fleeting moments of happiness are captured in moments of present time (Barker, 1989).

Future research

The consequence of the combination of relaxation and breathing control is a renewal of resource and energy for the individual. Thus so far the model concentrates on the needs of the nurse but these methods of renewal can equally apply to the patient and members of the family. If all the participants of the model achieve renewal at the same time then the resource and energy content of the model will be high. Similarly, asynchrony of positive and negative flows will cause different behaviours of the model.

Matrices which depict these combinations of resource and energy levels of the participants will identify the unique character of each situation. They will of necessity be complex in nature but a setting out of the balances will enable an understanding of the processes that underlie the interaction of the participants in the proposed model of palliative care.

Research is needed as to how these flows of energy and resource can be quantified and how they change over the course of time (Folkman and Lazarus, 1980; Folkman, 1984; Folkman and Lazarus, 1985).

It is necessary to know when the conservation of resource and energy is particularly important for the survival of model homeostasis, and equally important to know when inputs of resource and energy will enhance its function.

All the skills of the nurse are required to convert these forces into one that will carry the model through on a smooth path to its natural conclusion. Nurses in palliative care require the specialised training that will allow these objectives to be achieved (Barstow, 1980; Fisher, 1988; Manley, 1988). An understanding of a conceptual model of palliative care of this nature may go some way towards this end.

References

ADAMS, J. (1984). A prescription for coping failure. *Nursing Forum*, **21**(1), 28–30.

APPLEY, M. H. and TRUMBULL, R. (1986). Dynamics of stress and its control. In *Dynamics of Stress. Physiological, Psychological and Social Perspectives*, M. H. Appley and R. Trumbull (Eds), pp. 309–27. Plenum Press.

BAILEY, R. D. (1985). *Coping with Stress in Caring*. Blackwell Scientific Publications, Oxford.

BARKER, P. (1989). Zen and the art of pseudo-enlightenment. *Nursing Times*, **85**(38), 30–2.

BARSTOW, J. (1980). Stress variance in hospice nursing. *Nursing Outlook*, December 1980, 751–4.

BEISHON, P. and PETERS, G. (1972). *Systems Behaviour.* Open University Press, Harper & Row.

BERSTEIN, D. and BORKOVEC, T. (1973). *Progressive Relaxation Training: A Manual for the Helping Professions.* Research Press, Chicago.

BELLERT, J. L. (1989). Humour. A therapeutic approach in oncology nursing. *Cancer Nursing,* **12(2),** 65–70.

BROWN, B. B. (1978). *Stress and the Art of Biofeedback,* Bantam.

CATHCART, F. (1989). Coping with distress. *Nursing Times,* **85(42),** 33–5.

CHIRIBOGA, D., JENKINS, G. and BAILEY, J. (1983). Stress and coping among hospice nurses: tests of an analytic model. *Nursing Research,* **32(5),** 294–9.

CONBOY-HILL, S. (1986). Psychosocial aspects of terminal care. *International Nursing,* **33(1),** 19–21.

CORNER, J. L. (1988). Assessment of nurses attitudes towards cancer: a critical review of research methods. *Journal of Advanced Nursing,* **13,** 640–8.

DEROGATIS, L. R., LIPMAN, R. S., RICKELS, K., UHLEN HUTH, E. H. and COVI, L. (1974). The Hopkins Symptom Checklist (HSCL). In *Psychological Measurements in Psychopharmacology,* P. Pichot (Ed.). *Mod. Probl. Pharmacopsychiat.,* Vol. 7. pp. 79–110. Krager Basel.

DILLON, K. M., MINCHOFF, B. and BAKER, K. H. (1985). Positive emotional states and enhancement of the immune system. *International Journal of Psychiatry in Medicine,* **15(1),** 13–17.

FISHER, M. (1988). Hospice nursing. *Nursing,* **3(32),** 8–10.

FOLKMAN, S. (1984). Personal control and stress and coping processes. *Journal of Personality and Social Psychology,* **46(4),** 839–56.

FOLKMAN, S. and LAZARUS, R. S. (1980). An analysis of coping in a middle aged community sample. *Journal of Health and Social Behaviour,* **21,** 219–39.

FOLKMAN, S. and LAZARUS, R. S. (1985). If it changes, it must be a process: study of emotion and coping during three stages of a college examination. *Journal of Personality and Social Psychology,* **48(1),** 150–70.

HEIDT, P. (1981). Effect of therapeutic touch on anxiety level of hospitalised patients. *Nursing Research,* **30(1),** 32–7.

JACOBSON, E. (1938). *Progressive Relaxation.* University of Chicago Press, Chicago.

KARASEK, R. A. (1979). Job demands, job decision latitude and mental strain: implications for job redesign. *Administrative Science Quarterly,* **24,** 285–311.

KASTENBAUM, R. (1967). Multiple perspectives on a geriatric death valley. *Community Mental Healt Journal,* **3(1),** 21–9.

KNIGHT, M. and FIELD, D. (1981). A silent conspiracy: coping with dying cancer patients on an acute surgical ward. *Journal of Advanced Nursing,* **6,** 221–9.

KREIGER, D. (1986). *The Therapeutic Touch. How to use your hands to help or to heal.* Prentice Hall Press.

LAZARUS, R. S. and FOLKMAN, S. (1984). In *Stress, Appraisal and Coping.* Springer Publishing Company, New York.

LAZARUS, R. S. and LAUNIER, R. (1977). Stress related transactions between person and environment. In *Perspectives in Interactional Psychology,* L. A. Pervin and M. Lewis (Eds), pp. 287–327. Plenum Press.

LE MAY, A. (1986). The human connection. *Nursing Times,* **82(13),** 28–30.

LUCK, N. A. (1989). Transcending stress. *Nursing Times,* **85(15),** 40–1.

MANLEY, K. (1988). The needs and support of relatives. *Nursing,* **3(32),** 19–22.

MARTIN, R. A. and LEFCOURT, H. M. (1983). Sense of humour as a moderator of the relation between stressors and moods. *Journal of Personality and Social Psychology*, **45(6)** 1313–24.

MCCORKLE, R. (1974). Effects of touch on seriously ill patients. *Nursing Research*, **23(2)**, 125–32.

OSKINS, S. L. (1979). Identification of situational stressors and coping methods by intensive care nurses. *Heart and Lung*, **8(5)**, 953–60.

PENSON, J. M. (1979). Helping the bereaved. *Nursing Times*, April 5th, 593–5.

PENSON, J. M. (1984). Helping relatives cope with cancer. *Nursing Times*, April 11th, 24–6.

PITTS, F. N. (1969). The biochemistry of anxiety. *Scientific American*, February, 69–75.

POWER, K. G. and SHARP, G. R. (1988). A comparison of sources of nursing stress and job satisfaction among mental handicap and hospice nursing staff. *Journal of Advanced Nursing*, **13**, 726–32.

SELYE, H. (1974). *Stress without Distress*. Corgi.

SELYE, H. (1976). *Stress in Health and Disease*. Butterworths.

SELYE, H. (1980). The Stress Concept Today. In *Handbook on Stress and Anxiety*, I. L. Kutash and L. B. Schlesinger (Eds). Jossey Bass, San Francisco.

SIMS, S. (1986) Slow stroke back massage for cancer patients. Occasional Paper. *Nursing Times*, **82(13)**, 47–50.

SIMS, S. (1988). The significance of touch in palliative care. *Palliative Medicine*, **2**, 58–61.

SMITH, M. (1990). Healing through touch. *Nursing Times*, **86(4)** 31–2.

WALLACE, R. K. and BENSON, H. (1972). The physiology of meditation. *Scientific American*, February, 84–91.

Further reading

BOND, M. (1987). *Stress and Self-awareness: A Guide for Nurses*. Heinemann Nursing, London.

MADDERS, J. (1981). *Stress and Relaxation*. Martin Dunitz Limited, London.

MITCHELL, L. (1988). *Simple Relaxation. The Mitchell Method for Easing Tension.* John Murray (Publishers) Ltd.

WHICH BOOKS (1988). *Understanding Stress*. A Consumer Publication, Consumers Association.

17

Reflections

Olga M. Craig

> In the case of a friendless foreigner dying in a Public Hospital who was brought here, the most dreadful kind of death was at least at intervals freed from pain and even a smile from time to time rewarded those who were around her – to whom, *when assured of their sympathy*, she was able to express her thoughts and feelings.'
>
> *Reports to the Governors of her Nursing Home (1853–1854), Florence Nightingale*

When I look back through many years of being privileged to share closely with people life's problems, some incidents stay in my memory, and later I can see that they were really pointers in illuminating something profound, even if at the time I did not fully realise the significance.

I believe the practice of social work to be a creative art: social workers have no drugs, no syringe, nothing to offer but themselves, their own self awareness and experience. In their training they learn to look at themselves, their thoughts and feelings, their potential. They try to understand why they react in certain ways, why they may react to situations with anger, hostility, fear, withdrawal, aggression and, in looking at this human motivation, they try better to understand how patients and their relatives feel, to help them to face themselves and, in sharing, transmute their feelings. The patients and their relatives are facing the impact of cancer, possibly death, and the fear of this; and the fear of something is often more destructive than the thing itself. In expressing their fears the space between the patient, relatives and the carer, be they a social worker or a nurse, can be filled with something more positive and bearable, and many of the anxieties dissolve.

I remember the words of a philosopher:

> 'What you are speaks so loudly, I cannot hear what you say to the contrary.'

When you approach this type of caring you bring not only your professional self, but the person that you really are, the things you have achieved, your failures, your ideals, your total personality, and it is all this and more that you share with your patients, their families and your colleagues. I see patients as living, not dying, and my work is concerned with the living – not the length of time, but the quality of life in the period that they are still in this world. If we share with them closely, honestly, and compassionately, that time can sometimes be the most meaningful of their lives.

Some years ago I read, in a social work journal, a review of some of the works of Martin Buber, the Jewish philosopher. I do not know which were the words of Buber and which were those of the reviewer, but the following made sense to me.

> 'For this thinker the quality of the relationship between people is what brings about the healing process. *For Buber*, the therapist must be ready to be surprised by his patient and to be guided by what the patient brings him. The way to achieve this is by 'obedient listening'. It is much easier to impose oneself on the patient than it is to use the whole

force of one's soul to leave the patient to himself and not to touch him. The real master responds to uniqueness. The kind of healing Buber has in mind takes place through the meeting of one person with another rather than through insight and analysis. A situation is transformed when something in the other person comes alive in me.'

What we are trying to do with our patients and families is not new and not just related to cancer. It is to do with the sharing with anyone who is facing a deep, profound life experience because, in my view, illness is an experience, just as are birth, marriage, loss and love. It is what you make of the experience, how you learn about yourself and life, and how you can grow through it that is important, not the experience itself.

I completed my midwifery training, because that was the thing to do, and during that training I had some time working in the community. As I walked out of the gate of the hospital I realised that, for the first time, I was free to work as an individual and not as an adjunct to others. That was the final experience which led me to move into the Social Work field. For many years I worked in Child Care, with families, marriage problems, delinquency, children, and all the common traumas of life. However, when it all became too bureaucratic with too many people telling me what to do, I moved into Medical Social Work where this intense need to work as an individual and in a free way was still possible. However, soon this field was taken over by the same bureaucratic set-up. At that time, 'out of the blue', the first Macmillan unit was being built nearby. I was fortunate in being appointed as the only Social Worker and, as it was a pioneering venture, I felt I would be free to work creatively, face to face, with the patients. With much perseverance and 'battling' I succeeded.

As the unit, at that time, was the first under the National Health Service, it was seen to be different and controversial. We were prepared to face problems which, before, were often pushed under the carpet, or perhaps more correctly, behind the screens on many a ward round I have seen the retinue pass the rejected patient with 'terminal cancer' with hardly a word except to ask if I could hurry up the discharge. Although things are now different prejudice is still found, often born of fear, within many professional workers – they too need help.

From my diary of experiences I have recalled a few examples which you may meet from time to time.

Most of us end up with titles and qualifications, but these are just labels and we should perhaps be wary of 'labels'. There is a danger that we and our patients will turn into our 'labels'. He has cancer, he is terminal, hasn't long to live, I give him six months, he is difficult, uncooperative, daft as a brush, gone to the fairies, he has cerebral secondaries. I have seen many patients with the last label become quite rational and normal when someone spent time penetrating the barrier of fear. I remember a patient who had 'an ulcer that was leaking'. She was very depressed and was still running a temperature. I was asked to see her and I listened to her life story. She had always been the strength of the home and was now fearful for the future. She wept, and weeping for the right reason can be a marvellous release. 'You see', she said, 'the nurses and doctors keep telling me about my ulcer, that it is drying-up, getting smaller and so on. Sometimes I feel I am becoming a leaking abscess'. When we have to cope with the physical body it is very important that we do not forget the human being within.

I trained as a Nurse just before the advent of antibiotics. Patients were often in hospital for months, not days. We had time to get to know them, and because we couldn't just treat them with drugs, which remove the symptoms but not always the cause, we had to use our imagination and traditional bedside Nursing to treat and 'comfort' our patients. When I see someone in hospital who is ill, I do not see a patient, but a unique human being with a unique life history of which the illness is only a part.

As a second year nurse I came on duty one night to be told by the Sister that one of my patients, an elderly lady from the east end of London who had advanced cancer, was dying and unlikely to survive the night. The relatives were round the bed and the curtains were drawn. The night wore on and I looked frequently at my patient, with drips in her nose, and in her arms and hardly breathing. Some relatives were crying. At one point I sent them away to have a cup of tea and a rest, and tidied up and washed the old lady's face. About a half an hour later, as I passed the bed, I looked in astonishment as somehow she had hooked her spectacles over the tubes and her eyes were open. I leaned over, and in a broad Cockney accent, she said clearly, 'I want a cup of tea, Nurse!' Many weeks later she walked out of the ward. Of course it caused quite a commotion, when someone who should have died recovered, both for the staff and the relatives.

I remember another night with this same patient, as she was getting better, talking to her about her remarkable recovery. I did not understand then what I do now, but she looked me straight in the eye and said, 'I saw them all standing round my bed, wishing me away and dividing up my money and I thought, not yet you don't!' Now, one is aware that many factors apart from our care, are working to affect our patients. Perhaps not always for the best of reasons, but a shift in outlook can often change the course of an illness.

I can recall another significant happening. I was a staff nurse on a medical ward, at that time, an experiment was being tried of placing a few psychiatric patients in the ward. I was given the main charge of these patients. The Psychiatrist was very good and explained everything fully to me. It was a new experience, because all the social aspects were discussed, and then I began to feel I wanted to work with people before they were admitted, and I'm sure this is what ultimately led me to Social Work. One of the patients was a girl of limited intelligence who had a paralysed arm. She had had all the usual tests, and X-rays which showed nothing abnormal. In my presence the Psychiatrist hypnotised the girl, and while under hypnosis at his suggestion the arm became completely relaxed. However, he did now allow the arm to remain like this and when she woke, he explained that whatever trauma was causing it, must be found first or worse symptoms could follow. It was after many more sessions before, on one occasion, she became very disturbed and eventually admitted that her brother had raped her.

With each of the patients and families who come for our help, we feel like part of an extended family. It is perhaps the most profound experience of living to be facing the possibility of death, and experience of people in this dimension reminds me of when I was a midwife, and later when involved in placing babies for adoption, both emotive happenings, and in the case of adoption actually bringing the baby to the couple. I felt part of the whole family unit during the period that I was involved. It would seem the same with our patients with cancer, perhaps facing death.

Many patients and their families feel guilty and inadequate, and often react with aggression and project their uncomfortable feelings on others, including staff. As the women who placed her feelings about rape into her arm because it was too awful to face it in reality, so people will blame others for their distress. We have to remember it is no help being sentimental in this work, empathy not sympathy is needed. A young woman about whom I shall say more later, said to me one day 'Don't pity me, it is degrading, when I cry with pain you all go soft on me, it's no help'. I also remember her on another occasion. When I came on duty the staff said she had had a bad night in pain and very angry. I passed her bed, and seeing her expression I almost went past without stopping! However, I sat beside her and she said, 'What can you know about my pain, and you are only here because it is your job'. 'No', I replied 'I can never know your pain, it is yours alone, but I can sit beside you while you swear at me if it will help'. We sat together and talked, and after a time the pain eased. You see, pain of the body is often pain of the heart.

Relatives do not always feel loving towards themselves or the patient. For example, a daughter who had resentfully looked after her demanding elderly mother and sometimes 'wished her dead'. Now the mother is dying and the daughter is filled with guilt. Being able to voice these feelings before the death is the beginning of help towards the bereavement period.

The woman who refused to have her husband around when she was dying, 'He will only mess it up, as he has messed everything else up in my life'. When I saw the husband he wept, and admitted he was impotent and had never been able to satisfy his wife who despised him.

It is of value to a person to be able to voice these thoughts with someone who can accept but not necessarily condone – 'Acceptance' is one of the social workers prime casework principles. So this I found was part of my role, as someone a little outside the dependancy role, to whom people can voice their true feelings. To be able to sit with someone and look into their eyes, so that they can bring out what is in their heart, not what they think you want to hear.

Remember that because of the 'image' of a doctor, nurse, minister, or social worker, some people will only say what they think we expect. I came on a ward one day in my capacity as a social worker, and the Ward Sister said, 'You will have to see Mrs Smith, she has been restless all night, and refusing to go to another hospital for tests. I've told her that a bed will be kept for her here, and the Doctor has assured her the tests will not hurt, but she refuses to budge until she sees the Social Worker'. Needless to say, Sister was not too pleased! As soon as Mrs Smith saw me, she said, 'I'm not going in that ambulance without my knickers on, it isn't decent with them ambulance men, but I couldn't tell Sister, 'er being what she is.' She was a very good Sister, but she thought the patient was worried about her bed, the Doctor thought she was afraid the tests would be painful. I am not quite sure what it makes me, but there has to be someone around to whom you can literally or metaphorically talk about your 'knickers'. Like the husband of a woman whose face was slowly disintegrating and she had a long spell in our unit. He did not like to ask if there was a room where he could make love to her; 'I thought you might think it "dirty".' Of course we found a room without a glass panel. The spinster aged sixty years who, with great distress, told me her father had sexually abused her as a child, the shame was still deep within her and she had not told anyone till she became ill.

So often, when faced with something serious and profound, people find a need to bring out the hurts, disappointments and frustrations of their life which may have been bottled up for years. The illegitimate child, the wife he never really loved, the fact that someone was homosexual. The wife and mistress both in a man's life, and he wants both to visit him. The soldier who, in the last war, was a prisoner of the Japanese, had worked on the infamous railway and seen his comrades shot when they collapsed. Luckily, he had told me all this, and when one night he fell out of bed and was a little confused, he tried to strangle a nurse, but was distressed afterwards and said to me, 'I thought I was back on the track and the Japs would kill me'. At least this knowledge saved him from being considered a psychiatric case.

In social work we have always to look at the total person – physically, mentally, spiritually, emotionally, the home, work situation, family interaction, hobbies, the marriage, the children. The patients and family sense this and the kind of questions we ask seem to make them feel we are interested in them as people not patients. This results in comments like 'I've never spoken to anyone like this before, now I don't have to pretend, I feel so at ease now I have told you this'. With the bringing out of these deep seated things which laid hidden there often comes a release, with the release comes a lessening of tension which is sometimes followed by an easing of symptoms and consequently the ability to reduce drugs – it is like a human tranquilliser. One woman, after admitting that she had dreaded making love to her husband all her married life, took her hands and said 'This fear has sat like a hard lump here', and where she put her hands was just where the cancer had appeared. 'Now', she said, 'it is as if a cloud has been lifted'. Difficulties occur when professionals contemplate telling patients 'the Truth'. What the professional carer thinks and what the patients think are often very different. A man who had worked in the Police service was admitted and sat silently in the entrance of the ward for several days. Eventually he asked a Staff Nurse who had tired to talk to him to wheel him into the grounds, and then he point blank asked, 'Have I got cancer?' The nurse had never before told this to a patient, but she did on this occasion. She felt completely shaken and, because I knew her well, she came to talk to me. She said. 'I feel I cannot continue with this work, by telling him he has cancer I feel I have given him the disease'.

The nurse felt that the actuality of knowing would hasten the disease. In fact, the next day, there was a knock at my door and in came this man saying 'Well, I've at last been told I've got cancer, I knew something was up, because they are so damned kind here. Now we can get to grips with things, and I can do what has to be done'. I made sure that the nurse followed through with me what transpired next. The patient was an intelligent man, he wanted to see his employer, his minister and, most of all, he said 'Now my wife and I can discuss the future honestly'. He wanted to put his affairs in order, talk to his children, and a great deal of good positive work was done which, without the initial 'telling', might not have happened. And so the nurse saw that her act, far from being destructive, was the opening to something better.

There was an educated lady who had been a concert pianist. She had travelled the world, and now she was admitted because there was no-one at home to look after her. I went to see her soon after admission and she said, 'Have I got cancer?' As I did not know much about her I suggested she might like to see the Doctor. Three times the Doctor saw her, and tried to give her an opening to talk, but she did not ask. Then one day I again saw her and she said, 'No-one will tell me I have cancer, and I know I have, because I have read my notes!' I said, 'Do you want me to tell you that you have cancer', 'Oh no dear', she replied, 'I am a single woman, I have always had to plan my own life, and I want to know whether I should get my solicitor in and make my will, or should I buy a local paper and start looking for a flat.' I suggested she should put her affairs in order, as by now she was very ill. And she did this and died soon after.

A rough, tough man who had been a docker in Glasgow was admitted. At first, staff thought he was a bit 'peculiar', but I found he spoke with a broad Scottish dialect full of swear words, and hated being fussed over by all the nurses. As I came from his country I understood him, and tried to help him adjust. Eventually I traced a long lost daughter and grandchildren in Australia, and they all wrote to him. One day when he was near the end, he said to me, 'I'm not going to get better am I?' I knew he had been told 'the truth' by a doctor in a previous hospital, so I said, 'I think you know that you have cancer, and were told that before you came here'. 'Yes', he said, 'but I'm no having a young chit of a girl telling me something as serious as that, I don't mind you telling me, as you are a good woman' – by that he meant an old woman! But there is a time for telling, and there has sometimes to be a re-telling, when the patient is ready to face the full import.

There was also the young mother who was going to die. Her husband was a kind but uneducated man, who had been brought up in Children's Homes. 'I haven't got a way with words', he told me. He had told the elder daughter the truth, but couldn't tell his young son, as he had always been the mother's favourite. At first he asked me to tell him, but I helped him to see that this would solve nothing. When at last he plucked up courage and told him, he was shattered when the lad said, 'Oh, I've known Mother was going to "pop off" for ages, can I go and play now'. One can rarely hide the truth from children, they have their own radar system.

Communication is indeed an art. To be able to communicate not only in words but by look, touch and physical contact, is most important. When I was involved with foster children, often rejected and separated from their families, tiny children right up to teenage, they were so distressed, lonely and afraid they could not hear what you said. You had to hold them tight, so that they felt your thoughts and love. To be able to sit quietly relaxed, without fear, with a patient or relative, to stroke their forehead, hold their hands, and say nothing – they so often need this tangile expression of acceptance and understanding when they face this lonely journey. I remember, on a ward round, an elderly lady who had just lost her husband before being admitted, and she was particularly vulnerable. When the Doctor put out his hand, her eyes lit up, and she put out her hands to his. It was pushed aside with 'Let us see her abdomen, sister' and I can still see that arm slowly fall and the head droop.

Through all that nurses and social workers try to do there runs this special alchemy called LOVE, which nurses in particular, with their frequent intimate contact with people can evoke, sometimes without being aware of it. If it cannot always turn a person from sickness to health, then certainly it can turn them from distress to peace.

A man who had lost weight was admitted to a medical ward. He had all the tests including an interview with a psychiatrist, but with no results. As a last resort he was referred to me. After we had got to know one another he told me his only daughter had married a man he did not approve of, seven years ago. He told her he did not want to see her again, and in fact he never did because she died of cancer a year later. His guilt and distress were so deep he had not been able to share the event with his wife. The houseman on the ward was particularly sensitive and I suggested he follow up my talk, and the man again poured out his feelings. It was very therapeutic and eventually he was due to be discharged. I arranged for him to talk about his diet with the dietician and because he liked porridge, I suggested he sprinkle some wheat germ on it. Good for the nerves I said. Three months later I was walking through the out-patients department when this same man rushed up with bright eyes, and colour in his cheeks. 'Miss Craig, that wheat germ is marvellous, from the first mouthful I felt better!' Well, you can see, it was only a vehicle into which he projected what he felt was the love and understanding experienced in the hospital. But it worked.

A sad little spinster of uncertain years came in, she had no visitors and no family. She ultimately told me she had always 'missed' everything in life. She lost her job, she never had a boy-friend, and even her grandmother called her 'Miss one too many' when she was young. 'I never felt I belonged'. I shared with all the staff, who in their own special way gave her lot of TLC (tender loving care). After some months when the end was near, I brought some flowers to her which had been given to me. She looked up at me and said, 'All my life I have been looking for somewhere and someone who would love me for myself. Now that I have found it with you all, it does not matter any more whether I die'. She smiled, and I never saw her again.

Staff often have to spend a great deal of time dealing with unpleasant and distressing physical symptoms. One can get caught up and submerged in this. I have always shared and encouraged staff to see the very positive and happy things that may be occurring within the family while the body is being eaten away. The lady whose face was ultimately just a cavity, but she remained mentally intact to the end. She told me that she and her husband had become closer since the illness, than in all married life, and were able to share their real feelings. The husband who had never been very capable found he could cope with the children and home, and his self confidence improved.

When someone becomes seriously ill, close members of the family are affected in different ways, but all feel that they have a right to participate in the experience. A young woman who is dying, has a husband, parents, in-laws, children, brothers or sistes, and all have a part to play. The parents may blame the son-in-law for the illness, there may be squabbling as to who is going to look after the children. A young father may feel inadequate and be glad of help while his wife is ill, but later may want to care for the children himself, and be afraid he will offend the parents or inlaws if he insists. A young man was dying and his mother refused to come and visit him because she did not want to watch him die, and he felt she had rejected him. Three daughters and a grand-daughter arguing and rowing over the unconscious mother, and all the years of past jealousy and friction spilling out – perhaps it was no wonder the mother remained unconscious, sometimes death may be a blessed escape.

However, all these various people need to air their mixed feelings and often, with help, resolve many of the destructive consequences. This, again, is the start of bereavement process.

A pending death can precipitate past memories and hurts. I remember a daughter whose father was dying – she poured out a flood of resentment against him. 'He always made use of me, and was always criticising me, and yet my brother was his favourite and could do no wrong'. But now the brother couldn't find time to come and see his father. The bitterness poured out and although she was 40 years of age, she wept and even spoke like a hurt young child again.

There are difficulties when a family is prepared for someone to die and the patient improves. If a person is 'set' for bereavement it can be traumatic to have to switch their feelings again.

What of the children themselves? Special thought is required to help parents prepare their children for loss: the right word and moment is needed, and this depends on the ages of the children. Some children react to difficulties by becoming aggressive, or ignoring them, some become silent and withdrawn and take their tears to their pillow. If the truth is not spoken and shared with them they can build up a fantasy picture and fears which may be worse than is actually the case. Parents absorbed in their own grief may have little time or emotion left for the children and an aunt, grandparent or good friend can share the burden.

A young father who had a great deal of pain and discomfort sometimes shouted at his children when they were being noisy at home. One day he was sitting in his bedroom and heard one of his sons say, 'I wish daddy would die soon, I don't like him any more'. A single mother took a great deal of trouble to make sure that her daughter would have legal guardians after her death, and be protected from any argument as to who would look after her. These are just a few of the dilemmas which can occur.

Now, one or two of the more practical aspects of our patients care.

When someone becomes ill or they are admitted to hospital, they leave behind many worries and responsibilities. With patients who may die, it is especially important that they are helped to remain as involved as possible in their lives. Relatives or staff who try to shield patients from dealing with their affairs can make the patient feel that they have already been pushed aside. The patient is often more concerned that they will lose their mental faculties than about the physical symptoms. The professional career must be there to offer help, but self determination, another case work principle, is most important for both patient and relatives.

Help may be needed to arrange care for dependants left at home. Children may need the support of relatives, friends, schools or Social Services. Financial matters loom large. Assistance may be required in contacting a patient's employer regarding benefits, early retirement, pension schemes, etc., and finding sources of grants which might be appropriate. As I had a good knowledge of Community Resources, staff used me as a reservoir of information as to where to go and who to contact for help with a particular problem. Links with all people involved with a family should be maintained so that there is no overlapping and maximum efficient help and support can be offered.

Patients may wish to make or remake their will, or wish to cut somebody out of their will, and they do not always want the relatives involved. Hence there is a need for sensitive solicitors. One 'gentleman of the road' had nothing to leave but a wrist watch, but felt if he was going to die he should make a will. A very special solicitor spent an hour with him doing all that was necessary. Now, that is an example of what this word 'dignity' is all about.

Many people want to plan their own funeral. A patient who had had little peace in her life asked for the rose called 'Peace' to be planted in the garden. Many relatives have never been involved with a funeral and want to discuss all the details before the patient dies – the cost, how to pay, insurance, and whether burial or cremation. Some patients come from abroad, different religions, and special arrangements may be needed. Tactful talking about all these matters can relieve a great deal of anxiety when the patient actually dies.

Patients whose health improves may need alternative accommodation, some may need help to move to other parts of the country to be near relatives, or even to another country. Then there is the question of tracing relatives often out of the picture for years. This may also be a time for reconciliation. I remember a man who was admitted from a hostel for the homeless. I was told he had no next of kin, only a mate in the hostel. I saw the patient, and because I so often get an intuitive feeling about someone, I asked about himself. Eventually he admitted that he had a sister somewhere, but as he had been a 'black sheep' and had done nothing for her, he did not feel it was fair to bother her. After some persuasion, he agreed that I could try and trace her. This I did with the help of the Salvation Army. I found not only the sister, but three brothers, an ex-wife, a daughter, and a grandaughter he had never seen! They all came to see him, and the loose threads were gathered together, even if they did not all get on with one another!

We are not always successful – a young man longed to meet his real father before he died. Although we traced the father he would not come because he felt it would be too upsetting.

I will conclude with the story of a remarkable, courageous and special woman in her early twenties, who came under our care. She had been the rounds of several hospitals, had had many forms of treatment, and, eventually, had been sent home to the care of her parents because 'nothing' more could be done. She had lived apart from her famiy for some years, and it was not easy for either side to deal with the situation. She was not expected to live long, but in fact she lived two years. During that time she found her creative centre, perhaps because she could no longer avoid facing herself by being continually on the move. She taught us all a great deal.

When she was first admitted she was angry and resentful, and could see no point in living if it meant being in a wheel chair. She had many of the usual problems of a normal young woman, including a boy-friend who had let her down, and all these were as important to her as the illness. It was a long hard battle, and that is a story in itself. Suffice it to say that when she began to become close to her family and ourselves, she decided to write about her experiences, in order to help others. We sent her on a writing course, where the staff were marvellous and put a bed in the classroom. Her article was accepted by a magazine and she received her fee!

About this time, when she started to 'give of herself' to others (and when this happens it is often the beginning of true healing, not physical but healing of the soul), she pushed the following poem into my hands. When later I asked if I could use it for teaching she looked at me very directly – she was a very direct woman – and said, 'Yes, by all means use it, actually you ought to, you lot are just talking about it. I'm in it.'

Although it is addressed to me, it is written to all of us who try to help by taking a step into this other dimension into which many of our patients eventually move.

To Miss Craig – who always cared

A patient's feelings about her social worker
On my back, lying flat,
Looking up and staring at the ceiling.
You, your white coat, painted smile,
Thought you'd just drop by a while.
Do you know what I am feeling?

I'm a number in your book,
Come on have a damn good look,
Another problem to be solved
Better not get too involved.
Put me neatly in the filing.
Sorry I don't feel like smiling.

Do you want to know my name,
No – you lot, you're all the same
Helping me to know my rights?

Oh, my head, these bloody lights.
Disabled Persons pension schemes?
Bet it isn't all it seems.
You might think that I am thick,
To hell with it, you make me sick

Oh Hi! again, thought I'd seen
The last of you when you had been.
Always want it all my way,
But glad you came again to-day,
And you gave me food
for thought

Sorry I was rude.
I ought
to hold my tongue
I know you're only here to try
To help me out by and by,
To get back among Society.
Won't you stay and have some tea?

Want to have a heart to heart
God, I don't know where to start
Can't express how I feel,
All this pain, it can't be real.
The doctor says he'll do what's best
Take the pills and lots of rest.
Most of all I need some hope,
Please be the one to help me cope.

Now I'm home and so much better
Thought I'd write this little letter,
Just to wish you all the best,
Thanks a lot and all the rest
You know, you helped me very much
I'd like to try to keep in touch,
You helped me win this long hard fight,
And sometimes in the dead of night,
I lay back and think a while
Those things I said, that 'painted smile'
Knowing now that from the start,
It really did come from the heart.
Thanks again, and though I've cried
Please file me under 'satisfied'.

© *Olga M. Craig*

Useful addresses

There are many groups which offer help to people affected by cancer, either as a patient, or the family and friends of a patient. The following national groups will provide information and advice, as well as support and practical help. All the groups listed try to work alongside the health service professionals, and offer help other than medical advice and treatment.

The authors are grateful to the Cancer Relief Macmillan Fund for permission to reproduce this information which is included in their leaflet, Help is There, National Contacts for People with Cancer.

England

BACUP
121/123 Charterhouse Street
London EC1M 6AA
Tel: 071-608 1661
0800 181199 outside London (information linkline)
071-608 1785 (administration)

Helps patients, their families and friends, cope with cancer. Trained cancer nurses provide information, emotional support and practical advice by telephone or letter. A range of free publications and a newspaper are available. One-to-one counselling service in Greater London.

Breast Care and Mastectomy Association of Great Britain (BCMA)
26a Harrison Street
Kings Cross
London WC1H 8JG
Tel: 071-837 0908

A free service of practical advice, information and support to women concerned about breast cancer. Volunteers who have had breast cancer themselves assist the staff in providing emotional support, nationwide. The BCM complements medical and nursing care.

British Association for Counselling
37a Sheep Street, Rugby
Warks CV21 3BX
Tel: 0788 78328/9

BAC members are individuals and organisations concerned with counselling in a variety of settings. The Information Office publishes directories listing counselling services and will refer enquirers to an experienced local counsellor, free of charge. Please send SAE with enquiries.

British Colostomy Association
38–39 Eccleston Square
London SW1V 1PB
Tel: 071-828 5175

An information and advisory service, giving comfort, reassurance and encourage-ment to patients to return to their previous active lifestyle. Emotional support is given on a personal and confidential basis by helpers who have long experience of living with a colostomy. Free leaflets and list of local contacts available. Can arrange visits in hospitals or at home on request.

Cancer Aftercare and Rehabilitation Society (CARE)
21 Zetland Road
Redland, Bristol BS6 7AH
Tel: 0272 427419

An organisation of cancer patients formed into self-help groups who offer advice and support. Forty seven branches and contacts throughout the country provide social outlets as well as informative activities.

CancerLink
17 Britannia Street
London WC1X 9JN
Tel: 071-833 2451

Provides emotional support and information in response to telephone and letter enquiries on all aspects of cancer, from people with cancer, families and friends and professionals working with them. Resource to over 300 cancer support and self-help groups throughout Britain, and helps people who set up new groups. Various free publications available.

Cancer Relief Macmillan Fund
Anchor House
15/19 Britten Street
London SW3 3TZ
Tel: 071-351 7811

Supports and develops services to provide skilled care for people with cancer and their families. Macmillan nurses; Macmillan units for in-patient and day care; financial help through grants. Services usually part of the NHS. Information on Macmillan services available on request. Grant applications through community nurses, hospital or local authority social workers.

Carer's National Association
29 Chilworth Mews
London W2 3RG
Tel: 071-724 7776

Offers information and advice, inlcuding contacts for local groups, and links carers with each other. Encourages self-help and lobbies government, both local and national, on behalf of carers.

The Compassionate Friends
6 Denmark Street
Bristol BS1 5DQ
Tel: 0272 292778

A self-help group of parents who have lost a son or daughter of any age, including adult. Quarterly newsletter, postal library, range of leaflets. Personal and group support. Befriending, rather than counselling.

CRUSE
Bereavement Care
Cruse House, 126 Sheen Road
Richmond, Surrey TW9 1UR
Tel: 081-940 4818

Helps any bereaved person by providing counselling individually and in groups by trained counsellors. Advice and information on practical problems, and social contact. Training courses for professionals and counsellors. Publications list available.

Headway–National Head Injuries Association Ltd.
200 Mansfield Road
Nottingham NG1 3HX
Tel: 0602 622382

Provides help, advice and support for patients who suffer the devastating effects of head injury, and their families. The aim is to help them come to terms with the enormous responsibilities of home care and rehabilitation.

Hodgkin's Disease Association
PO Box 275, Haddenham
Aylesbury, Bucks HP17 8JJ
Tel: 0844 291500

Provides information and emotional support for lymphoma (Hodgkin's Disease and non-Hodgkin's Lymphoma) patients and their families. Literature and video available. National network of helpers with experience of the disease, with whom enquirers may be linked, usually by telephone.

Hospice Information Service
St Christopher's Hospice
51–59 Lawrie Park Road
Sydenham, London SE26 6 DZ
Tel: 081-778 9252

The Hospice Information Service publishes a directory of hospice services which provides details of Hospices, Home Care Teams, and Hospital Support Teams in the UK and the Republic of Ireland. For copies of the directory or details of local services, write or telephone.

Hysterectomy Support
c/o WHRIC
52 Featherstone Street
London EC1Y 8RT
Tel: 071-251 6332/6580 (11.00–17.00 Mon, Wed–Fri)

Refers women (and family or partners) concerned about hysterectomy to former patients in their area, who will provide encouragement, advice and support through the informal sharing of experiences and information. Membership of local support groups (details from above). Contact by letter, over the telephone, or through group meetings. Booklet available.

Institute for Complementary Medicine
21 Portland Place
London W1N 3AF

Can supply names of reliable practitioners of various kinds of complementary medicine, such as homeopathy, relaxation techniques, and osteopathy. Also has contact with other support groups. Please send SAE for information, stating area of interest.

Institute of Family Therapy
43 New Cavendish Street
London W1M 7RG
Tel: 071-935 1651

The Institute's Elizabeth Raven Memorial Fund offers free counselling to recently bereaved families, or those with seriously ill family members. Works with the whole family. While the service is free, voluntary donations to the Fund are welcomed to help other families.

Let's Face It
Christine Piff
10 Wood End, Crowthorne
Berks RG11 6DQ
Tel: 0344 774405

A contact point for people of any age coping with facial disfigurement. Provides a link for people with similar experiences. Telephone and letter contact; meetings for self-help or social contact.

Leukaemia Care Society
PO Box 82, Exeter
Devon EX2 5DP
Tel: 0392 218514

Promotes the welfare of people with leukaemia and allied blood disorders. Offers family caravan holidays and friendship and support via unpaid Area Secretaries throughout Great Britain. Limited financial assistance. Membership is free.

The Malcolm Sargent Cancer Fund for Children
14 Abingdon Road
London W8 6AF
Tel: 071-937 4548

Can provide cash grants for parents of children up to the age of 21 with cancer, to help pay for clothing, equipment, travel, fuel bills, etc. Apply through a hospital social worker anywhere in the UK, who will fill in a form on patient's behalf.

Marie Curie Cancer Care
28 Belgrave Square
London SW1X 8QG
Tel: 071-235 3325

Nursing care available in eleven Marie Curie homes throughout the UK. Admission details through the individual Matrons. Day and night nursing can be provided in patient's home through the Community Nursing Service, administered by the appropriate local health authority. Welfare grant schemes; applications through the district nursing service.

National Association of Laryngectomee Clubs
4th Floor, 39 Eccleston Square
London SW1V 1PB
Tel: 071-834 2857

Promotes the welfare of laryngectomees within the British Isles. Encourages the formation of clubs with objective of assisting rehabilitation through speech therapy, social support and monthly meetings. Advises on speech aids and medical supplies. Offers referral service.

The Neuroblastoma Society
Neville and Janet Oldridge
Woodlands, Ordsall Park Road
Retford, Notts DN2 7PJ
Tel: 0777 709238

Information and advice by telephone or letter for patients and their families. Provides contact where possible with others who have experienced the illness in the family, for mutual support.

Oesophageal Patients' Association
16 Whitefields Crescent
Solihull, W. Midlands B91 3NU
Tel: 021 704 9860

Leaflets, telephone advice and support, before and during treatment. Visits, where possible, by former patients to people with oesophageal cancer.

Retinoblastoma Society
Mrs Kaye Balmforth
c/o Children's Department
Moorfields Eye Hospital
City Road, London EC1V 2PD
Tel: 071-253 3411 X2345

Links families in the same situation and area, to give moral support and practical help. Creates an opportunity for parents to exchange information and share experiences.

Save Our Sons (SOS)
Shirley Wilcox
Tides Reach, 1 Kite Hill
Wooton Bridge
Isle of Wight PO33 4LA
Tel: 0983 882876 (evenings preferred)

Information and emotional support for men and boys with testicular cancer. Advice given by qualified nurse, who will listen and offer help where possible. Leaflet on self-examination techniques available.

The Sue Ryder Foundation
Cavendish, Sudbury
Suffolk CO10 8AY
Tel: 0787 280252

Six Sue Ryder Homes in England specialise in cancer care. Visiting nurses care for patients in their own homes. Advice and bereavement counselling.

Urostomy Association
(Central Office)
'Buckland', Beaumont Park
Danbury, Essex CM3 4DE
Tel: 024 541 4294

Assists patients before and after surgery with counselling on appliances, housing, work situations or marital problems. Helps them to resume as full a life as possible with confidence. Branch and house meetings held. Can also arrange hospital and home visits by former patients on request.

Northern Ireland

The Ulster Cancer Foundation
40–42 Eglantine Avenue
Belfast BT9 6DX
Tel: 0232 663281/2/3
Helpline: 0232 663439 (9.30–12.30 weekdays)

Involved in many aspects of cancer, from prevention to patient support. Operates an information helpline for cancer-related queries for patients and their families, staffed by experienced cancer nurses, who can arrange counselling by personal appointment at the Centre. Rehabilitation support services include: mastectomy advice (volunteer visiting by former patients); laryngectomee club (monthly activities, support in hospitals and at home); lymphoma support (patient and family link-up).

Republic of Ireland

Irish Cancer Society
5 Northumberland Road
Dublin 4
Tel: 0001 681855 or Dial 10 and ask for 'Freefone Cancer' (Ireland only)

Information on all aspects of cancer from nurses via Freefone service. Funds home care and rehabilitation programmes run by voluntary groups, for all cancer patients. Support groups for mastectomy, colostomy and laryngectomy patients, and Hodgkin's Disease advice. Home night nursing service available on request of patient's doctor or public health nurse.

Scotland

Breast Care and Mastectomy Association
Cancer Relief Macmillan Fund
CancerLink
9 Castle Terrace
Edinburgh EH1 2DP
Tel: 031 228 6715 (BCMA)
Tel: 031 229 3276 (CRMF)
Tel: 031 228 5557 (CancerLink)

Details for these associations are given above.

Tak Tent
Cancer Support Organisation
G Block, Western Infirmary
Glasgow GI1 6NT
Tel: 041 332 3639

Gives emotional support, counselling and information on cancers and treatments. Has support groups throughout Scotland, plus a one-to-one counselling service at Centre by appointment. Runs various 'Coping with Cancer' courses.

Wales

Tenovus Cancer Information Centre
142 Whitchurch Road
Cardiff CF4 3NA
Tel: 0222 619846

Although the primary concern is prevention, the Centre provides information and advice on all cancer-related concerns. Contact by telephone, letter, or personal visit.

Further useful address

The Joseph Rowntree Family Fund
Joseph Rowntree Memorial Trust
PO Box 50
York YO1 1UY

Index